Global Infections and Child Health

Editor

JAMES P. NATARO

PEDIATRIC CLINICS
OF NORTH AMERICA

www.pediatric.theclinics.com

Consulting Editor
BONITA F. STANTON

August 2017 • Volume 64 • Number 4

ELSEVIER

1600 John F. Kennedy Boulevard • Suite 1800 • Philadelphia, Pennsylvania, 19103-2899

http://www.theclinics.com

THE PEDIATRIC CLINICS OF NORTH AMERICA Volume 64, Number 4
August 2017 ISSN 0031-3955, ISBN-13: 978-0-323-53251-8

Editor: Kerry Holland
Developmental Editor: Casey Potter

The Pediatric Clinics of North America (ISSN 0031-3955) is published bimonthly by Elsevier Inc., 360 Park Avenue South, New York, NY 10010-1710. Months of issue are February, April, June, August, October, and December. Periodicals postage paid at New York, NY and additional mailing offices. Subscription prices are $208.00 per year (US individuals), $589.00 per year (US institutions), $281.00 per year (Canadian individuals), $784.00 per year (Canadian institutions), $338.00 per year (international individuals), $784.00 per year (international institutions), $100.00 per year (US students and residents), and $165.00 per year (international and Canadian residents and students). To receive students/resident rare, orders must be accompanied by name of affiliated institution, date of term, and the signature of program/residency coordinator on institution letterhead. Orders will be billed at individual rate until proof of status is received. Foreign air speed delivery is included in all *Clinics* subscription prices. All prices are subject to change without notice. **POSTMASTER:** Send address changes to *The Pediatric Clinics of North America*, Elsevier Health Sciences Division, Subscription Customer Service, 3251 Riverport Lane, Maryland Heights, MO 63043. **Customer Service: 1-800-654-2452 (US and Canada). From outside of the US and Canada: 1-314-447-8871. Fax: 1-314-447-8029. For print support, E-mail: JournalsCustomerService-usa@elsevier.com. For online support, E-mail: JournalsOnlineSupport-usa@elsevier.com.**

Reprints. For copies of 100 or more, of articles in this publication, please contact the Commercial Reprints Department, Elsevier Inc., 360 Park Avenue South, New York, NY 10010-1710. Tel.: 212-633-3874; Fax: 212-633-3820; E-mail: reprints@elsevier.com.

The Pediatric Clinics of North America is also published in Spanish by McGraw-Hill Inter-americana Editores S.A., Mexico City, Mexico; in Portuguese by Riechmann and Affonso Editores, Rua Comandante Coelho 1085, CEP 21250, Rio de Janeiro, Brazil; and in Greek by Althayia SA, Athens, Greece.

The Pediatric Clinics of North America is covered in *MEDLINE/PubMed (Index Medicus)*, *Excerpta Medica*, *Current Contents*, *Current Contents/Clinical Medicine*, *Science Citation Index*, *ASCA*, *ISI/BIOMED*, and *BIOSIS*.

PROGRAM OBJECTIVE
The goal of the *Pediatric Clinics of North America* is to keep practicing physicians and residents up to date with current clinical practice in pediatrics by providing timely articles reviewing the state-of-the-art in patient care.

TARGET AUDIENCE
All practicing pediatricians, physicians and healthcare professionals who provide patient care to pediatric patients.

LEARNING OBJECTIVES
Upon completion of this activity, participants will be able to:
1. Review global issues in childhood nutrition, growth, and development.
2. Discuss subclinical infection, diarrheal illnesses, and other infectious diseases in children.
3. Recognize current updates in global infections and child health.

ACCREDITATION
The Elsevier Office of Continuing Medical Education (EOCME) is accredited by the Accreditation Council for Continuing Medical Education (ACCME) to provide continuing medical education for physicians.

The EOCME designates this enduring material for a maximum of 15 *AMA PRA Category 1 Credit*(s)™. Physicians should claim only the credit commensurate with the extent of their participation in the activity.

All other healthcare professionals requesting continuing education credit for this enduring material will be issued a certificate of participation.

DISCLOSURE OF CONFLICTS OF INTEREST
The EOCME assesses conflict of interest with its instructors, faculty, planners, and other individuals who are in a position to control the content of CME activities. All relevant conflicts of interest that are identified are thoroughly vetted by EOCME for fair balance, scientific objectivity, and patient care recommendations. EOCME is committed to providing its learners with CME activities that promote improvements or quality in healthcare and not a specific proprietary business or a commercial interest.

The planning committee, staff, authors and editors listed below have identified no financial relationships or relationships to products or devices they or their spouse/life partner have with commercial interest related to the content of this CME activity:
Zulfiqar A. Bhutta, MBBS, FRCPCH, FAAP, PhD; Lauren M.S. Cohee, MD; Donna M. Denno, MD, MPH; Rebecca Dillingham, MD, MPH; Anjali Fortna; Megan E. Gray, MD; Richard L. Guerrant, MD; Kerry Holland; Peter J. Hotez, MD, PhD; Eric R. Houpt, MD, PhD; Amira M. Khan, MBBS, DCH; Beena Koshy, MD, MBBS; Miriam K. Laufer, MD, MPH; Angelina Maphula, PhD; G. Paul Matherne, MD, MBA; Rojelio Mejia, MD; Blandina T Mmbaga, MD, MMed, PhD; Shaun K. Morris, MD, MPH; James P. Nataro, MD, PhD, MBA; Kathleen M. Neuzil, MD, MPH; Phillip Nieberg, MD, MPH; Shadae L. Paul; Paige C. Pullen, PhD; Elizabeth T. Rogawski, PhD, MSPH; Reeba Roshan, PhD; Elizabeth T. Rotrosen, BA; Rebecca J. Scharf, MD, MPH; Debbie-Ann T. Shirley, MBBS, MPH; Rita Shrestha, PhD; Bonita F. Stanton, MD; Parminder S. Suchdev, MD, MPH; Tania A. Thomas, MD, MPH; Vignesh Viswanathan; Linda A. Waggoner-Fountain, MD; Jill E. Weatherhead, MD; Katie Widmeier; Anne M. Williams, PhD, MPH.

The planning committee, staff, authors and editors listed below have identified financial relationships or relationships to products or devices they or their spouse/life partner have with commercial interest related to the content of this CME activity:
Karen L. Kotloff, MD has research support from Merck & Co., Inc.

UNAPPROVED/OFF-LABEL USE DISCLOSURE
The EOCME requires CME faculty to disclose to the participants:
1. When products or procedures being discussed are off-label, unlabelled, experimental, and/or investigational (not US Food and Drug Administration [FDA] approved); and
2. Any limitations on the information presented, such as data that are preliminary or that represent ongoing research, interim analyses, and/or unsupported opinions. Faculty may discuss information about pharmaceutical agents that is outside of FDA-approved labelling. This information is intended solely for CME and is not intended to promote off-label use of these medications. If you have any questions, contact the medical affairs department of the manufacturer for the most recent prescribing information.

TO ENROLL

To enroll in the *Pediatric Clinics of North America* Continuing Medical Education program, call customer service at 1-800-654-2452 or sign up online at http://www.theclinics.com/home/cme. The CME program is available to subscribers for an additional annual fee of USD 290.

METHOD OF PARTICIPATION

In order to claim credit, participants must complete the following:

1. Complete enrolment as indicated above.
2. Read the activity.
3. Complete the CME Test and Evaluation. Participants must achieve a score of 70% on the test. All CME Tests and Evaluations must be completed online.

CME INQUIRIES/SPECIAL NEEDS

For all CME inquiries or special needs, please contact elsevierCME@elsevier.com.

Contributors

CONSULTING EDITOR

BONITA F. STANTON, MD
Founding Dean, Seton Hall-Hackensack Meridian School of Medicine, Professor of Pediatrics, Seton Hall University, South Orange, New Jersey

EDITOR

JAMES P. NATARO, MD, PhD, MBA
Benjamin Armistead Shepherd Professor, Chair, Department of Pediatrics, University of Virginia School of Medicine, Charlottesville, Virginia

AUTHORS

ZULFIQAR A. BHUTTA, MBBS, FRCPCH, FAAP, PhD
Professor, Peter Gilgan Centre for Research and Learning (PGCRL), Robert Harding Chair in Global Child Health and Policy, Co-Director, Centre for Global Child Health, The Hospital for Sick Children, Toronto, Ontario, Canada; Founding Director, Centre for Excellence in Women and Child Health, Aga Khan University, Karachi, Pakistan

LAUREN M. COHEE, MD
Fellow, Division of Malaria Research, Institute for Global Health, University of Maryland School of Medicine, Baltimore, Maryland

DONNA M. DENNO, MD, MPH
Department of Pediatrics, University of Washington School of Medicine, Departments of Global Health, and Health Services, University of Washington School of Public Health, Seattle, Washington

REBECCA DILLINGHAM, MD, MPH
Director of the Center for Global Health, Associate Professor, Division of Infectious Diseases and International Health, Department of Medicine,University of Virginia, Charlottesville, Virginia

MEGAN E. GRAY, MD
Division of Infectious Diseases and International Health, Department of Medicine, University of Virginia, Charlottesville, Virginia

RICHARD L. GUERRANT, MD
Division of Infectious Diseases and International Health, Department of Medicine, University of Virginia, Charlottesville, Virginia

PETER J. HOTEZ, MD, PhD
Professor, Departments of Pediatrics and Molecular Virology and Microbiology, Sabin Vaccine Institute, Texas Children's Hospital (TCH), Center for Vaccine Development, Dean, National School of Tropical Medicine, Baylor College of Medicine (BCM), Houston, Texas

ERIC R. HOUPT, MD
Division of Infectious Diseases and International Health, Department of Medicine,
University of Virginia, Charlottesville, Virginia

AMIRA M. KHAN, MBBS, DCH
Peter Gilgan Centre for Research and Learning (PGCRL), Research Analyst II, Centre for
Global Child Health, The Hospital for Sick Children, Toronto, Ontario, Canada

BEENA KOSHY, MD, MBBS
Professor, Developmental Paediatrics, Christian Medical College, Vellore, Tamil Nadu,
India

KAREN L. KOTLOFF, MD
Professor of Pediatrics and Medicine, Division of Infectious Disease and Tropical
Pediatrics, Center for Vaccine Development, Institute for Global Health, University of
Maryland School of Medicine, Baltimore, Maryland

MIRIAM K. LAUFER, MD, MPH
Associate Professor, Division of Malaria Research, Institute for Global Health, University
of Maryland School of Medicine, Baltimore, Maryland

ANGELINA MAPHULA, PhD
Professor, Department of Psychology, University of Venda, Thohoyandou, South Africa

GAYNELL PAUL MATHERNE, MD, MBA
Professor of Pediatrics, Division of Pediatric Cardiology, University of Virginia Children's
Hospital, Charlottesville, Virginia

ROJELIO MEJIA, MD
Assistant Professor of Pediatrics, Section of Tropical Medicine, National School of
Tropical Medicine, Baylor College of Medicine (BCM), Houston, Texas

BLANDINA T. MMBAGA, MD, MMed, PhD
Department of Pediatrics, Kilimanjaro Christian Medical Centre, Kilimanjaro Clinical
Research Institute, Moshi, Tanzania

SHAUN K. MORRIS, MD, MPH
Clinician-Scientist, Division of Infectious Diseases, Assistant Professor, Department of
Pediatrics, The Hospital for Sick Children, University of Toronto, Toronto, Ontario, Canada

JAMES P. NATARO, MD, PhD, MBA
Benjamin Armistead Shepherd Professor, Chair, Department of Pediatrics, University of
Virginia School of Medicine, Charlottesville, Virginia

KATHLEEN M. NEUZIL, MD, MPH
Professor of Medicine and Pediatrics, Director, Center for Vaccine Development, University of Maryland, Baltimore, Maryland

PHILLIP NIEBURG, MD, MPH
Visiting Associate Professor of Pediatrics, University of Virginia, Charlottesville, Virginia

SHADAE L. PAUL
Department of Global Health, University of Washington School of Public Health, Seattle,
Washington

PAIGE C. PULLEN, PhD
Associate Professor of Education and Pediatrics, Department of Pediatrics, University of
Virginia, Charlottesville, Virginia

ELIZABETH T. ROGAWSKI, PhD, MSPH
Department of Public Health Sciences, Division of Infectious Diseases and International Health, Department of Medicine, University of Virginia, Charlottesville, Virginia

REEBA ROSHAN, PhD
Professor of Psychology, Developmental Paediatrics, Christian Medical College, Vellore, Tamil Nadu, India

ELIZABETH T. ROTROSEN, BA
Clinical Research Assistant, Center for Vaccine Development, University of Maryland, Baltimore, Maryland

REBECCA J. SCHARF, MD, MPH
Assistant Professor, Developmental Pediatrics, University of Virginia Children's Hospital, Charlottesville, Virginia

DEBBIE-ANN T. SHIRLEY, MBBS, MPH
Assistant Professor, Department of Pediatrics, University of Virginia School of Medicine, Charlottesville, Virginia

RITA SHRESTHA, PhD
Professor, Department of Psychology, Tribhuwan University, Kirtipur, Kathmandu, Nepal

PARMINDER S. SUCHDEV, MD, MPH
Department of Pediatrics, Emory University School of Medicine, Hubert Department of Global Health, Rollins School of Public Health, Emory University, Atlanta, Georgia

TANIA A. THOMAS, MD, MPH
Assistant Professor, Division of Infectious Diseases and International Health, Department of Medicine, University of Virginia, Charlottesville, Virginia

LINDA A. WAGGONER-FOUNTAIN, MD
Professor, Department of Pediatrics, Division of Infectious Diseases, University of Virginia School of Medicine, Charlottesville, Virginia

JILL E. WEATHERHEAD, MD
Adult and Pediatric Infectious Disease Clinical Fellow, Department of Pediatrics, Section of Tropical Medicine, National School of Tropical Medicine, Baylor College of Medicine (BCM), Houston, Texas

ANNE M. WILLIAMS, PhD, MPH
Adjunct Assistant Professor, Hubert Department of Global Health, Emory University, Atlanta, Georgia

Contents

Ninety-nine percent of the 5.9 million annual child deaths occur in low and middle-income countries. Undernutrition underlies 45% of deaths. Determinants include access to care, maternal education, and absolute and relative poverty. Socio-political-economic factors and policies tremendously influence health and their determinants. Most deaths can be prevented with interventions that are currently available and recommended for widespread implementation. Millennium Development Goal 4 was not achieved. Sustainable Development Goal 3.2 presents an even more ambitious target and opportunity to save millions of lives, and requires attention to scaling up interventions, especially among the poorest and most vulnerable children.

Improving maternal and child nutrition is central to global development goals and reducing the noncommunicable disease burden. Although the process of becoming malnourished starts in utero, the consequences of poor nutrition extend across the life cycle and into future generations. The global nutrition targets for 2025 include reducing infant and young child growth faltering, halting the increase of overweight children, improving breastfeeding practices, and reducing maternal anemia. In this review, we address nutritional assessment, discuss nonnutritive factors that affect growth, and endorse the evidence-based interventions that should be scaled up to improve maternal and child nutrition.

Worldwide, children are often not meeting their developmental potential owing to malnutrition, infection, lack of stimulation, and toxic stress. Children with disabilities are more likely to experience poverty, neglect, and abuse, and are less likely to have adequate access to education and medical care. Early childhood developmental stimulation can improve language, learning, and future participation in communities. Therapeutic supports and endeavors to reduce stigma for people of all abilities strengthen communities and allow for human thriving.

Lack of success in achieving considerable reductions in neonatal mortality is a contributory factor in failing to achieve Millennium Development Goal 4.2.6 million neonates still die each year, with preterm birth and infections the two leading causes. Maternal infections and environmental and infant factors influence acquisition of viral and bacterial infections in the perinatal and neonatal period. Scaling up evidence-based interventions addressing maternal risk factors and underlying causes could reduce neonatal infections by 84%. The emergence of new infections and increasing antimicrobial resistance present public health challenges that must be addressed to achieve substantial reductions in neonatal mortality.

Reductions in mortality from diarrheal diseases among young children have occurred in recent decades; however, approximately 500,000 children continue to die each year. Moreover, similar reductions in disease incidence have not been seen, episodes that impact the growth and development of young children. Two recent studies, MAL-ED and GEMS, have more clearly defined the burden and cause of diarrhea among young children, identifying four leading pathogens: rotavirus, *Cryptosporidium Shigella*, and heat stable toxin–producing enterotoxigenic *Escherichia coli*. Global introduction of rotavirus vaccine is poised to substantially reduce the incidence of rotavirus infection. Interventions are needed to reduce the burden that remains.

Environmental enteropathy is a chronic condition of the small intestine associated with increased intestinal permeability, mucosal inflammation, malabsorption, and systemic inflammation. It is commonly accompanied by enteric infections and is misleadingly considered a subclinical disease. Potential effects of enteric infections and enteropathy on vaccine responses, child growth, cognitive development, and even later life obesity, diabetes, and metabolic syndrome are increasingly being recognized. Herein, we review the evolving challenges to defining environmental enteropathy and enteric infections, current evidence for the magnitude and determinants of its burden, new assessment tools, and relevant interventions.

Diarrheal disease remains the second leading cause of mortality in children in developing countries. *Cryptosporidium* is a leading cause and its importance stands to increase as rotavirus vaccine becomes used around the world. *Cryptosporidium* is particularly problematic in children younger than 2 years old and in the immunocompromised. *Giardia lamblia* is a common intestinal protozoan that is associated with diarrhea and, perhaps, growth faltering in impoverished settings. This review establishes the current prevalence of these infections in global settings and reviews current diagnosis and management approaches.

Malaria is a leading cause of morbidity and mortality in endemic areas, leading to an estimated 438,000 deaths in 2015. Malaria is also an important health threat to travelers to endemic countries and should be considered in evaluation of any traveler returning from a malaria-endemic area who develops fever. Considering the diagnosis of malaria in patients with potential exposure is critical. Prompt provision of effective treatment limits the complications of malaria and can be life-saving. Understanding *Plasmodium* species variation, epidemiology, and drug-resistance patterns in the geographic area where infection was acquired is important for determining treatment choices.

Helminth infections, including soil-transmitted helminths and schistosomiasis, remain one of the most common infections in the world with over 1 billion people infected. These infections cause significant morbidity, particularly in young children, that may last a lifetime, including growth and cognitive stunting. There is an urgent need for the control and elimination of helminth infections from areas of poverty to reduce morbidity in children. Mass drug administration programs were adopted by the World Health Assembly in 2001 and have evolved to provide coverage with multiple anthelmintic medications in a single rapid impact package and more extensive coverage within a community.

Children and adolescents living with human immunodeficiency virus (HIV) represent a population that requires a unique approach to HIV care. Prevention, testing, initiation of antiretroviral therapy (ART), and retention and engagement in care are critical steps. Each step requires providers to address age-specific barriers, so that successful and prolonged viral suppression can occur. Adherence to ART, disclosure of HIV-positive status, and stigma are examples of struggles faced by youth, their families, and health care providers. A multifaceted approach and thoughtful transitions of care are needed, but with sustained ART, youth living with HIV can survive and thrive with the expectation of a normal lifespan.

PEDIATRIC CLINICS OF NORTH AMERICA

THE CLINICS ARE AVAILABLE ONLINE!
Access your subscription at:
www.theclinics.com

Foreword

Global Infections and Child Health

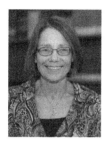

Bonita F. Stanton, MD
Consulting Editor

Despite much progress in their control, infectious diseases remain a global concern. The number of under-five deaths worldwide has declined from 12.7 million in 1990 to 5.9 million in 2015 (http://www.who.int/mediacentre/factsheets/fs178/en/). Globally, approximately half of under-five deaths are due to infectious diseases.[1] Although numbers are substantially lower in industrialized nations including the United States, infectious causes remain among the top 10 causes of childhood mortality and cause significant morbidity (http://www.kidsdata.org/topic/659/childdeathrate-age-cause). Moreover, infectious diseases are continually emerging as new pathogens, as more virulent pathogens, and/or in new settings. In the past few years, the World Health Organization has noted the appearance of a Crimean Congo hemorrhagic fever, Ebola virus disease, Marburg virus, Lassa fever, Middle East respiratory syndrome, severe acute respiratory syndrome, coronavirus diseases, Nipah and Rift Valley fever (http://www.who.int/medicines/ebola-treatment/WHO-list-of-top-emerging-diseases/en/). Over the past year, Zika virus has emerged as a major threat in the Americas, including the United States (https://www.cdc.gov/zika/index.html).

Thus, there are many reasons it is important for every pediatrician to be familiar with extant and emerging pathogens from across the globe. First, we are a single globe, and health and wellness is our concern worldwide. Second, whether or not the pathogen is currently in the United States, it could easily arrive here—and thrive.

This issue of *Pediatric Clinics of North America* effectively summarizes a vast literature updating the health care provider on familiar infectious diseases and describing those that are newly recognized, emerging, and/or migrating. The issue is both fasci-

Pediatr Clin N Am 64 (2017) xv–xvi
http://dx.doi.org/10.1016/j.pcl.2017.05.002
0031-3955/17/© 2017 Published by Elsevier Inc.

nating and very helpful, written by true leaders in the world of childhood infectious diseases.

Bonita F. Stanton, MD
Seton Hall-Hackensack Meridian School of Medicine
Seton Hall University
400 South Orange Street
South Orange, NJ 07079, USA

E-mail address:
bonita.stanton@shu.edu

REFERENCE

1. Liu L, Oza S, Hogan D, et al. Global, regional, and national causes of child mortality in 2000–13, with projections to inform post-2015 priorities: an updated systematic analysis. Lancet 2015;385:430–40.

Preface

Global Infections and Child Health

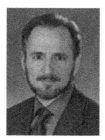

James P. Nataro, MD, PhD, MBA
Editor

At the Millennium Summit in 2000, world leaders articulated an ambitious agenda to reduce extreme poverty, improve child and maternal health, reduce gender disparities, and improve environmental sustainability. The framers proposed specific measureable goals that were to be met by the end of 2015. Examining the trajectory of these efforts over this 15-year span reveals impressive progress in some areas, with remaining large disparities.[1] Among the successes include reduction of the number of people living in extreme poverty by an estimated 130 million, reduction of child mortalities from 103 deaths per thousand live births per year to 88, and improvement of life expectancy from 63 years to nearly 65 years globally.[1] Child deaths from infection have also improved, as fewer children than ever succumb to malaria and diarrheal diseases. HIV diagnosis and therapy is now available in much of the world, and HIV itself could become a manageable chronic disease where resources are available.

In light of the relative success controlling infectious diseases, some have called for a redirection of emphasis toward noncommunicable diseases. While it is true that non-communicable diseases are on the rise in developing countries, accounting for an increasing proportion of overall deaths since 1990, most children continue to succumb to infectious diseases, perinatal morbidity, and nutritional disorders.[2] Moreover, a health economics focus on disability-adjusted-life-years-lost from death and disease continues to demonstrate that morbidity and mortality in children account for the greatest loss of productive years.[3] Therefore, now and for the foreseeable future, it is appropriate to maintain a focus on our most vulnerable pediatric populations.

Beyond the social imperative of caring for populations in greatest need, the globalization of infectious disease has never been a greater threat. With growing penetration into hitherto remote areas and rapid transportation across the globe, the movement of infected individuals and the migration of infectious agents have become urgent threats. Experience in this decade with Ebola virus and Zika virus illustrates these principles.

Pediatr Clin N Am 64 (2017) xvii–xviii
http://dx.doi.org/10.1016/j.pcl.2017.05.001
0031-3955/17/© 2017 Published by Elsevier Inc.

pediatric.theclinics.com

Migration of peoples is also occurring in dramatic fashion. Refugees now move from country to country and continent to continent with prodigious volume and speed. International adoption, clearly a blessing for a child in compromised circumstances, represents a challenge to a family and a health care provider in an industrialized setting.

With these considerations in mind, we focus this issue of the *Pediatric Clinics of North America* on global infections and child health. We present a consideration of the overall state of children's health after the endpoint of the Millennium Development Goals. We also focus on specific infectious diseases that continue to afflict children in developing countries, and which can be seen by providers who treat adoptees, migrants, and travelers. We consider as well the global ecology of infectious diseases, including such agents as Zika virus and influenza, so as to provide an overall appreciation of the influence of infectious diseases on man and vice versa.

My thanks to the *Pediatric Clinics of North America* and the outstanding authors who have committed their time to this endeavor.

James P. Nataro, MD, PhD, MBA
Department of Pediatrics
University of Virginia School of Medicine
Box 800386
Charlottesville, VA 22908, USA

E-mail address:
Jpn2r@virginia.edu

REFERENCES

1. United Nations. The millenium development goals report 2014. New York: United Nations; 2014.
2. Institute for Health Metrics and Evaluation, 2015. Results. Available at: http://healthdata.org/results. Accessed December 29, 2016.
3. Wiseman V, Mitton C, Doyle-Waters MM, et al. Using economic evidence to set healthcare priorities in low-income and lower-middle-income countries: a systematic review of methodological frameworks. Health Econ 2016;25(Suppl 1):140–61.

Child Health and Survival in a Changing World

Donna M. Denno, MD, MPH[a,b,c],*, Shadae L. Paul[b]

KEYWORDS

- Global child health • Low and middle-income countries
- Sustainable development goals • Child mortality • Socio-political-economic factors
- Health interventions • Social determinants

KEY POINTS

- The vast majority of child deaths occur in low and middle-income countries; most are preventable with interventions already available and recommended for implementation.
- If the Sustainable Development Goal child health target is to be met, increased investment in scaling up lifesaving interventions, with proactive attention to reaching the most vulnerable and marginalized populations, is needed.
- Tracking national mortality levels (and other outcome indicators and coverage rates) is important but insufficient; within-country disaggregation also is necessary to monitor equity in intervention coverage and health outcomes.
- Addressing the determinants of health, including limited maternal education, absolute poverty, and relative poverty, is needed for deeper and sustained gains in child survival and health. This will require attention to socio-political-economic policies that drive health and their determinants.

INTRODUCTION

Each year, millions of children die, the vast majority in poor countries. Tragically, most of these deaths are preventable with technologies that are currently available and recommended for universal implementation. Progress is being made: 5.9 million children younger than 5 years died in 2015, down from 12.4 million in 1990. This reduction,

Disclosure Statement: The authors have no financial relationships relevant to this article to disclose. This commentary does not contain a discussion of an unapproved/ investigative use of a commercial product/device.

[a] Department of Pediatrics, University of Washington School of Medicine, Box 354920, 6200 Northeast 74th Street, Suite 110, Seattle, WA 98115, USA; [b] Department of Global Health, University of Washington School of Public Health, Box 357965, Harris Hydraulics Building, 1510 Northeast San Juan Road, Seattle, WA 98195, USA; [c] Department of Health Services, University of Washington School of Public Health, Seattle, WA 98195, USA
* Corresponding author. Department of Pediatrics, University of Washington, Box 354920, 6200 Northeast 74th Street, Suite 110, Seattle, WA 98118.
E-mail address: ddenno@uw.edu

Pediatr Clin N Am 64 (2017) 735–754
http://dx.doi.org/10.1016/j.pcl.2017.03.013
pediatric.theclinics.com

although substantial, was insufficient to meet Millennium Development Goal (MDG) 4: reduce child mortality by two-thirds between 1990 and 2015. In 2000, 189 countries endorsed the MDGs, which consisted of 8 specific goals to reduce poverty and improve health and development. In addition to MDG4, the other 2 health-related goals, MDG3 (reduce maternal mortality) and MDG6 (reduce infectious diseases), were not met. The "post MDG era" has ushered in the Sustainable Development Goals (SDGs), a much broader array of 17 ambitious goals with 169 targets. One of the 17 SDGs specifically relates to health: SDG3, and its 9 targets cover a much wider scope of problems (eg, injuries, mental health, and chronic noncommunicable diseases) than was tackled by the MDGs. SDG3.2, the target related to child health, calls for ending "preventable deaths of newborns and children under 5 years of age, with all countries aiming to reduce neonatal mortality to at least as low as 12 per 1000 live births and under-5 mortality to at least as low as 25 per 1000 live births" by 2030.[1]

This article provides an overview of the scope and causes of childhood deaths, interventions currently recommended to combat these killers, trends in child mortality, and potential reasons for these trends through the lens of the global potential to meet SDG3.

SCOPE OF THE PROBLEM

Health is defined by the World Health Organization as "a state of complete physical, mental and social well-being and not merely the absence of disease or infirmity."[2] Health is clearly more than just survival; however, as a starting point, it is hard to avoid the fact that more than 16,000 children are estimated to die each day.[3] "Child," as used in this article and as typically defined in the global health field, includes persons younger than 5 years because of their particular biologic and social vulnerability. The under-5 mortality rate (U5MR), defined as the number of deaths among children younger than 5 years per 1000 live births, is often used as an indicator of the health of a population more broadly. If conditions favor the health and welfare of this vulnerable group, the situation generally can be considered favorable for the overall society.

Age-specific mortality rates decline appreciably beyond 5 years. Ninety-nine percent of child deaths occur in low-income and middle-income countries (LMICs). A child born in sub-Saharan Africa (SSA) faces a 1 in 12 chance of dying before his or her fifth birthday compared with 1 in 140 for a child born in the United States and 1 in 167 for high-income countries (HICs) on average. The global child health community has started to focus on the broader picture of health, including morbidity, developmental disability, and long-term impacts on adult chronic disease and economic capacity. Unfortunately, child mortality remains as a tenacious problem requiring confrontation.

MAJOR CAUSES OF CHILD MORTALITY

Forty-five percent of child mortality occurs in the neonatal period (first 28 days of life) (**Fig. 1**). These deaths are largely preventable and their causes are discussed in detail in the article by Zulfiqar A. Bhutta and colleagues, "Neonatal and perinatal infections," in this issue. Four problems are responsible for approximately 60% of postneonatal deaths: pneumonia, diarrhea, injuries, and malaria. Mortality from these causes is also mostly preventable with sustainable implementation of available interventions as described later in this article. Undernutrition, including lack of sufficient macronutrients (eg, protein, calories), micronutrient-deficient diets (eg, vitamin A, zinc, iron), and suboptimal breastfeeding practices, contributes to 45% of all child deaths.[4] Undernutrition increases susceptibility to infectious diseases, reduces recovery from

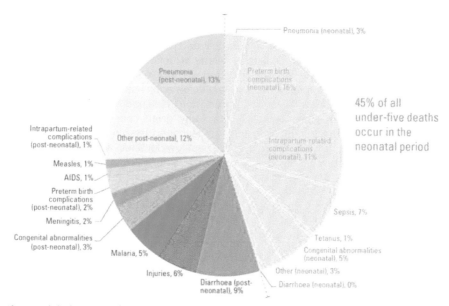

Fig. 1. Global causes of under-5 deaths in 2015. (Reproduced with permission from Liu L, Oza S, Hogan D, et. al. Global, regional, and national causes of under-5 mortality in 2000-15: an updated systematic analysis with implications for the Sustainable Development Goals. Lancet 2016; 0140-6736.)

disease and injury, and is associated with longer-term sequelae, such as cognitive impairment, poor school performance, and noncommunicable diseases in adulthood.

Undernutrition and the common direct causes of child deaths are not exotic tropical diseases, but rather diseases of poverty, brought under control a century ago in the United States and other HICs before the advent of vaccinations and antimicrobials, through social changes addressing crowding, sanitation, nutrition, and basic living conditions. Medical breakthroughs, such as antibiotics, immunizations, and insecticides (to prevent malaria, which was endemic in parts of the United States, for example) further accelerated gains in controlling disease and preventing childhood mortality.

Although less proximate, the social determinants of health, are perhaps even more important underlying causes of mortality. Children in rural areas have a 1.7-fold increased risk of dying compared with their urban counterparts. With increasing urbanization, however, urban slum dwellers face survival challenges. Services may not be available in rural areas, but urban slum dwellers may lack *access* due to cost, discrimination, and other factors and suffer overcrowded and unsanitary living conditions. Race, ethnicity, and gender are other important determinants.

Maternal education is arguably the most important determinant of child survival. Children whose mothers have no formal education are, on average, 2.8 times as likely to die before their fifth birthday compared with those with mothers with secondary or higher education. This is not categorical: for each additional year of maternal schooling, deaths drop by 9%.[5] Although literacy and health literacy are important outcomes of women's education, they do not fully explain the effect on child health; agency and decision-making power likely play important roles.[6]

Approximately 10% of the world lives below the international poverty line: $1.90 per day.[7] Absolute poverty is an extreme hardship, limiting access to the basic necessities to support survival (eg, essential medicines and health care, water, sanitation, adequate nutrition, education). Relative poverty is defined as large gaps between rich and poor within a society and is associated with worse societal health outcomes, especially among the poorer segments. This phenomenon has been demonstrated in both rich and poor countries.[8] Overall, children living in the poorest fifth of households compared with the wealthiest quintile within any given country, face a 1.9-fold increased risk of mortality.[9] Unfortunately, as described later in this article, income inequality has dramatically increased over the past few decades, along with increases in health disparities in many countries. For example, among 36 countries experiencing national declines in U5MR, half had an increased gap in child mortality between the wealthiest and poorest quintiles.[10]

INTERVENTIONS TO REDUCE CHILD MORTALITY

The following section reviews currently recommended prevention and treatment interventions for tackling the leading childhood killers beyond the neonatal period and provides an overview of intervention coverage rates, defined as the proportion of individuals needing an intervention who receive it. For example, if the condition is diarrheal disease and the intervention is oral rehydration solution (ORS), the denominator would be children younger than 5 years with diarrhea, and the numerator all children with diarrhea who received ORS.

PNEUMONIA

Pneumonia is the leading cause of death after the neonatal period, killing more than 900,000 children annually. Pneumococcus and *Haemophilus influenzae* type b (Hib) are prevalent causes of childhood pneumonia, the most important etiologies of severe pneumonia in young childhood, and the cause of about half of childhood pneumonia deaths globally.[11,12] Other common microbes include viruses, especially respiratory syncytial virus; other bacteria, particularly *Staphylococcus aureus* and *Klebsiella pneumoniae*; and *Mycobacterium tuberculosis*, especially among individuals infected with the human immunodeficiency virus (HIV). Where HIV prevalence is high, *Pneumocystis jiroveci* is an important cause of childhood pneumonia deaths, despite recommendations for cotrimoxazole among HIV-infected individuals as an inexpensive and effective prophylaxis against *P jiroveci* pneumonia.

Prevention measures are important in reducing pneumonia incidence and case fatality. Undernutrition leads to reduced immunity and increased difficulty in clearing secretions due to weakened respiratory muscles. Optimal breastfeeding practices and adequate complementary feeding, including adequate micronutrients (especially those involved in immune protection, such as zinc), are important interventions to prevent the incidence of and case fatality from respiratory infections.[4,13] For example, infants have a 15-fold and 2-fold greater risk of death from pneumonia if not breastfed or partially breastfed, respectively, in first 6 months of life compared with exclusively breastfed. Currently, only 43% of young infants globally are exclusively breastfed, and only 74% and 46% continue to breastfeed through the first and second years of life, respectively. Furthermore, only 19% of those 6 to 23 months old receive a minimally acceptable diet of complementary foods.[14]

Household air pollution is associated with a 1.8-fold risk of contracting pneumonia and is largely caused by burning of solid fuels (eg, wood, charcoal, dung, crop waste) in dwellings for heat and cooking. These polluting fuels are used by 40% of the world's population and primarily by poor households. Chimney stoves have been shown to reduce household air pollution by half and severe pneumonia by approximately 30%.[15] Hand hygiene (washing with soap) is important for preventing the spread of respiratory infection and requires water security: access to sufficient quantities of water. This is a challenge for the many women and children who walk long distances to collect water for their households.

Vaccinations play a vital prevention role. Secondary bacterial pneumonia is a common sequelae of measles and pertussis infections. Measles and diphtheria-pertussis-tetanus (DPT) vaccines are inexpensive and effective; they were rolled out in 1976 as part of the original Expanded Program on Immunizations. The largest pneumococcus and Hib disease burden has been and continues to be in LMICs.[12] Immunizations against these pathogens were incorporated into routine immunization schedules in HICs toward the end of the twentieth century. Cost and immunization system (eg, cold chain) expansion have impeded rapid scale-up in poor countries. Furthermore, serotype coverage in pneumococcal vaccines has favored markets in HICs.[12] Hib vaccine was first introduced in an LMIC in 1997; 191 countries now incorporate Hib vaccine into national immunization schedules and global coverage is 64% (**Fig. 2**). Pneumococcal vaccine rollout commenced less than a decade ago in LMICs; it is part of routine schedules in 129 countries and global coverage is 37%.[16] Although coverage rates for measles and DPT (data not shown) vaccines are 85% and 86%, respectively, and have increased substantially over decades, their coverage rates have virtually stagnated since 2008 and are below the World Health Organization (WHO) and United Nations International Children's Emergency Fund (UNICEF) goal of achieving 90% coverage by 2010 for routine vaccines.[17] Furthermore, global and national coverage estimates mask variations and disparities in coverage *within* countries. A recent analysis demonstrated pro-rich and pro-urban inequities in immunization coverage in most LMICs and pro-male inequities in Southeast Asian LMICs. Some countries substantially reduced these inequities; however, they have increased in other countries.[18] Differences between the wealthiest and poorest quintiles for immunization and other intervention coverage rates as global averages are depicted in **Fig. 3**.

Although prevention plays an important role in pneumonia control, appropriate antibiotic treatment is critical for reducing case fatality. Despite increasing resistance to readily accessible and inexpensive first-line amoxicillin, in vivo efficacy continues to be good, at least at this time. Prompt and appropriate case management hinges on the following: (1) parent/caretaker recognition of symptoms, especially tachypnea and retractions, for which prompt health care should be sought, (2) access to appropriate care without delay (ie, services are available, geographically proximate, affordable, good quality, and nondiscriminatory), (3) accurate diagnosis and treatment by health workers, and (4) availability and affordability of treatment and completion of a full therapeutic course. However, parental recognition that fast breathing and retractions require urgent medical attention is inadequate[19] and fewer than 65% of children with pneumonia symptoms are taken for appropriate health care.[14] Fewer still actually receive antibiotics. Tragically, there has been little improvement in these coverage statistics over the past decade (see **Fig. 3**), especially in SSA.

Use of lay health workers (LHWs) to diagnose and treat pneumonia in the communities where children live, especially in rural areas with lack of access to health facilities, is increasingly showing promise. Studies have consistently shown that LHWs trained in pneumonia case management can accurately identify and effectively treat pneumonia.[20,21] However, in 2010 fewer than one-third of SSA countries had policies in place that allow LHWs to treat children with pneumonia, fewer than 20% had

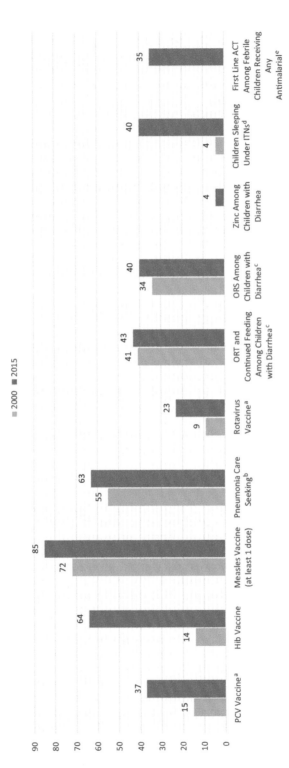

Fig. 2. Data represent percent coverage globally except where indicated. [a] The 15% and 9% figures in the first blue bars represent data from 2011; wide-scale adoption into immunization schedules in LMICs commenced more recently, hence 2000 data are not available or negligible. [b] Excludes data from China. [c] Excludes data from China and India. [d] Based on data from SSA. [e] The 4% figure is data from 2005. [e] Based on data from SSA. (*Data from* Refs.[14,56,57])

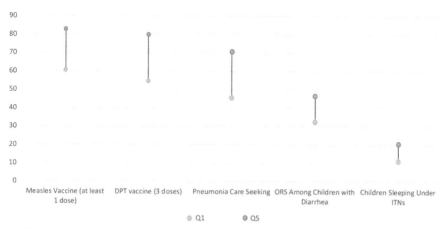

Fig. 3. Coverage of select interventions comparing highest to lowest wealth quintiles. Q1 is the poorest wealth quintile. Q5 is the richest wealth quintile. (Data represent percent coverage and are global estimates. Immunization and ITN data are from Barros AJ, Ronsmans C, Axelson H, et al. Equity in maternal, newborn, and child health interventions in Countdown to 2015: a retrospective review of survey data from 54 countries. Lancet 2012;379(9822):1225–33; and The remainder are from UNICEF Data: Monitoring the Situation of Children and Women. Available at: data.unicef.org. Accessed November 25, 2016.)

programs in place to implement community case management, and fewer than 10% had scaled up such programs to a national level.[19] Policies and programs conducive to improving access to and quality of care in communities and in health facilities and efforts to educate families about danger signs for which to seek care, in addition to improved coverage of prevention interventions, are critical to reducing pneumonia mortality.

DIARRHEAL DISEASE

The number of children dying from diarrhea has declined dramatically over the past couple of decades; however, diarrhea remains the second leading cause of child mortality beyond the neonatal period, causing more than 500,000 child deaths annually. These deaths are almost exclusively in LMICs. Indeed, a death from diarrhea in the United States would justifiably raise alarm; it should be no less acceptable elsewhere.

The decline in diarrhea mortality is unlikely due to prevention measures, as incidence rates have remained stable over the past couple of decades and account for nearly 1.7 billion child episodes annually.[22] The important impacts of childhood enteric diseases on morbidity are increasingly being recognized. Specifically, environmental enteric dysfunction (EED) is thought to be caused by enteric infections (clinically apparent or asymptomatic) and/or exposure to a preponderance of nonpathogenic intestinal microbes due to exposure to fecally contaminated environments, which is common in settings without adequate sanitation facilities.[22,23] EED contributes to undernutrition, itself a risk factor for infectious disease acquisition and mortality; thus the vicious cycle of malnutrition, infections, and EED (**Fig. 4**).

There is much overlap between the interventions to combat pneumonia and diarrhea, such as hand hygiene, adequate nutrition, and improved care seeking and case management. Rotavirus, *Shigella*, *Cryptosporidium*, and enterotoxigenic *Escherichia coli* are important microbiologic causes of moderate-to-severe diarrhea, and the

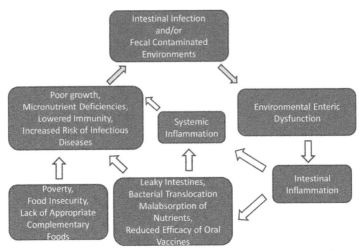

Fig. 4. The vicious cycle of intestinal infection, EED, and undernutrition. (*Adapted from* Denno D. Global child health. Pediatr Rev 2011;32(2):e25–38.)

latter 2 organisms plus typical enteropathogenic *E coli* are predominant causes of mortality.[24] These microbes are spread by the fecal-oral route via hands, food, utensils, flies, and water. Improvements in handwashing with soap, sanitation (ie, safe feces disposal), and water quality could reduce diarrhea risk by 48%, 36%, and 17%, respectively,[25] and prevent other water-related diseases. "Moreover, water, hygiene and sanitation have other important benefits, including the emancipation of women from drudgery and the enhancement of human dignity."[25]

At 91%, the 2015 global coverage rate for improved water sources (those protected from fecal contamination, such as piped water, boreholes, protected wells, and rainwater) met the MDG7 water target.[14] However, more than 663 million people still use unimproved sources; nearly half in SSA and one-fifth in South Asia.[26] Moreover, this indicator does not describe water security or quality. For example, at least 1.8 billion people worldwide are estimated to drink water that is fecally contaminated.[27] The situation is more dire for sanitation, an intervention of even greater import for preventing enteric infections. Only 68% of the world's population has access to improved sanitation facilities (those that hygienically separate human waste from human contact, such as units that flush or pour-flush into sewer or septic systems or pit latrines); the MDG7 sanitation target was not achieved.[27] The situation is worse for rural dwellers, and South Asian and SSA individuals where coverage is 51%, 47%, and 30%, respectively.[26] SDG6 contains 8 targets and covers the water cycle, water quality, and waste management more broadly. However, both MDG7 and SDG6 lack any within-country equity measures, by socioeconomic status, for example. Furthermore, neither include hygiene targets, which, as described previously, are arguably the most important "WaSH" (water, sanitation, and hygiene) interventions for preventing diarrheal and other infections.

Vaccines hold promise for preventing diarrhea due to specific agents. In 2006, Mexico was one of the first LMICs to rollout rotavirus vaccine; coverage rates there are currently 81% compared with 23% globally[16,28] (see **Fig. 2**). Eighty-four countries have incorporated rotavirus vaccine into routine schedules. Vaccines against cholera and enterotoxigenic *E coli* are under development.

Oral rehydration therapy (ORT) is a key treatment intervention: the sugar-salt composition prevents and corrects dehydration and electrolyte losses. ORT is estimated to save the lives of 1 million children annually. ORT uses prepackaged ORS mixed with water or the use of appropriate other fluids, such as homemade solutions. The recommendation to continue feeding through illness has replaced the old medical notion of "rest the gut." Continued feeding promotes gut recovery and mitigates the impact of infection on growth. International guidelines also recommend an oral zinc course for all children who contract diarrhea and live in areas with a presumed high prevalence of zinc deficiency (ie, most low-income countries). Treatment with zinc reduces illness severity and duration and decreases the likelihood of diarrheal episodes in subsequent months.[29] Antibiotics play a limited role in current diarrhea treatment guidelines, with the rationale that most illnesses are viral, that outcomes of some bacterial enteric infections can be worsened by antibiotics (eg, prolonged carrier state for some *Salmonella* infections), and due to concerns about promotion of antibiotic resistance. Antibiotics are currently recommended only for dysentery, previously a sensitive marker of *Shigella* infections, which does warrant antimicrobial treatment. However, with shifting *Shigella* serotype patterns and waning *Shigella dysenteriae* prevalence, dysentery is no longer a reliable indicator of shigellosis.[24,30] Reconsideration of indications for antibiotics may be warranted.

ORS has been the cornerstone of diarrhea treatment for decades. Despite this, coverage rates are low, especially among the poorest quintile, and improvements have been sluggish (see **Figs. 2** and **3**). Zinc treatment was first recommended in 2004, but only 3 countries have coverage rates exceeding 20%: Bangladesh (44%), Nepal (31%), and Malawi (28%). The unacceptable death toll from diarrhea is a tragic reminder of the work that remains in delivering known, effective prevention and treatment to children most in need.

INJURIES

This article is situated within a series on global infectious diseases. However, coverage of child health and survival would not be complete without discussion of injuries, which are the third leading cause of child mortality beyond the neonatal period and responsible for 354,000 under-5 deaths annually. More than 95% of all injury-related deaths in children occur in LMICs, are largely preventable, and disproportionately affect children from poorer households. Ninety percent of child injuries are unintentional; drowning, burns, and fire-related injuries are the leading cause of deaths due to injuries among children younger than 5 years. For every death, thousands of children suffer disability from injuries.[31]

Combinations of multidisciplinary approaches have been most effective for reducing child injuries. Examples include civil and transportation engineers designing and building traffic calming structures (eg, speed bumps) or barriers to separate pedestrians from traffic, product safety engineers and manufacturers developing tamper-resistant products to prevent poisoning, law enforcement personnel enforcing drunk driving and speed containment laws, social scientists developing behavior change strategies, educators and community leaders sensitizing the public to increase uptake of prevention measures (eg, vehicle safety restraints), multiple disciplines of medicine providing care to injured children (eg, physical therapists to ensure optimal function after fractures or burns involving joints), and victim/family advocacy groups serving as powerful change agents. In countries in which the greatest child injury reductions have been recorded, combination approaches have been used based on local epidemiology. For example, in Bangladesh, the environmental risk profile translates to drowning as a leading cause of child mortality; researchers and program implementers have focused on drowning prevention by teaching "survival swimming" and safe rescue skills as one strategy.[32,33] By working with relevant stakeholders, health care and public health professionals can advance prevention initiatives and care practices to reduce injury-related mortality and disability.

MALARIA

Almost 50% of the world's population lives in malaria-endemic areas. Infection with any of the 4 malaria-causing species (*Plasmodium falciparum*, *Plasmodium vivax*, *Plasmodium malariae*, and *Plasmodium ovale*), through the bite of the *Anopheles* mosquito can cause significant morbidity, although the vast majority of malaria deaths are due to *P falciparum*. Asymptomatic and "uncomplicated" malaria primarily presents with flulike symptoms. Malaria parasites replicate in and lyse red blood cells, causing anemia, which exacts a toll on physical and mental development in children. Untreated uncomplicated malaria can rapidly lead to life-threatening "complicated" malaria in young children due to lack of acquired immunity in *P falciparum*–endemic areas. Severe hemolytic anemia and cerebral malaria are the most common forms of complicated malaria and are associated with high fatality rates.

Malaria control requires a multipronged approach consisting of prevention and treatment interventions. Insecticide-treated nets (ITNs) are one of the most effective methods of preventing transmission. Regular ITN use in malaria-endemic areas has been shown to reduce all-cause child mortality by 17%.[34] Not only do ITNs protect sleeping individuals with a physical barrier against mosquitoes, the insecticide also offers protection to nonusers up to several hundred meters away. Early on, ITN implementation strategies were geared toward generating demand for purchase. However, even at subsidized prices, nets were unaffordable for those in most need and at highest risk, and coverage rates were low. Implementation strategies shifted to a pro-poor approach through free mass distribution (eg, during antenatal and immunization services) (**Fig. 5**). Use rates increased multifold, although much more progress is required to move current 40% coverage rates to the 80% goals set by the WHO World Health Assembly in 2005 for achievement by 2010.

Rapid diagnostic tests for malaria have revolutionized access to malaria diagnosis, previously dependent on microscopy, which is not feasible in most clinic and community settings. However, implementation of testing is lagging; only one-fifth of febrile children treated with an antimalarial were tested for malaria between 2010 and 2014; regions with the highest child malaria–related mortality burden have the weakest coverage.[35]

Malaria parasites can quickly develop drug resistance; conventional therapies (eg, chloroquine, sulfadoxine-pyrimethamine) are no longer effective in *P falciparum*–endemic areas. Artemisinin combination therapy (ACT), once deemed too costly for wide-scale use, is now the recommended first-line treatment for uncomplicated malaria in areas characterized by high resistance to conventional therapies. Artemisinin is an effective antimalarial, and when used in combination with another antimalarial, progression to resistance is substantially reduced. Unfortunately, its use remains too low: only 35% of children treated with an antimalarial for fever in SSA received ACT (see **Fig. 2**).

TRENDS IN CHILD MORTALITY AND RELATIONSHIP TO MILLENNIUM DEVELOPMENT GOAL 4 AND SUSTAINABLE DEVELOPMENT GOAL 3.2

Tracking of health data globally started in the 1960s. There has been a continual decline in rates and numbers of child deaths annually over the intervening decades

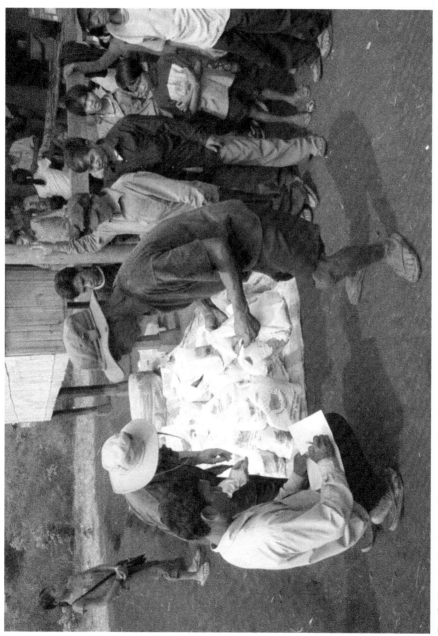

Fig. 5. ITN distribution in Cambodia. (*Courtesy of S. Hollyman; and Reproduced from* http://www.who.int/campaigns/world-health-day/2014/photos/malaria/en/. Accessed November 26, 2016, with permission.)

(**Fig. 6**). However, mortality reductions have been uneven between countries, within countries (often with more rapid gains among children from wealthier households for example), and over time. Remarkable gains were made in the first couple of decades after commencement of data monitoring, followed by a marked diminution in progress starting in the mid-1980s, with stagnating and sometimes increasing mortality rates in some countries, followed by improved U5MR deceleration at the start of this century, albeit at a more moderate pace compared with earlier decades and insufficient for MDG4 attainment.

This prompts the question: was MDG4 realistic? MDG4 was agreed on in 2000 and was based on earlier trends in U5MRs (see **Fig. 6**) coupled with data demonstrating that two-thirds of child deaths could be averted with interventions, such as ORS and ITNs, that are proven effective, available, and recommended for wide-scale implementation.[36] MDG4 was not "pie in the sky"; with concerted effort, it is an achievable goal. Lessons can be learned from the 24 (of 81) LMICs that met MDG4 as we move toward more aggressive fixed (as opposed to percent reduction) target of SDG3.2.[37] One example is Malawi, which, despite a current U5MR of 64 that is 1.5-fold higher than the global average, started with a staggering U5MR of 242 in 1990. By 2013, Malawi was able to achieve MDG4 primarily through the scale-up of interventions against the major causes of child deaths in this country (malaria, pneumonia, and diarrhea), programs to reduce child undernutrition and mother-to-child HIV transmission, and some improvements in the quality of care provided around birth to reduce poor neonatal outcomes.[38] It is unclear if Malawi will be able to achieve the SDG3.2 target of 25 by 2030.

The broader SDG agenda could prove beneficial to promoting an environment favorable to the determinants of health. However, child health is now dwarfed as only 1 of 169 targets: it will be important for stakeholders to continue to closely monitor child mortality trends at national and subnational levels. The drivers of child mortality shift over time, are complex, and are multifactorial. Some of these factors are described as follows.

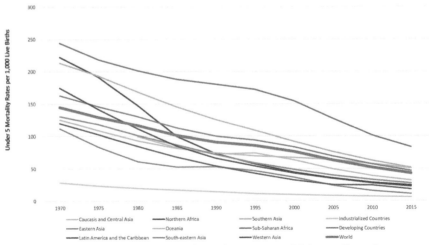

Fig. 6. Under-5 mortality rate by region. (*Data from* UNICEF. Child mortality estimates: country specific under-5 mortality rates. Available at: http://data.unicef.org. Accessed October 19, 2016.)

FACTORS WITHIN THE HEALTH SYSTEM

The 1970s Primary Health Care (PHC) movement takes a human rights approach to universal access to essential medicines and health services and addresses underlying environmental (eg, water and sanitation) and social determinants of health (eg, education): PHC is referred to as a comprehensive and horizontal approach.[39] PHC was supplanted by a narrower, disease-focused approach, termed Selective PHC. Selective PHC uses a vertical approach that focuses on one disease and a limited number of interventions at a time and shifted away from improving health systems that support the health care and public health delivery more broadly. There is a resurgence of interest in the PHC model; for example, the topic of WHO's 2008 annual World Health Report was "Primary Health Care (Now More Than Ever)."

The Global Fund to Fight AIDS, Tuberculosis and Malaria and the US President's Emergency Plan for AIDS Relief (PEPFAR), established in 2002 to 2003, continued in the disease-specific approach. The initiatives poured millions of dollars into combatting these important scourges with impressive gains in reducing mortality from HIV and malaria with approaches that did not invest in building up health systems to address broader problems.[40] However, PEPFAR and Global Fund applicants are now being encouraged to include "diagonal" strategies to strengthen health systems through disease-specific programming.

In the 1990s, in response to single disease programs, WHO and UNICEF developed the Integrated Management of Childhood Illness (IMCI), which focuses on caring for the whole child. IMCI includes treatment algorithms to target the most common child mortality causes (excluding injuries) as well as screening and prevention elements, such as monitoring growth and immunization status during sick visits. Effective IMCI implementation includes 3 components: (1) improving health worker case management skills, (2) improving health practices within families and communities, and (3) improving overall health systems.

IMCI evaluations have demonstrated improved clinical performance by health workers by those trained in IMCI. However, the evaluations also showed that less attention has been focused on implementing the family/community and health systems components. To achieve any significant reduction in child mortality through IMCI, full attention to all 3 components is needed as well as implementation on a larger scale.[41]

Attention is being focused on universal access to health interventions and pro-poor implementation strategies as a means to accelerate progress. Implementation approaches have traditionally relied on universal implementation strategies; that is, not specifically targeting those in most need. Better-off segments of the population generally uptake interventions first, followed by a trickling down of use among more vulnerable segments. Recent data demonstrate that with the same investment level, pro-poor implementation strategies result in more effective overall coverage rates and reductions in inequities.[42,43] An analysis of 63 countries representing 90% of the global child mortality burden reveals that one-quarter of deaths could be averted if national coverage rates of essential health interventions were brought up to the level of the wealthiest households, thereby averting 1.3 million child deaths.[35]

FACTORS OUTSIDE OF THE HEALTH SYSTEM

Sociopolitical and economic issues and policies are estimated to account for half of the gains in reducing child mortality since 1990.[44] Some are described as follows.

Conflict

Most countries experiencing U5MR increases are embroiled in conflict. The tragedy of Syria is a recent example whereby infant death rose by 9% a year from 2010 to 2013, compared with an average 6% per annum decline before 2010.[45] Since World War II, civilian deaths, including those of women and children, outnumber combatant deaths, accounting for 90% of conflict-related mortality. Most child deaths in conflict settings are not trauma-related because of overwhelming increases in common infectious childhood killers. The destruction of and disruptions to civilian infrastructure, including public health services and water and sanitation systems for example, result in decreased vaccine delivery, and increases in vaccine-preventable and diarrheal-disease prevalence. Health care facilities can be unsafe to access, and suffer lack of upkeep due to resource diversion or destruction from bombing.

International Economic Policies

Austerity measures are neoliberal policies intended to rein in government spending. They can be enacted internally, for example, as a means to grow the private sector. When they are imposed externally by international actors or stakeholders, such as the International Monetary Fund or the World Bank, they are referred to as condition-alities. Conditionalities are often exacted as part of borrowing packages and debt-relief initiatives (see the next section). Austerity measures/conditionalities can include slashing funds for the construction, improvement, and even upkeep of hospitals and clinics, leading to crumbling health facilities and a lack of essential medicines and sup-plies.[46] Civil service workforce (eg, health professionals, teachers) layoffs and/or salary cuts have many knock-off effects including "under-the-table charges" for health services, health workers reducing hours in the public sector to accommodate second private sector jobs, and "brain drain" to HICs for better remuneration. These policies contribute to health workforce shortages, long wait times for health services (**Fig. 7**), and reduced service quality. Imposition of user fees and/or reduced subsidies for pub-lic services directly affect those who most need the services (eg, fee-based health care and education and water privatization).

Debt

Many low-income countries are servicing debt burdens from high-interest-rate loans owed to international lending agencies, such as the International Monetary Fund and World Bank, diverting sorely needed funds from infrastructure, health, and educa-tion investments. For example, African countries pay more than twofold in debt than they receive in donor aid. It is not unusual for countries to face paying more in debt service than they spend on health and education services.[47]

Global Free-Trade Policies

Free-trade policies can affect health and the determinants of health, especially among the poor in LMICs, in different ways. For example, trade treaties have resulted in weak-ened investments and regulations in health care, and drug patent policies limit access to medicines.[47]

Unmet Development Aid Promises and Aid Effectiveness

Since 1970, HICs within the Organization for Economic Cooperation and Development (OECD) have pledged and continue to reiterate their pledge to give 0.7% of their gross national income as donor aid.[48] However, only 6 OECD countries have actually met this pledge. The United States gives the most in total dollar terms, but the least in

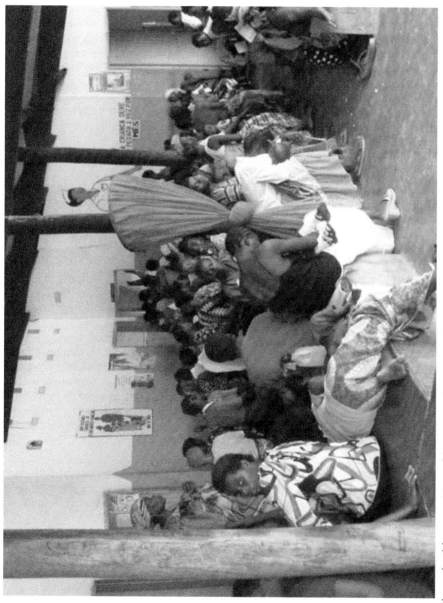

Fig. 7. Sussundenga health center, Mozambique, 1995. (*Courtesy of Stephen Gloyd MD, MPH, Seattle, WA; with permission.*)

relation to the pledge, donating 0.17% of gross national income (compared with 0.3% for 28 OECD donor countries overall).[49]

Donor aid without aid effectiveness measures can translate to wasted dollars, or worse, negative impact. Approximately half of funding is through international nongovernmental organizations (NGOs) (for-profit or not-for-profit) based in donor countries instead of directly to recipient countries' governmental or nongovernmental institutions. International NGO operations are relatively expensive for several reasons, including high overhead costs (eg, to maintain a headquarters in an HIC) and expenses related to hiring of expatriate professionals, such as physicians, for field positions, including salaries, benefits, and travel. Furthermore, international NGOs often work outside of national health systems; that is, not contributing to building local health systems' capacity. Projects tend to concentrate in capital cities, not necessarily reaching those communities that are most in need. A group of international NGOs have penned an "International Code of Conduct" as a guiding principle to mitigate these problems.[50]

Unmet Government Commitment to Health

LMICs also have pledged to provide resources for the health sector. For example, in 2001, African heads of state agreed to devote at least 15% of domestic expenditures to the health sector. Seven and 27 countries have decreased and increased health sector funding since 2001, respectively, with no change in another 12 (S.S. Gloyd, personal communication, 2016).

Skewed Research Priorities

In 1998, the term "10/90 gap" was coined by the Global Forum for Health Research to express that only 10% of health research funding was directed toward the 90% of the disease burden that affects the poor globally.[51] The term continues to be relevant as a reflection of continued wide gaps, despite recent increases in global health research spending. Furthermore, 97% of child health research funding goes toward the development of new technologies (eg, new drugs or immunizations) that have the potential to reduce child mortality by 22%. Only 3% of child health research dollars are spent on research to determine how to get services delivered to those in most need and increase coverage rates of interventions with the potential to reduce child mortality by 63%.[52]

Rising Income Inequality

Economic stability and growth generates resources to build and maintain health and education systems, but does not necessarily translate to improvements in child survival. For example, India experienced unprecedented economic growth from 2000 to 2006, but only weak reductions in child mortality. This is in contrast to neighboring Bangladesh, which during the same period made weak economic strides but strong improvements in child survival (indeed Bangladesh achieved MDG4).[53] National wealth and economic growth without equity-oriented strategies do not translate to improved child health, especially among the poor. As noted previously, relative poverty is an important health determinant; unfortunately, global income inequality is at an all-time high.

Climate Change

Climate change poses an increasing threat to health in many ways, including effects on clean air, safe drinking water, sufficient food, secure shelter, and vector-borne diseases, such as malaria. These health consequences disproportionately impact LMICs.[54]

WHAT WILL IT TAKE TO MEET SUSTAINABLE DEVELOPMENT GOAL 3.2?

The SDG child health target requires accelerating reductions in child mortality. Of the 79 countries that have U5MRs in excess of the 25 per 1000 target, only 32 will reach SDG3.2 if current rates of progress are sustained. Thirty countries must at least double their current rate of reduction and 11 of the 30 must at least triple their current reduction rate. Two-thirds of low-income countries must accelerate their rates of reduction in under-5 mortality if they are to achieve SDG3.2. If the pace of progress increases such that the SDG3.2 target is met globally, an additional 13 million child lives will be saved between 2016 and 2030.[35]

So, What Needs to Be Done? and What Can We, as US-Based Health Care and Public Health Professionals Do?

American health care and public health professionals can and do play an important role in improving the lives of children in LMICs: most of the children in the world. Many are working to improve child survival and health through overseas work or are supporting organizations that are on the ground in resource-limited settings. Through careful consideration of ethical engagement in participatory and sustainable global health work to address local needs and build local health institution and health professional capacity, individuals and organizations can avoid unintended negative consequences and provide maximal benefit.[50,55] Research on new innovations, such as new diagnostics, vaccines, and medicines have potential to reset the bar on the number of deaths that can be prevented. We must scale-up coverage of existing interventions, especially to those who need them the most: the poorest and most vulnerable and marginalized populations. Continued research and evaluation on effective implementation strategies is critical to inform effective approaches for existing and new innovations. Assessment of health indicators and coverage rates must be disaggregated to identify and eliminate disparities.

Perhaps the most impactful approach for American health professions is to advocate for policies conducive to attaining the SDGs, such as meeting donor aid pledges, effective aid allocation based on need, debt relief, mitigation of austerity measures, transparent trade proceedings, and trade policies that are fair to poor countries. Working for policies that address the underlying determinants of health, including those that address poverty, both absolute poverty and income inequality or relative poverty, can help us achieve deeper and more long-lasting gains in child health. We can play an important educational role to assist and catalyze others in the community in becoming better informed and effective advocates for children; in light of the current political climate, this role may be more important now than ever.

REFERENCES

1. United Nations. UN sustainable development goals: 17 goals to transform our world. Available at: http://www.un.org/sustainabledevelopment/sustainable-development-goals/. Accessed November 23, 2016.
2. Constitution of the World Health Organization. Geneva (Switzerland): World Health Organization; 1948.
3. Liu L, Oza S, Hogan D, et al. Global, regional, and national causes of under-5 mortality in 2000-15: an updated systematic analysis with implications for the Sustainable Development Goals. Lancet 2016;388(10063):3027–35.

4. Black RE, Victora CG, Walker SP, et al. Maternal and child undernutrition and overweight in low-income and middle-income countries. Lancet 2013;382: 427–51.
5. Gakidou E, Cowling K, Lozano R, et al. Increased educational attainment and its effect on child mortality in 175 countries between 1970 and 2009: a systematic analysis. Lancet 2010;376:959–74.
6. Caldwell J, McDonald P. Influence of maternal education on infant and child mortality: levels and causes. Health Policy Educ 1982;2:251–67.
7. World Bank, International Monetary Fund. Global monitoring report 2015/2016: development goals in an era of demographic change. Washington, DC: World Bank; 2016.
8. WHO. Closing the gap in a generation: health equity through action on the social determinants of health: Commission on Social Determinants of Health final report. Geneva (Switzerland): World Health Organization, Commission on Social Determinants of Health; 2008.
9. Bucher K. Progress for children: beyond averages: learning from the MDGS. New York: UNICEF; 2015.
10. O'Malley J. An equity focus on MDG4 and MDG5. UNICEF; 2015. Available at: https://data.unicef.org/wp-content/uploads/2015/12/Progress-on-Sanitation-and-Drinking-Water_234.pdf.
11. Rudan I, Boschi-Pinto C, Biloglav Z, et al. Epidemiology and etiology of childhood pneumonia. Bull World Health Organ 2008;86:408–16.
12. Adegbola RA. Childhood pneumonia as a global health priority and the strategic interest of the Bill & Melinda Gates Foundation. Clin Infect Dis 2012;54:89–92.
13. Hambidge KM. Zinc and pneumonia. Am J Clin Nutr 2006;83:991–2.
14. UNICEF. UNICEF data: monitoring the situation of children and women. 2016. Available at: https://data.unicef.org/. Accessed November 23, 2016.
15. Smith KR, McCracken JP, Weber MW, et al. Effect of reduction in household air pollution on childhood pneumonia in Guatemala (RESPIRE): a randomised controlled trial. Lancet 2011;378:1717–26.
16. WHO. Immunization coverage. Secondary immunization coverage. 2016. Available at: http://www.who.int/mediacentre/factsheets/fs378/en/. Accessed November 22, 2016.
17. GIVS: global immunization vision and strategy, 2006-2015. Geneva: UNICEF/WHO; 2005.
18. Restrepo-Mendez MC, Barros AJ, Wong KL, et al. Inequalities in full immunization coverage: trends in low- and middle-income countries. Bull World Health Organ 2016;94:794–805B.
19. W.H.O. Pneumonia and diarrhea: Tackling the deadliest diseases for the world's poorest children. Geneva (Switzerland): WHO; 2012.
20. Theodoratou E, Al-Jilaihawi S, Woodward F, et al. The effect of case management on childhood pneumonia mortality in developing countries. Int J Epidemiol 2010; 39(Suppl 1):155–71.
21. Bhutta ZA, Das JK, Walker N, et al. Interventions to address deaths from childhood pneumonia and diarrhoea equitably: what works and at what cost?". Lancet 2013;381(9875):1417–29.
22. Fischer Walker CL, Perin J, Aryee MJ, et al. Diarrhea incidence in low- and middle-income countries in 1990 and 2010: a systematic review. BMC Public health 2012;12:220.
23. Humphrey JH. Child undernutrition, tropical enteropathy, toilets, and handwashing. Lancet 2009;374:1032–5.

24. Keusch GT, Denno DM, Black RE, et al. Environmental enteric dysfunction: pathogenesis, diagnosis, and clinical consequences. Clin Infect Dis 2014;59:207–12.

25. Kotloff KL, Nataro JP, Blackwelder WC, et al. Burden and aetiology of diarrhoeal disease in infants and young children in developing countries (the Global Enteric Multicenter Study, GEMS): a prospective, case-control study. Lancet 2013;382: 209–22.

26. Cairncross S, Hunt C, Boisson S, et al. Water, sanitation and hygiene for the prevention of diarrhoea. Int J Epidemiol 2010;193–205.

27. UNICEF. 25 years' progress on sanitation and drinking water. UNICEF; 2015.

28. WHO. WHO UNICEF review of national immunization coverage, 1980-2014. 2013. Available at: http://apps.who.int/immunization_monitoring/globalsummary/wucoveragecountrylist.html. Accessed November 23, 2016.

29. Walker CL, Black RE. Zinc for the treatment of diarrhoea: effect on diarrhoea morbidity, mortality and incidence of future episodes. Int J Epidemiol 2010;63–9.

30. Pavlinac PB, Denno DM, John-Stewart GC, et al. Failure of syndrome-based diarrhea management guidelines to detect *Shigella* infections in Kenyan children. J Pediatric Infect Dis Soc 2016;5:366–74.

31. WHO guidelines approved by the guidelines review committee. In: Peden M, Oyegbite K, Ozanne-Smith J, et al, editors. World report on child injury prevention. Geneva (Switzerland): World Health Organization; 2008.

32. Linnan H, Rahman A, Scarr J, et al. Child drowning: evidence for a newly recognized cause of child mortality in low and middle income countries in Asia. Florence (Italy): UNICEF Office of Research; 2012.

33. Linnan M, Rahman A, Scarr J, et al. Child drowning: evidence for a newly recognized cause of child mortality in low and middle income countries in Asia, working paper 2012-07, special series on child injury No. 2. Florence (Italy): UNICEF Office of Research; 2012.

34. Lengeler C. Insecticide-treated bed nets and curtains for preventing malaria. Cochrane Database Syst Rev 2004;(2):CD000363.

35. UNICEF. Committing to child survival: a promise renewed progress report 2015. New York: UNICEF; 2015.

36. Jones G, Steketee RW, Black RE, et al. How many child deaths can we prevent this year? Lancet 2003;362:65–71.

37. WHO, UNICEF, UN, et al. Levels & trends in child mortality: report 2015: estimates developed by the UN Inter-Agency Group for Child Mortality Estimation. 2015.

38. Kanyuka M, Ndawala J, Mleme T, et al. Malawi and millennium development goal 4: a countdown to 2015 country case study. Lancet 2016;4:201–14.

39. Declaration of the 1978 Alma-Ata International Conference on Primary Health Care. Available at: www.who.int/publications/almaata_declaration_en.pdf. Accessed November 18, 2016.

40. Biesma RG, Brugha R, Harmer A, et al. The effects of global health initiatives on country health systems: a review of the evidence from HIV/AIDS control. Health Policy Plan 2009;24(4):239–52.

41. Bryce J, Victora CG, Habicht JP, et al. Programmatic pathways to child survival: results of a multi-country evaluation of integrated management of childhood illness. Health Policy Plan 2005;5–17.

42. Carrera C, Azrack A, Begkoyian G, et al. The comparative cost-effectiveness of an equity-focused approach to child survival, health, and nutrition: a modelling approach. Lancet 2012;380:1341–51.

43. Victora CG, Barros AJ, Axelson H, et al. How changes in coverage affect equity in maternal and child health interventions in 35 countdown to 2015 countries: an analysis of national surveys. Lancet 2012;380:1149–56.

44. Kuruvilla S, Schweitzer J, Bishai D, et al. Success factors for reducing maternal and child mortality. Bull World Health Organ 2014;92:533–544B.

45. Mokdad AH, Forouzanfar MH, Daoud F, et al. Health in times of uncertainty in the eastern Mediterranean region, 1990-2013: a systematic analysis for the Global Burden of Disease Study 2013. Lancet 2016;4:704–13.

46. Fort MP, Mercer MA, Gish O. Sickness and Wealth: The Corporate Assault on Global Health. Cambridge (MA): South End Press; 2004.

47. Birn A-E, Pillay Y, Holtz TH. Globilization, trade, work, and health. In: Textbook of international health: global health in a dynamic world. New York: Oxford University Press; 2009. p. 418–63.

48. OECD. History of the 0.7% ODA target. DAC J 2002;3. III-9–11. Available at: http://www.oecd.org/dac/stats/ODA-history-of-the-0-7-target.pdf. Accessed November 17, 2016.

49. OECD. Official development assistance 2015. 2015. Available at: http://www2.compareyourcountry.org/oda?cr=oecd&lg=en. Accessed November 24, 2016.

50. NGO Code of Conduct for Health Systems Strengthening. Available at: http://ngocodeofconduct.org/. Accessed November 23, 2016.

51. The Secretariat of the Global Forum for Health Research. 10/90 report on health research 2003-2004. Geneva (Switzerland): Global Forum for Health Research; 2004.

52. Leroy JL, Habicht JP, Pelto G, et al. Current priorities in health research funding and lack of impact on the number of child deaths per year. Am J Public Health 2007;97:219–23.

53. Save the Children UK. Saving children's lives: why equity matters. Available at: https://www.savethechildren.org.uk/sites/default/files/docs/saving-childrens-lives_1.pdf. Accessed November 23, 2016.

54. WHO. Climate Change and Health. 2016. Available at: http://www.who.int/mediacentre/factsheets/fs266/en/. Accessed November 28, 2016.

55. Suchdev P, Ahrens K, Click E, et al. A model for sustainable short-term international medical trips. Ambul Pediatr 2007;7:317–20.

56. WHO. Global immunization profile. Available at: http://www.who.int/immunization/monitoring_surveillance/data/gs_gloprofile.pdf?ua=1. Accessed November 24, 2016.

57. WHO. World health statistics 2010. 2010, Available at: http://www.who.int/gho/publications/world_health_statistics/EN_WHS10_Full.pdf. Accessed November 18, 2016.

Assessing and Improving Childhood Nutrition and Growth Globally

Anne M. Williams, PhD, MPH[a],*, Parminder S. Suchdev, MD, MPH[b,c]

KEYWORDS

- Anthropometry • Overweight • Obesity • Micronutrient malnutrition • Infant feeding
- Inflammation • Food security • Preschool children

KEY POINTS

- Linear growth faltering is the most common measurement used to assess child growth and affects numerous neurodevelopmental outcomes, such as cognition and motor skill development.
- Breastfeeding is a critical component of child nutrition with substantial health benefits. Improved breastfeeding practices could reduce child death, improve maternal health, and reduce the noncommunicable disease burden.
- Dietary diversity is a proxy for diet quality; measuring and improving diet quality deserves greater attention globally. Resource-constrained and resource-rich environments share a high prevalence of childhood obesity.
- Consequences of poor infant and maternal nutrition affect society through reduced capacity for work, diminished earnings, and stymied development.
- There are numerous proven interventions to alleviate malnutrition and optimize child growth and development that, when integrated with disease reduction interventions, will yield maximum effectiveness.

Disclosures and Conflicts of Interest: Authors have no conflicts of interest. A.M. Williams is supported in part by grants from the Emory Global Health Institute, Marcus Foundation and Centers for Disease Control & Prevention (CDC). P.S. Suchdev receives salary support from the CDC Nutrition Branch.
[a] Hubert Department of Global Health, Emory University, 1518 Clifton Road, Atlanta, GA 30322, USA; [b] Department of Pediatrics, Emory University School of Medicine, 1760 Haygood Drive, Atlanta, GA 30322, USA; [c] Hubert Department of Global Health, Rollins School of Public Health, Emory University, Atlanta, GA 30322, USA
* Corresponding author.
E-mail address: anne.williams@emory.edu

INTRODUCTION
Nutrition Is the Foundation of Child Health and Well-Being

Improving maternal and child nutrition is central to global development goals and reducing the noncommunicable disease burden.[1,2] Undernutrition, characterized by poor growth and micronutrient deficiencies, is responsible for a substantial burden of mortality and loss of disability-adjusted life-years in children under 5 years of age.[3,4] In fact, approximately one-half of all childhood deaths globally are caused directly or indirectly by malnutrition.[1] Neurodevelopment and productivity also require adequate nutrition and are associated with linear growth and nutrient intake early in life.[5,6]

The first thousand days encapsulates the time from conception to when a child turns 2 years old and is when consequences of malnutrition are thought to be irreversible.[4] Robust observational studies report that poor linear growth at age 2 is associated with lower earning, less schooling, and a greater chance of living in poverty compared with children who grow normally.[4,7] Although the process of becoming malnourished often starts in utero, the consequences of poor nutrition extend across the life cycle and also into future generations.

The Etiologies of Malnutrition are Multifactorial and Interrelated

There are multiple, overlapping causes of malnutrition including individual or patient-level factors, community-level factors, and conditions at the societal level (**Fig. 1**).[8] Given the interrelated causes of malnutrition, no single "magic bullet" intervention exists to eradicate it. Subtypes of malnutrition include growth faltering, overweight and obesity, and micronutrient malnutrition, also known as "hidden hunger"; these conditions often coexist and are considered a double or triple burden of malnutrition.[3] At the basis of nutrition is food, which constitutes much more than nutrients and includes the culture and ecology surrounding food patterns and availability, as well as the individual ability to use food via ingestion, absorption, utilization, and excretion. Child nutrition is unique, in that requirements change rapidly alongside the demands for tissue accrual. Given that intake in children is often demand driven, once a child is malnourished, it may be difficult to reverse.

Malnutrition Remains Widespread Globally

Chronic malnutrition or stunting affects more than 160 million children, the global prevalence of obesity in children is approximately 13%, and 43% of preschool children live

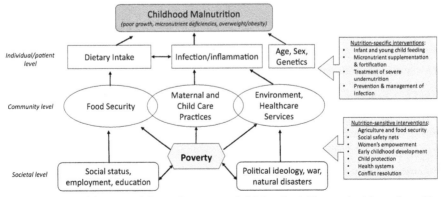

Fig. 1. Conceptual framework for major causes of child malnutrition and evidence-based interventions. (*From* Suchdev PS. What pediatricians can do to address malnutrition globally and at home. Pediatrics 2017:139(2); with permission.)

with anemia.[1,9] There is significant regional variation among these figures, and some regions face all 3 nutritional challenges. We are approaching 10 years since the 2008 *Lancet* series on Maternal and Child Undernutrition stated that "Nutrition is a desperately neglected aspect of maternal, newborn and child health"[10] and the progress is not sufficient. The 2013 *Lancet* series revised the title from Undernutrition to Nutrition, introducing overweight and obesity as malnutrition with global scale.[1] In this review, we summarize recent evidence on child growth and nutrition and present opportunities to act both at the individual (clinical) and population (public health) levels.

ASSESSMENT OF CHILDHOOD NUTRITION
Assessment of Growth

Anthropometry is the assessment of physical size and tissue density to assess body composition, and poor growth is defined by statistical comparisons of anthropometric measurements to sex-specific population reference growth curves. The primary anthropometric indices used to define malnutrition are underweight (below –2 standard deviations from median weight for age of reference population), stunting (below –2 standard deviations from median height for age of reference population), and wasting (below –2 standard deviations from median weight for height of reference population).[11] In children 2 years and older, body mass index for age can be used to classify children as overweight or obese. Overnutrition often coexists with micronutrient deficiencies,[1] especially when energy-dense, nutrient-poor foods dominate the diet. Additional anthropometric measurements that may be used include head circumference (to track brain growth), mid-upper arm circumference (to identify severe acute malnutrition in community settings), and skinfold assessment of fat mass and dual-energy x-ray absorptiometry to assess body composition.

Considerable effort went into standardizing anthropometric measurements and ensuring a globally representative sample of healthy, breast-fed infants to generate the World Health Organization (WHO) Child Growth Standards,[11] which provides a global yardstick for growth assessment. In contrast, the Centers for Disease Control and Prevention growth reference charts, developed in 2000, were based on a nonrepresentative sample of predominately formula-fed children in the United States.[12] Individual- or population-level anthropometric data can be plotted and analyzed using software available from the WHO (www.who.int/childgrowth/software) or Centers for Disease Control and Prevention (www.cdc.gov/epiinfo).

Although severe malnutrition, categorized as marasmus (severe wasting) and kwashiorkor (malnutrition with edema), may have distinctive clinical manifestations, physical examination and laboratory features of severe malnutrition are generally not reliable. Thus, anthropometric measurements by trained personnel should be emphasized for the identification of malnutrition.

Assessment of Micronutrient Status

Assessment of micronutrient status is more challenging than assessment of growth, because biological indicators of nutrition typically require blood collection and access to a laboratory. Collection of biomarkers is often expensive, invasive, and logistically cumbersome in a most population settings. In clinical settings, some nutritional biomarkers are not reliable at diagnosing individual status and therefore are only beneficial in representative population-based sampling. For example, WHO recommends median urinary iodine concentration to monitor population iodine status, but does not recommend urinary iodine to detect individual status because its concentration varies between days and from hour to hour.[13] Similarly challenging is the assessment of zinc status, which fluctuates based on time since last meal and with diurnal variations; further, specimens can be easily contaminated, therefore requiring sophisticated collection techniques.[14] In general, nutrient biomarker concentrations change with age, are affected by physiologic factors, and can differ by gender. For example, inflammation can directly affect concentrations of nutrients, because some nutrient biomarkers are themselves acute phase proteins (eg, serum ferritin and retinol). The confounding effects of inflammation can result in an incorrect diagnosis of malnutrition in individuals, as well as overestimation or underestimation of the prevalence of deficiency in a population. Strategies to account for inflammation when interpreting nutritional biomarkers have been proposed but have yet to be endorsed by the WHO.[15,16] With the increasing burden of noncommunicable diseases, accounting for inflammation may be even more important for estimating micronutrient malnutrition.

The Biomarkers of Nutrition for Development (BOND), the Inflammation and Nutrition Science for Programs and Interpretation of Research Evidence (INSPIRE), and Biomarkers Reflecting Inflammation and Nutrition Determinants of Anemia (BRINDA) projects, organized by the National Institute of Child Health and Human Development and other partners, have compiled evidence to guide researchers, clinicians, and policymakers on micronutrient assessment in various settings.[17] Given the high cost and challenge of collecting biomarkers, cost-effective nutrient biomarkers are needed, as well as those that better measure changes in exposure or status in response to nutrition interventions.[18]

Assessment of Diet

Dietary assessment methods are required to more comprehensively assess child nutrition. Dietary assessment at the population level relies heavily on assumptions and estimated availability rather than intake, and is based on national food supply data. Individual-level food availability and dietary intake patterns are more challenging to assess at scale. Food frequency questionnaires, weighed food records, and 24-hour dietary recall methods are available to assess individual consumption patterns, but have not been considered practical for national surveys. However, tablet-based data collection has improved the potential to collect quantitative dietary data at scale using camera-enabled technologies to identify foods and estimate portion sizes that can be linked directly to nutrient databases.[19] The challenge that single-day dietary intake records are not sensitive for assessing usual intakes of nutrients,[20] and confounding factors such as seasonality, will continue to complicate dietary assessment. As such, dietary diversity is a metric that is useful for assessing nutrient adequacy, although it too has limitations because most dietary diversity tools do not capture quantity.[21–23] Another noteworthy limitation of dietary diversity tools is that they often do not account for nutrient-poor, energy dense foods, such as sugar-sweetened beverages, that contribute to obesity. Dietary assessment of women and young children is now standardized across settings based on extensive research by the WHO and the Food and Nutrition Technical Assistance (FANTA) project.[24,25]

Assessment of Infant Feeding Practices

In 2008, the WHO published 3 technical documents pertaining to global infant and young child feeding practices: definitions, measurements, and country profiles.[25] More recently, the infant and young child feeding framework has been expanded to include maternal nutrition. These population-level indicators allow for standardized assessment and monitoring, as well as providing a basis for formulating program targets. The practice of these recommended infant feeding practices are correlated with better growth and child survival.[26] In addition to exclusive breast-feeding for the first 6 months of life, continued breastfeeding is recommended for up to 2 years of age.[25] The introduction of foods at 6 months of age to complement breastfeeding is assessed by feeding frequency and dietary diversity. The 7 food groups considered in the WHO infant and young child feeding package for infants 6 to 24 month old are (1) grains, roots, and tubers, (2) legumes and nuts, (3) dairy, (4) flesh foods, (5) eggs, (6) vitamin A–rich fruits and vegetables, and (7) other fruits and vegetables. Consuming at least 4 of these 7 food groups in the previous 24 hours is considered sufficient as a population indicator for dietary diversity.[27] The cutoff of 4 food groups was chosen because it requires that either an animal source food or a high-protein source (legumes or nuts) would have been included in the child's diet. Other context-specific health eating indices have been developed, but there are no global dietary guidelines outside of recommended nutrient intakes. The recommended nutrient intakes for infants and young children are often set as adequate intakes, which means that there is insufficient evidence to designate a recommended allowance for this age group. A lack of evidence for recommended feeding practices of children 2 to 5 years of age persists throughout the school age period.

NONNUTRITIVE CONSIDERATIONS FOR CHILD GROWTH AND DEVELOPMENT

The interactions between child nutrition and growth, infection, and neurodevelopment are complex and multidirectional.[18] Chronic and acute infection impairs growth and may cause micronutrient deficiencies through reduced appetite and increased losses via diminished absorption and direct loss through diarrhea or vomiting, as well as the heightened metabolic requirements associated with infection.[28] Further, malnutrition inhibits the body's defense system to fight infections.[29,30] Nonnutritive factors known or suggested to affect child growth and development include environmental exposures, the gut microbiota, maternal characteristics, home environment, and toxic stress, and have been reviewed recently.[18]

Environmental Exposures

Mycotoxins are a form of fungal food contamination, the most common being aflatoxins, that are implicated to negatively affect child growth.[31–33] A primary concern with aflatoxin exposure is the ubiquitous nature of this contamination in regions that are already plagued with food insecurity and poor crop diversity.[34] Maize and groundnuts are 2 staple food items that are commonly infected with aflatoxins. Groundnuts, along with milk powder, is a vital component of ready to use therapeutic food, and the control of aflatoxins could enable safe locally available production of ready to use therapeutic food for community-based treatment of malnutrition.[35]

Environmental enteropathy, also called tropical enteropathy, is an obscure condition of blunted intestinal villi that is also implicated in poor growth and nutritional status.[36] The reduced mucosal surface area prevents optimal nutrient absorption. Environmental enteropathy is difficult to characterize, and the current array of biomarkers include those that identify intestinal inflammation, such as myeloperoxidase and alpha-1 antitrypsin.[37] Ongoing studies assessing environmental enteropathy and growth show a negative relationship.[38–40] For example, in a pilot study in Bangladesh, cleaner household environments were associated with less environmental enteropathy and improved growth.[41] The widespread environmental contamination and resulting inflammation that prevents optimal child growth suggests that more programs promoting clean environments are warranted.

Gut Microbiota

The emerging field of discovery surrounding the gut microbiome is enabling powerful investigations to elucidate the mechanisms between poor environmental health and growth faltering. The Breastmilk, Gut Microbiome, and Immunity (BMMI) project is focused on understanding the role of nutrient intake in early life on microbiome diversity and subsequent health conditions.[42,43] Experimental investigations of gut microbiota and human milk oligosaccharides reveal unique patterns of diversity among the microbial and oligosaccharide communities when comparing healthy and malnourished infants.[44,45]

Maternal Characteristics

Maternal stature is a primary predictor of child length for age.[1] Well-nourished mothers are more likely to give birth to children who do not suffer from intrauterine growth restriction or are small for their gestational age.[1,46] Maternal illness during pregnancy is also a negative predictor of child growth,[31] similar to maternal depression on child growth[47] and neurodevelopment.[48–50] Maternal depression can affect child behavior and academic functioning at all stages, starting prenatally through adolescence. There is also limited evidence suggesting that maternal time constraints detract from child nutrition.[51] Improved child feeding has been documented through more paid leave, allowing parents to best feed their children.[52]

Home Environment

The home environment is a critical component of childhood growth and developmental success.[5] Although specific nutrient deficiencies can be tied to developmental delays, such as iodine or vitamin B_{12}, adequate and appropriate stimuli are also required for children to reach their development potential.[5,53] Underlying drivers of adequate intake of nutrient-rich foods, like access to animal source foods and the likelihood of having books at home, for example, may be economically driven.[54] However, the level of nurturance and stimulation provided within a child's environment can have a significant effect on a child's development. There is growing evidence that interventions focused on parenting and responsive stimulation can positively affect parent–child interactions and child outcomes in low- and middle-income countries.[55–57]

Toxic Stress

Toxic stress refers to the stress response resulting from "strong, frequent, or prolonged activation of the body's stress response systems in the absence of the buffering protection of a supportive adult relationship" and is considered the result of cumulative adverse childhood experiences, including such things as abuse and parental alcoholism, divorce, and mental illness.[58] There are now extensive data demonstrating the deleterious effects of toxic stress on children's health and development, summarized in a 2012 technical report for the American Academy of Pediatrics.[58]

CLINICAL MANAGEMENT AND POPULATION INTERVENTIONS TO ADDRESS MALNUTRITION

Evidence-based interventions for child malnutrition can be generalized as nutrition specific (address immediate causes, often at the individual level) or nutrition sensitive (address underlying causes, often at the community or societal level; see **Fig. 1**). Effective nutrition-specific interventions include management of severe protein-energy malnutrition using the WHO 10-step approach and ready-to-use therapeutic foods, promotion of breastfeeding and appropriate complementary feeding practices, and micronutrient supplementation and food fortification.[59] Nutrition-sensitive interventions include conditional cash transfer programs, promoting the education of girls and the social status of women, health care infrastructure improvements, and focusing on nutrition when planning agriculture. The impact of these interventions results in hundreds of thousands of lives saved annually, and most of these interventions are considered highly cost effective.[59–62] In addition to saving lives, the impact of these interventions on child growth, improved micronutrient status, and developmental potential are summarized in **Table 1**.

Breastfeeding Promotion and Complementary Feeding Education

Infant feeding promotion is an evidence-based intervention known to improve child growth and optimize development.[63,64] Breastfeeding is advantageous for the mother and the child, and comes at a relatively low cost captured by increased maternal caloric needs and time to feed the child. Mothers benefits from a reduced risk of cancer and children incur the nutritive and nonnutritive benefits of breastmilk as well as increased intelligence and reduced burden of infections.[65] Maternal nutrition influences milk composition, specifically with respect to the fat composition of breastmilk, which accounts for approximately 50% of the kilocalories in breastmilk. Moms with low-fat diets generate fat de novo or recruit stored lipids. De novo generation of fat for breastmilk results in short to medium chain fatty acids. Long chain polyunsaturated fatty acids are known to be antiinflammatory agents and are most easily recruited into breastmilk from maternal dietary sources.[66,67] There is wide regional variation of breastmilk fatty acid composition, which impacts infant health and development, more dramatically among preterm infants.[68] The fat composition of breastmilk and general dietary nutrient composition of complementary foods predisposes children to a myriad of health outcomes. Optimal complementary feeding guidance promotes dietary diversity and improves feeding frequency, and can be done at a low cost, promoting women in communities to share knowledge and gain employment as health workers, which also plays a positive role in women's empowerment.[69,70] Knowledge that infant nutrition alters the risk for noncommunicable diseases and that obesity is more common among nonbreastfed infants demands that child nutrition be prioritized.[71]

Maternal Nutrition

It is negligent to discuss infant growth and nutrition without discussing maternal health and nutrition as well. Maternal diet influences fetal development,[72,73] can affect methylation patterns that lead to epigenetic programming,[74] and maternal nutritional status is correlated with breastmilk nutrient composition.[75] Often overlooked, the maternal diet is also important for maternal health itself, which is paramount for children's well-being. Mothers tend to be the primary caregiver to children in most settings. Maternal nutrition directly affects child nutrition from conception throughout breastfeeding, and maternal and child dietary patterns are correlated at the time of introduction of household foods,[76] further emphasizing the importance of maternal nutrition on child nutrition and growth.

Summary and Call to Action

Evidence indicates that supoptimal nutritional and environmental conditions during the developmental window of time from conception up to 5 years of age can have lifelong lasting consequences.[4] As a scientific community and engaged citizens, it is our duty to advocate for improved child and maternal nutrition. There is evidence of

Table 1
Summary of effects of evidence-based nutrition interventions on child nutrition and growth

Intervention	Estimated Effect on Child Micronutrient Deficiency or Morbidity	Estimated Effect on Child Survival, Growth, or Development
Preconception nutrition		
Multiple micronutrient supplementation	No difference in anemia and iron deficiency anemia[80]	11%–13% reduction in low birthweight and SGA births[59,80]
Iron and folic acid supplementation	Reduced anemia by 27%; increased hemoglobin 4.6 g/L and serum ferritin 8.3 μg/L (mean differences)[81]	19% reduction in low birthweight[82]
Calcium supplementation	No data available	24% reduction in preterm births[83]
Iodine supplementation or fortification	73% reduction in cretinism; 10%–20% increase in developmental scores (among iodine deficient populations)[84]	No data available
Infant and young child feeding		
Early initiation of breastfeeding promotion	No data available	44%–45% reduction in all-cause and infection-related neonatal mortality[85]
Breastfeeding promotion	No data available	Increased exclusive breastfeeding by 90% for 1–5 mo[86]
Complementary feeding promotion	No data available	Increased height (HAZ standard mean difference 0.22) among food secure populations; reduced stunting by 32% in food insecure populations
Micronutrient supplementation and fortification		
Iron supplementation	Reduce anemia by 49% and iron deficiency by 76%	No effect on growth Increased mental development score (0.30, 0.15–0.46)
Vitamin A supplementation	Reduce all-cause mortality by 24% (0.17–0.31)	No effect
Zinc supplementation[87]	Reduce diarrhea by 13% and pneumonia by 19%	Improved mean height of 0.37 cm
Multiple micronutrients	Reduction of iron deficiency anemia by 57% and retinol deficiency by 21%[88]	Increased length (0.13, 0.06–0.21)
Home fortification	Reduce anemia by 31%; Reduce iron deficiency by 51%[89]	No effect[89]

(continued on next page)

Table 1
(continued)

Intervention	Estimated Effect on Child Micronutrient Deficiency or Morbidity	Estimated Effect on Child Survival, Growth, or Development
Treatment of severe undernutrition	No data available	RUTF compared with standard care has similar effect on mortality but faster rate of weight gain[59]
Prevention and management of infection		
WASH (water, sanitation, hygiene)	Reduce diarrhea by 48%[90]	Increase in HAZ score 0.08[91]
Deworming	No effect on anemia[59]	No effect on growth[59]
Malaria prevention	Reduce anemia by 29%[92]	Reduced malaria-attributable mortality by 55% in Africa[93]

Abbreviations: HAZ, height for age z-score; RUTF, ready to use therapeutic food; SGA, small for gestational age.

effective interventions, both at the individual and population levels, and the cost is modest relative to other diseases that have a comparable morbidity and mortality burden. For example, every $1 invested in child micronutrient interventions can yield $30 in benefits.[77] It is unclear why the demonstrated benefits from nutrition-specific and nutrition-sensitive interventions have not generated more demand for implementation of such interventions at scale. This must change.

The importance of nutrition for child growth and development is not an international topic—it is global[1]; for example, the United States has a large burden of childhood obesity[78] and food insecurity, which disproportionately affect children. There is some evidence of improved dietary quality and improved rates of childhood obesity through federal social assistance programs, such as the Special Supplemental Nutrition Program for Women, Infants, and Children.[79] Interventions to improve maternal and child nutrition need to receive ample support to ensure the health and well-being of future generations, which will benefit the greater society as a whole.

REFERENCES

1. Black RE, Victora CG, Walker SP, et al. Maternal and child undernutrition and overweight in low-income and middle-income countries. Lancet 2013; 382(9890):427–51.
2. World Health Organization (WHO). World Health Assembly nutrition targets. 2015. Available at: http://www.who.int/nutrition/topics/nutrition_globaltargets2025/en/. Accessed February 10, 2015.
3. Muthayya S, Rah JH, Sugimoto JD, et al. The global hidden hunger indices and maps: an advocacy tool for action. PLoS One 2013;8(6):e67860.
4. Black RE, Allen LH, Bhutta ZA, et al. Maternal and child undernutrition: global and regional exposures and health consequences. Lancet 2008;371(9608):243–60.
5. Prado EL, Dewey KG. Nutrition and brain development in early life. Nutr Rev 2014;72(4):267–84.
6. Prado EL, Abbeddou S, Adu-Afarwuah S, et al. Linear growth and child development in Burkina Faso, Ghana, and Malawi. Pediatrics 2016;138(2).

7. Hoddinott J, Behrman JR, Maluccio JA, et al. Adult consequences of growth failure in early childhood. Am J Clin Nutr 2013;98(5):1170–8.
8. Suchdev PS. What pediatricians can do to address malnutrition globally and at home. Pediatrics 2017;139(2):1666–9.
9. Kassebaum NJ, GBD 2013 Anemia Collaborators. The global burden of anemia. Hematol Oncol Clin North Am 2016;30(2):247–308.
10. Horton R. Maternal and child undernutrition: an urgent opportunity. Lancet 2008; 371(9608):179.
11. Group WMGRS. WHO Child Growth Standards based on length/height, weight and age. Acta Paediatr Suppl 2006;450:76–85.
12. Kuczmarski RJ, Ogden CL, Guo SS, et al. 2000 CDC Growth Charts for the United States: methods and development. Vital Health Stat 11 2002;(246):1–190.
13. Rohner F, Zimmermann M, Jooste P, et al. Biomarkers of nutrition for development–iodine review. J Nutr 2014;144(8):1322S–42S.
14. King JC, Brown KH, Gibson RS, et al. Biomarkers of Nutrition for Development (BOND)-Zinc review. J Nutr 2016;146(9):1816S–48S.
15. Suchdev PS, Namaste SM, Aaron GJ, et al. Overview of the Biomarkers Reflecting Inflammation and Nutritional Determinants of Anemia (BRINDA) Project. Adv Nutr 2016;7(2):349–56.
16. Thurnham DI, Northrop-Clewes CA. Inflammation and biomarkers of micronutrient status. Curr Opin Clin Nutr Metab Care 2016;19(6):458–63.
17. Raiten DJ, Raghavan R, Kraemer K. Biomarkers in growth. Ann Nutr Metab 2013; 63(4):293–7.
18. Suchdev, PS, Forsyth BW, Georgieff MK, et al. Assessment of neurodevelopment, nutrition and inflammation from fetal life to adolescence in low-resource settings. Pediatrics. Available at: http://pediatrics.aappublications.org/content/139/Supplement_1/S23.
19. International Dietary Data Expansion Project. Tufts University. Available at: http://inddex.nutrition.tufts.edu/. Accessed December 1, 2016.
20. Carriquiry AL. Estimation of usual intake distributions of nutrients and foods. J Nutr 2003;133(2):601S–8S.
21. Ruel MT. Operationalizing dietary diversity: a review of measurement issues and research priorities. J Nutr 2003;133(11 Suppl 2):3911S–26S.
22. Arimond M, Wiesmann D, Becquey E, et al. Simple food group diversity indicators predict micronutrient adequacy of women's diets in 5 diverse, resource-poor settings. J Nutr 2010;140(11):2059S–69S.
23. Kennedy G, Fanou-Fogny N, Seghieri C, et al. Food groups associated with a composite measure of probability of adequate intake of 11 micronutrients in the diets of women in urban Mali. J Nutr 2010;140(11):2070S–8S.
24. FAO and FHI360. Minimum Dietary Diversity for Women: A Guide for Measurement. Rome: FAO; 2016.
25. World Health Organization (WHO). Indicators for assessing infant and young child feeding practices: conclusions of a consensus meeting. Washington, DC, November 6–8, 2007. 2008.
26. Marriott BP, White A, Hadden L, et al. World Health Organization (WHO) infant and young child feeding indicators: associations with growth measures in 14 low-income countries. Matern Child Nutr 2012;8(3):354–70.
27. Arimond M, Ruel MT. Dietary diversity is associated with child nutritional status: evidence from 11 demographic and health surveys. J Nutr 2004;134(10):2579–85.

28. Dewey KG, Mayers DR. Early child growth: how do nutrition and infection interact? Matern Child Nutr 2011;7(Suppl 3):129–42.

29. Prentice AM, Darboe MK. Growth and host-pathogen interactions. Nestle Nutr Workshop Ser Pediatr Program 2008;61:197–210.

30. Prentice AM, Ghattas H, Cox SE. Host-pathogen interactions: can micronutrients tip the balance? J Nutr 2007;137(5):1334–7.

31. Wirth JP, Rohner F, Petry N, et al. Assessment of the WHO stunting framework using Ethiopia as a case study. Matern Child Nutr 2016;13(2):1–16.

32. Wu F, Groopman JD, Pestka JJ. Public health impacts of foodborne mycotoxins. Annu Rev Food Sci Technol 2014;5:351–72.

33. Khlangwiset P, Shephard GS, Wu F. Aflatoxins and growth impairment: a review. Crit Rev Toxicol 2011;41(9):740–55.

34. Wild CP, Gong YY. Mycotoxins and human disease: a largely ignored global health issue. Carcinogenesis 2010;31(1):71–82.

35. Manary MJ. Local production and provision of ready-to-use therapeutic food (RUTF) spread for the treatment of severe childhood malnutrition. Food Nutr Bull 2006;27(3 Suppl):S83–9.

36. Keusch GT, Denno DM, Black RE, et al. Environmental enteric dysfunction: pathogenesis, diagnosis, and clinical consequences. Clin Infect Dis 2014;59(Suppl 4):S207–12.

37. Arndt MB, Richardson BA, Ahmed T, et al. Fecal markers of environmental enteropathy and subsequent growth in Bangladeshi children. Am J Trop Med Hyg 2016;95(3):694–701.

38. Arnold BF, Null C, Luby SP, et al. Cluster-randomised controlled trials of individual and combined water, sanitation, hygiene and nutritional interventions in rural Bangladesh and Kenya: the WASH Benefits study design and rationale. BMJ Open 2013;3(8):e003476.

39. Prendergast AJ, Humphrey JH, Mutasa K, et al. Assessment of environmental enteric dysfunction in the shine trial: methods and challenges. Clin Infect Dis 2015;61(Suppl 7):S726–32.

40. Humphrey JH, Jones AD, Manges A, et al. The sanitation hygiene infant nutrition efficacy (shine) trial: rationale, design, and methods. Clin Infect Dis 2015; 61(Suppl 7):S685–702.

41. Lin A, Arnold BF, Afreen S, et al. Household environmental conditions are associated with enteropathy and impaired growth in rural Bangladesh. Am J Trop Med Hyg 2013;89(1):130–7.

42. Dewey K. Diet, child nutrition, and the microbiome. Available at: https://www.genome.gov/multimedia/slides/humanmicrobiomescience2013/28_dewey.pdf. Accessed January 12, 2016.

43. Ravel J, Braun J, et al. Human microbiome science: vision for the future, Bethesda, MD, July 24 to 26, 2013. Microbiome 2014;2:16.

44. Blanton LV, Charbonneau MR, Salih T, et al. Gut bacteria that prevent growth impairments transmitted by microbiota from malnourished children. Science 2016; 351(6275).

45. Charbonneau MR, O'Donnell D, Blanton LV, et al. Sialylated milk oligosaccharides promote microbiota-dependent growth in models of infant undernutrition. Cell 2016;164(5):859–71.

46. Abu-Saad K, Fraser D. Maternal nutrition and birth outcomes. Epidemiol Rev 2010;32(1):5–25.

47. Surkan PJ, Kennedy CE, Hurley KM, et al. Maternal depression and early child-hood growth in developing countries: systematic review and meta-analysis. Bull World Health Organ 2011;89(8):608–15.

48. Wachs TD, Black MM, Engle PL. Maternal depression: a global threat to children's health, development, and behavior and to human rights. Child Dev Perspect 2009;3(1):51–9.

49. Society CP. Maternal depression and child development. Paediatr Child Health 2004;9(8):575–98.

50. Center for the Developing Child, Harvard University. Maternal depression can undermine the development of young children: working paper No. 8. 2009. Available at: www.developingchild.harvard.edu. Accessed August 25, 2015.

51. Popkin BM. Time allocation of the mother and child nutrition. Ecol Food Nutr 1980; 9(1):1–14.

52. Walters D, Horton S, Siregar AY, et al. The cost of not breastfeeding in Southeast Asia. Health Policy Plan 2016;31(8):1107–16.

53. Richter LM, Daelmans B, Lombardi J, et al. Investing in the foundation of sustainable development: pathways to scale up for early childhood development. Lancet 2016;389(10064):103–18.

54. Dror DK, Allen LH. Effect of vitamin B12 deficiency on neurodevelopment in infants: current knowledge and possible mechanisms. Nutr Rev 2008;66(5):250–5.

55. Knerr W, Gardner F, Cluver L. Improving positive parenting skills and reducing harsh and abusive parenting in low- and middle-income countries: a systematic review. Prev Sci 2013;14(4):352–63.

56. Yousafzai AK, Rasheed MA, Rizvi A, et al. Effect of integrated responsive stimulation and nutrition interventions in the Lady Health Worker programme in Pakistan on child development, growth, and health outcomes: a cluster-randomised factorial effectiveness trial. Lancet 2014;384(9950):1282–93.

57. Singla DR, Kumbakumba E, Aboud FE. Effect of a parenting intervention to address maternal psychological wellbeing and child development in rural Uganda: a community-based, cluster-randomised trial. Lancet Glob Health 2015;3:458–69.

58. Shonkoff JP, Garner AS, Committee on Psychosocial Aspects of Child and Family Health. The lifelong effects of early childhood adversity and toxic stress. Pediatrics 2012;129(1):e232–46.

59. Bhutta ZA, Das JK, Rizvi A, et al. Evidence-based interventions for improvement of maternal and child nutrition: what can be done and at what cost? Lancet 2013; 382(9890):452–77.

60. Victora CG, Barros FC, Assuncao MC, et al. Scaling up maternal nutrition programs to improve birth outcomes: a review of implementation issues. Food Nutr Bull 2012;33(2 Suppl):S6–26.

61. Ruel MT, Alderman H, Maternal, Child Nutrition Study Group. Nutrition-sensitive interventions and programmes: how can they help to accelerate progress in improving maternal and child nutrition? Lancet 2013;382(9891):536–51.

62. Perez-Escamilla R. Evidence based breast-feeding promotion: the Baby-Friendly Hospital Initiative. J Nutr 2007;137(2):484–7.

63. Bhutta ZA, Ahmed T, Black RE, et al. What works? Interventions for maternal and child undernutrition and survival. Lancet 2008;371(9610):417–40.

64. Gillespie S, Allen L. What works, and what really works. Public Health Nutr 2002; 5(4):513–4.

65. Ip S, Chung M, Raman G, et al. Breastfeeding and maternal and infant health outcomes in developed countries. Evid Rep Technol Assess (Full Rep) 2007;(153): 1530–4396.

66. Brenna JT, Varamini B, Jensen RG, et al. Docosahexaenoic and arachidonic acid concentrations in human breast milk worldwide. Am J Clin Nutr 2007;85(6): 1457–64.

67. Yuhas R, Pramuk K, Lien EL. Human milk fatty acid composition from nine countries varies most in DHA. Lipids 2006;41(9):851–8.

68. Molloy C, Doyle LW, Makrides M, et al. Docosahexaenoic acid and visual functioning in preterm infants: a review. Neuropsychol Rev 2012;22(4):425–37.

69. Lutter CK, Iannotti L, Creed-Kanashiro H, et al. Key principles to improve programmes and interventions in complementary feeding. Matern Child Nutr 2013; 9(Suppl 2):101–15.

70. Stewart CP, Iannotti L, Dewey KG, et al. Contextualising complementary feeding in a broader framework for stunting prevention. Matern Child Nutr 2013;9(Suppl 2):27–45.

71. Singhal A. The role of infant nutrition in the global epidemic of non-communicable disease. Proc Nutr Soc 2016;75(2):162–8.

72. Christian P, Stewart CP. Maternal micronutrient deficiency, fetal development, and the risk of chronic disease. J Nutr 2010;140(3):437–45.

73. Christian P. Micronutrients, birth weight, and survival. Annu Rev Nutr 2010;30: 83–104.

74. Dominguez-Salas P, Moore SE, Baker MS, et al. Maternal nutrition at conception modulates DNA methylation of human metastable epialleles. Nat Commun 2014; 5:3746.

75. Allen LH. B vitamins in breast milk: relative importance of maternal status and intake, and effects on infant status and function. Adv Nutr 2012;3(3):362–9.

76. Nguyen PH, Avula R, Ruel MT, et al. Maternal and child dietary diversity are associated in Bangladesh, Vietnam, and Ethiopia. J Nutr 2013;143(7):1176–83.

77. Hoddinott JRM, Torero M. Investments to reduce hunger and undernutrition. Cambridge (United Kingdom): Cambridge University Press; 2013.

78. Lobstein T, Jackson-Leach R, Moodie ML, et al. Child and adolescent obesity: part of a bigger picture. Lancet 2015;385(9986):2510–20.

79. Gu X, Tucker KL. Dietary quality of the US child and adolescent population: trends from 1999 to 2012 and associations with the use of federal nutrition assistance programs. Am J Clin Nutr 2016;105(1):194–202.

80. Haider BA, Bhutta ZA. Multiple-micronutrient supplementation for women during pregnancy. Cochrane Database Syst Rev 2012;11:CD004905.

81. Fernández-Gaxiola AC, De-Regil LM. Intermittent iron supplementation for reducing anaemia and its associated impairments in menstruating women. Cochrane Database Syst Rev 2011;(12):CD009218.

82. Peña-Rosas JP, De-Regil LM, Dowswell T, et al. Daily oral iron supplementation during pregnancy. Cochrane Database Syst Rev 2012;(12):CD004736.

83. Imdad A, Bhutta ZA. Effects of calcium supplementation during pregnancy on maternal, fetal and birth outcomes. Paediatr Perinat Epidemiol 2012;26(Suppl 1):138–52.

84. Zimmermann MB. The effects of iodine deficiency in pregnancy and infancy. Paediatr Perinat Epidemiol 2012;26(Suppl 1):108–17.

85. Debes AK, Kohli A, Walker N, et al. Time to initiation of breastfeeding and neonatal mortality and morbidity: a systematic review. BMC Public Health 2013; 13(Suppl 3):S19.

86. Haroon S, Das JK, Salam RA, et al. Breastfeeding promotion interventions and breastfeeding practices: a systematic review. BMC Public Health 2013; 13(Suppl 3):S20.
87. Imdad A, Bhutta ZA. Effect of preventive zinc supplementation on linear growth in children under 5 years of age in developing countries: a meta-analysis of studies for input to the lives saved tool. BMC Public Health 2011;11(Suppl 3):S22.
88. Salam RA, MacPhail C, Das JK, et al. Effectiveness of Micronutrient Powders (MNP) in women and children. BMC Public Health 2013;13(Suppl 3):S22.
89. De-Regil LM, Suchdev PS, Vist GE, et al. Home fortification of foods with multiple micronutrient powders for health and nutrition in children under two years of age. Cochrane Database Syst Rev 2011;(9):CD008959.
90. Cairncross S, Hunt C, Boisson S, et al. Water, sanitation and hygiene for the prevention of diarrhoea. Int J Epidemiol 2010;39(Suppl 1):i193–205.
91. Dangour AD, Watson L, Cumming O, et al. Interventions to improve water quality and supply, sanitation and hygiene practices, and their effects on the nutritional status of children. Cochrane Database Syst Rev 2013;(8):CD009382.
92. Meremikwu MM, Donegan S, Sinclair D, et al. Intermittent preventive treatment for malaria in children living in areas with seasonal transmission. Cochrane Database Syst Rev 2012;(2):CD003756.
93. Lengeler C. Insecticide-treated bed nets and curtains for preventing malaria. Cochrane Database Syst Rev 2004;(2):CD000363.

Global Disability
Empowering Children of all Abilities

Rebecca J. Scharf, MD, MPH[a],*, Angelina Maphula, PhD[b], Paige C. Pullen, PhD[c], Rita Shrestha, PhD[d], Gaynell Paul Matherne, MD, MBA[e], Reeba Roshan, PhD[f], Beena Koshy, MD, MBBS[f]

KEYWORDS

- Disability • Child development • Neurodevelopmental disability
- Developmental stimulation

KEY POINTS

- Great disparities exist between children with and without disabilities with regard to education, health resources, participation in community life, and sometimes even access to basic necessities such as food and water.
- Children who receive early screening and diagnosis of neurodevelopmental disabilities have greater opportunities for treatment, therapies and learning opportunities.
- Early developmental screening of children is critical to identify those who will benefit from intervention.
- We sincerely believe there is reason for optimism. Around the world, children of all ability levels are increasingly included in health, education and social systems.
- Care for children with unique health care needs is improving and interdisciplinary teams are working together to care for all children.

GLOBAL BURDEN

Early childhood is the most effective time to prepare children to reach their full potential. The returns on investment in early child development cannot be matched across populations."[1–3] Studies estimate that more than 250 million children do not reach

---

None of the authors have any financial conflicts of interest to report. R.J. Scharf is funded by a Doris Duke Clinical Scientist Development Award (DDCF CSDA GF15030).

[a] Developmental Pediatrics, University of Virginia Children's Hospital, Box 800828, Stacey Hall, Charlottesville, VA 22903, USA; [b] Department of Psychology, University of Venda, Private Bag X5050, Thohoyandou 0950, South Africa; [c] Department of Pediatrics, University of Virginia, Box 400273, Charlottesville, VA 22903, USA; [d] Department of Psychology, Tribhuwan University, TU Road, Kirtipur, Kathmandu 44618, Nepal; [e] Division of Pediatric Cardiology, University of Virginia Children's Hospital, Box 800386, Charlottesville, VA 22908-0386, USA; [f] Developmental Paediatrics, Christian Medical College, Ida Scudder Road, Vellore, Tamil Nadu 632004, India
* Corresponding author.
E-mail address: rebeccascharf@virginia.edu

their developmental potential owing to nutrition, infection, lack of developmental stimulation, and early life adverse events.[4] Worldwide, disability is more likely to be acquired than congenital, and much owing to the influences of poverty. About 10% to 25% of the world's population lives with a disability, making this the largest minority group in the world.[5,6] People with disabilities are most likely to reside in the lowest resources settings where risk factors for stress, inequity, and lack of medical care or education may be very high.[6] Poverty often contributes to disabling conditions, and disabling conditions may contribute to people living in poverty. The World Bank estimates that people with disabilities make up 1 in 5 of the poorest people in the world—those living on less than a dollar per day, who lack basic provisions such as clean water, clothing, and shelter.[7]

A limited number of children with disabilities are able to attend school around the world.[8] Even fewer have access to high-quality early childhood care and intervention. Research is clear that early interventions provided before the school years can result in remarkable outcomes in cognitive, social and behavioral, and academic domains before children enter school.[9] Universal education, particularly early childhood education, has not yet been adopted and limited resources often dictate that only children who are healthy, mobile, and ready to learn are able to attend school. Great disparities exist between children with and without disabilities with regard to the type of education, resources provided, participation in community life, and sometimes even access to basic necessities such as food and water.[5,6,10] In addition, access to medical care may also be limited for people with disabilities. Owing to stigma, cost, physical barriers, and lack of education for medical providers, the children most in need of health care may be the ones least able to access it.[7] Unfortunately, children and adults with disabilities are much more likely to be victims of violence, abuse, and neglect than those without disabilities.[11–14]

Lack of access to education for school-age children with disabilities not only affects their overall development and well-being, but it often prevents them from entering the workforce and maintaining stable employment.[15] Without adequate employment, people with disabilities are relegated to a poor quality of life and continued cycle of poverty. Around the world, children with disabling conditions may be hidden from daily society owing to stigma, discrimination, and lack of education about causes and treatments of disabilities.

> *Unless disabled people are brought into the development mainstream, it will be impossible to cut poverty in half by 2015 or to give every girl and boy the chance to achieve a primary education by the same date - goals agreed to by more than 180 world leaders at the UN Millennium Summit in September 2000.*
> —James Wolfensohn

DEFINITIONS

When discussing childhood disability, it can be helpful to define a few terms. Disability may be used as an overarching term to describe motor, sensory, cognitive, or emotional differences that present challenges during activities of daily living. Disabilities are often thought of as conditions that limit movement, senses, or activities. However, disability is not only a physical or biological construct; it is the interaction between medical conditions, development, and the environment. Some children are born with an impairment or medical diagnosis affecting health and function, whereas others acquire disability as a result of injuries, poor nutrition, adverse experiences, or illness.[16] Some children have a single impairment and others may have multiple impairments. One helpful framework for discussion of disability is the International Classification of Functioning, Disability and Health (ICF),[17,18] created by the World Health Organization.

The ICF is an overarching framework developed by the World Health Organization to describe health states (**Fig. 1**).[19] The World Health Organization uses the ICF to measure health and disability at both individual and population levels, as well as to measure research outcomes. In a pediatric context, the ICF is useful in describing patient function at a body structure, personal activity, and community participation level. It describes capacity—or what a person with a health condition can do in a standard environment, as well as performance—what a person actually does in their usual environment.[20] Using the domains from the ICF can be useful in helping a child achieve the highest potential in body function, daily activity, and community participation. Disability is described using the ICF as (1) impairments in body function, (2) limits in activities, and (3) restrictions to participation, all taking into account environmental factors that interact in these domains.

When referencing childhood disability, it is important to remember that children with disabilities are first and foremost children. They need to be thought of in this context first; all children have the need for appropriate development, education, and emotional support so that they can mature and develop. The point of discussing disability is not to limit expectations, label children, or place them into silos of capabilities, but instead to describe conditions so that the best supports can be put in place to ensure each child is living to his or her fullest. The ICF seeks to highlight that all people have various functions and abilities based on changing states of health, wellness, or disability, within an environmental context, and this is part of the typical human experience as we move from childhood into maturity.

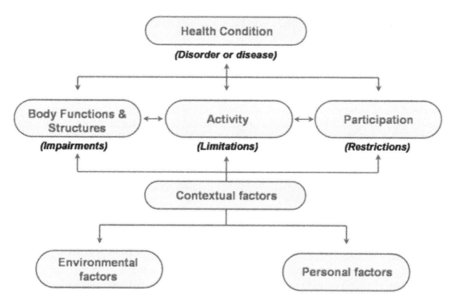

Fig. 1. The international classification of functioning, disability, and health (ICF). (*From* World Health Organization. International Classification of Functioning, Disability and Health [ICF]). Available at: http://www.who.int/classifications/icf/en/. Accessed December 1, 2016.)

While the challenges ahead are steep, the imperative for universal early childhood development is clear: every child has the right to develop to her or his fullest potential, and to contribute fully to society. Our responsibility to pursue this goal is just as clear.[21]

—Anthony Lake, UNICEF Executive Director.

COMMON ETIOLOGIES

The foundations of human brain development begin at conception, and neurodevelopmental disabilities may present anywhere from conception to childhood. Several etiologies of childhood disability are most prevalent around the world, and some are found with higher frequencies in low-resource settings. It may be helpful to discuss common etiologies in terms of antenatal, perinatal, and postnatal.

Prenatal Influences

Maternal health affects fetal development and mothers who are malnourished, who suffer from high rates of infections, who undergo severe stress, or who are exposed to high levels of toxins and pollutants are at increased risk for having an infant with poor health or a disability. Mothers living in poverty are at increased risk for all of these concerns, and this may transfer to the next generation through adverse consequences to a fetus of a mother in poor health. Genetic influences of child development may occur via spontaneous difference, heritability, consanguinity, or epigenetic effects of healthy and poverty.[22] Genetic influences act within an environmental context. Thus, genetic causes of neurodevelopmental disabilities may present along a broad spectrum, given environment–gene interactions and the influences of the social environment.

Birth/Perinatal

Worldwide, unattended birth rates are declining, but such births still happen in high numbers.[23] Several factors predispose mother–child dyads to risk for birth injury or complications. Very young or older maternal age influences birth patterns. Maternal malnutrition, illness, poor health, and emotional trauma are more likely associated with birth complications. When mothers deliver their babies without the presence of a skilled birth attendant or without access to emergency cesarean section or respiratory resuscitation for newborns, infants have higher odds of birth injury, asphyxia, or trauma. Additionally, the prevalence of prematurity is on the rise. More infants who are born prematurely are surviving worldwide, thus increasing the incidence of children with cerebral palsy, vision impairment, hearing impairment, and other developmental delays.[24] In addition, inattention and learning challenges resulting from early birth are common, and are often more difficult to diagnose and treat than more obvious medical or physical challenges.

Infection

Several infections around the world are associated with risk for longer term neurodevelopmental disability. Infections may be acquired prenatally, perinatally, and postnatally.[25] Overwhelming systemic infections that cause fatigue, anemia, sepsis, or lethargy may inhibit a child from participating in developmentally stimulating activities; children who are too tired to interact in family relationships are at risk for delayed developmental progress. Children with chronic infections may have some cognitive concerns, and these may be signs that the nervous system is not developing to the full extent.[26] The full neurodevelopmental consequences of chronic inflammatory states owing to pathogen carriage are still being studied.[27–29] Infections that specifically target the nervous system, and the developing nervous system in particular, are associated with a high risk of neurodevelopmental disability. Early childhood infections with cerebral malaria, neurocystercicosis, human immunodeficiency virus, and related infections of the neural axis such as cryptococcal meningitis, and TORCH infections (toxoplasmosis, rubella, cytomegalovirus, herpes simplex virus) all may have serious consequences for the developing nervous system and lead to cognitive, language, or motor disabilities.[30–33]

Helminths present a unique risk to the growth and development of children worldwide through loss of nutrients, inflammation, and disruption of the intestinal barrier. These infections are among some of the most widespread chronic infections in humans with billions of infections worldwide, and school-aged children are the most likely to be infected.[34] Accurately quantifying the burden of disease from intestinal helminths is an extraordinary challenge, owing to variability in clinical symptoms, difficulty in diagnosis and lack of epidemiologic and surveillance data.[35] Studies in the 1980s and 1990s found that worm infection had adverse implications for cognitive development in children.[36–43]

Childhood vaccines are one of the great triumphs of modern medicine. Indeed, parents whose children are vaccinated no longer have to worry about their child's death or disability from whooping cough, polio, diphtheria, hepatitis, or a host of other infections.

—Ezekiel Emanuel

Malnutrition

Malnutrition is a serious contributor to early childhood illness, as well as mortality, and several developmental disabilities are affected by malnutrition. Children who do not have adequate nutrition are at higher risk for infections, and children with infections are at higher risk for malnutrition (**Fig. 2**).[28,44]

Additionally, iron deficiency anemia can cause fatigue, learning challenges, and difficulty remembering things in school.[45,46] Vitamin A deficiency is a worldwide leading cause of night blindness.[47] Iodine deficiency, while becoming rarer, remains the leading cause of preventable intellectual disability.[45] Worldwide, insufficient macronutrients and micronutrients contribute to decreased growing and brain development potential.[48–50]

Developmental Stimulation

Recent evidence is accumulating that children who grow up without responsive, caring interactions are more likely to have emotional, cognitive, and learning challenges in the future.[51,52] To promote language, learning, and insight, children must be spoken to, and receive interactions that are responsive to their leading.[53] In settings of poverty and limited resources, children who do not receive opportunities to promote play, creative learning, and language are more likely to face challenges in school and work in the future.[2] Although both genetic and environmental factors influence child development, environmental factors seem to have their greatest influence in the early years, and early life neglect, toxic stress, adversity, or lack of reciprocal attachment can set the stage for future learning, behavior, and emotional concerns.[54,55]

Trauma

Unfortunately, all around the world, young children are exposed to trauma, whether broad conflicts and wars, local fighting or displacement, or domestic violence. It is

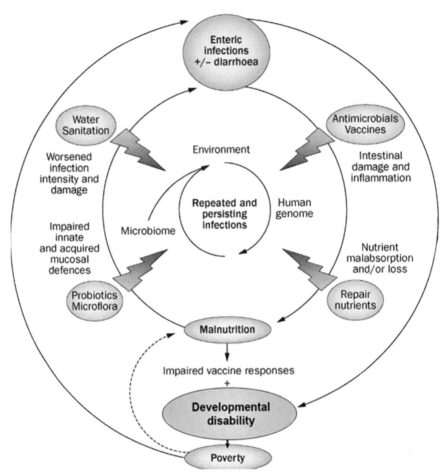

Fig. 2. Vicious cycle of enteric disease and malnutrition that has long-term implications for cognitive development and disability. Yellow circles indicate potential interventions. (*Adapted from* Guerrant RL, Deboer MD, Moore SR, et al. The impoverished gut-a triple burden of diarrhoea, stunting and chronic disease. Nat Rev Gastroenterol Hepatol 2013;10(4):221; with permission.)

estimated that 1 billion children worldwide have been exposed to violence. Exposure to trauma places children at risk for mental health concerns, socioemotional behavioral concerns, and lack of developmental opportunities.[56] Although children with disabilities are more likely to suffer violence, children who suffer violence are also likely to experience disability.[57–59]

SCREENING AND EARLY DIAGNOSIS

Children who receive early screening and diagnosis of neurodevelopmental disabilities have greater opportunities for treatment, therapies, and learning opportunities. Early developmental screening of children is critical to identify those who will benefit from intervention.[2,60,61]

Surveillance involves examining population trends in disease, whereas screening involves administering specific assessments to detect deficits in individual children at a period when intervention would improve developmental opportunities. Screening is not intended for diagnosis, but rather the quick identification of children who require further evaluation.[62] Children identified via screening as positive for a particular disorder can be referred for further evaluation which may involve more comprehensive history, examination, or assessment to more clearly describe diagnoses, depending on what is available.[61] Even when full diagnostic testing is not available, supportive measures, therapies, and education can be put in place to support children with developmental delays.[51]

TREATMENT AND SUPPORT

Since fewer children are dying from malnutrition and preventable diseases, the international community should now start to focus on the potential of children, and not just their survival.... We're now moving into an era where we can not only help children to survive, but really focus on helping them to thrive.
—Dana McCoy, PhD

Despite increased vulnerability to developmental challenges, children with disabilities may be excluded from the social and community programs that typically benefit children in early developmental stages. Several conventions have sought to elucidate the importance of caring for children with disabilities in the same ways we care for all children. The Convention on the Rights of the Child and Convention on the Rights of Persons with Disabilities[63] note that health care, nutrition, protection from violence and neglect, and inclusion in education systems are important for all children. There are many ways that communities can come together to provide support and therapeutic treatments to children with disabilities and their families. *Disabled Village Children* by David Werner provides many examples of ways families and communities can work together to promote developmental progress in children with disabilities or medical challenges. **Fig. 3** illustrates an example of a way to provide opportunities for therapy in a community setting.

Caregiver and Parent Training

Teaching caregivers about developmental stimulation and responsive caregiving has been found to be an effective way to improve child developmental outcomes.[64–68] Studies find that, when parents are given the opportunity to see these skills in practice, they are more likely to put them into effect, and when they have had the chance to practice them and positive, encouraging coaching from a supportive child development coach, the success is greater.[69–71] Positive, reciprocal, responsive caregiving can be taught and learned, and provides an excellent foundation for future learning and success as an adult.

Center-Based Therapies

Children may receive therapies at home, in centers, in schools, or in community group settings. Oftentimes services are coordinated in centers so ideally multiple children can have access to teachers and therapists who are trained to provide therapeutic support, rehabilitation or training to children with special health care, physical, or learning needs.[68,72] Teachers with experience in special education adapt lessons to a child's specific learning needs; for example, children with hearing impairment may benefit from use of sign language for communication. Children with reading disabilities may need support and extra time to learn early phonemic awareness. Physical

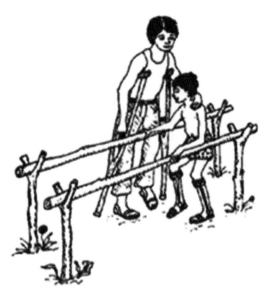

Fig. 3. Hesperian Health Guides published *Disabled Village Children*, a very helpful guide to rehabilitation that provides examples of ways to promote child development in resource-limited settings. (*From* Disability Information Resources. Available at: http://www.dinf.ne.jp/doc/english/global/david/dwe002/dwe00201.html. Accessed December 1, 2016.)

therapists can help children with mobility needs and may be instrumental for positioning, and prevention of pain and contractures. Several examples of organizations providing center-based therapies are given in **Table 1**.

School Readiness

The early years are critical to child development in cognitive and social domains that help to prepare children to be ready for success in school. Particularly for children living in poverty who are at risk for school failure, early childhood interventions can help to ensure a smooth transition into schools where more formal instruction in academic areas takes place. Programs that help to bridge this divide include skilled daycare, early childhood programs, home visiting programs, and early preschool programs.[9] Each of these has been shown to provide early skills that set critical foundations for future learning and the ability to enter a productive workforce. Because a strong start in life is one of the best ways to work toward a sustainable future for all,[73]

Table 1		
Examples of center-based therapeutic programs for children with disabilities around the world		
Name	**Website**	**Location**
Tesoros del Dios	http://www.tesorosdedios.org/	Nicaragua
Whole Child	http://www.wholechild.org/	El Salvador
Special Hope Network	http://specialhopenetwork.org/	Zambia
Mehnaz Fatima Educational & Welfare Organization	http://mehnazfatima.org/	Pakistan

resources must be invested in early childhood to promote sustainable social and economic development around the world.[74] In the United States, the RAND Corporation analyzed early intervention programs, including school-based, home-based, and combination programs.[75] According to their report, parents and children benefitted from participation in the early intervention programs. Outcomes included increased academic achievement and employment, and reduction of poverty, special education placements, delinquency, and crime. Furthermore, the program costs/benefit analysis indicated that the savings to society range from $1.80 to $17.07 per dollar spent.[76] Quality of life improvements along with the economic advantage to society underscore the importance of increasing access to early childhood programming for children with disabilities and their families across the globe. Around the world, organizations and governments are seeking to provide developmental skills, early learning, and foundations for education (see the *International Association for Early Intervention*, available at: https://depts.washington.edu/isei/). Early childhood programs can help children to be best prepared for a lifetime of learning.

Community Support and Working Against Stigma

It has been said that it takes a village to raise a child, and community support for children with disabilities and their families is invaluable. In many locations where there is high stigma toward having a child with a disability, finding support and services can be very challenging. Groups that seek to intentionally show kindness and hospitality to families affected by disability can have a large influence toward reducing stigma and mistreatment of children with disabilities. Organizations that purposefully include children with all abilities in community activities and social gatherings help to provide human dignity for these children and their families, and work toward reducing discrimination.[77] Measuring the impact of this on a family and local community is difficult, but is important to develop understanding of the benefits of these programs beyond meeting a child's individual needs.

Integration into School

Work is being done around the world to ensure access to education for all children. In fact, the United Nation's *Convention of the Rights of Persons with Disabilities* states explicitly that children with disabilities shall not be excluded from free and compulsory education.[63] However, access to school is often impaired by many factors, including, but not limited to, mobility, toilet training, malnutrition affecting cognitive functioning and attention, and medical needs. Additionally, hidden costs of school are significant barriers for children with disabilities to have access to schools. Although in many countries education is free, expenses such as uniforms, books, and other supplies prevent children living in poverty, including those with disabilities, from attending school.

In addition to barriers related directly to children with disabilities and their families, governments often lack the infrastructure to oversee programs and to ensure that children with disabilities have access to education. For example, the identification of students with disabilities is critical to providing special education services, yet assessment instruments are not available in many countries owing to the lack of resources and culturally appropriate assessment measures.[78] Furthermore, legislation in some countries (eg, Zambia) provides services to individuals with disabilities, but local areas may be without resources for actual implementation, whereas other countries (eg, Kenya) do not have legislation and funding but are making strides in providing services for children with disabilities in some areas. Lack of appropriate facilities, teacher education, and special education programming may contribute to the inaccessibility of providing appropriate education to children with disabilities.

Workplace Policies

There is need for workforce policies to protect caregivers in need of time to care for dependent family members, and particularly those caring for loved ones with disabilities. The flexible work arrangements, such as flextime programs that permit employees to vary their workday start and stop times, flexible week opportunities, job sharing, and telecommuting can enable a family to provide improved care and help to protect young children with disabilities or medical needs from being left alone during the day by family members who need to attend work. Allowing reentry after an absence for caregiving, as well as flexible work hours to enable a caregiver to provide care for those in need, is highly recommended.

Additionally, workplace policies that promote inclusion of workers with all level of abilities have improved diversity in the workplace, as well as promoting work skills for individuals with disabilities. Programs that provide incentives or set minimums for persons employed with disabilities can help to provide employment opportunities and advocate for continued learning.

KEYS TO PREVENTION

Prevention can been described in 2 broad categories: first, preventing the development of health, social and environmental challenges that lead to disabling conditions, and second, preventing unnecessary progression and further impairment of function in children with disabilities. Children with disabilities around the world present many unique strengths and gifts. Advocating for their worth and inclusion, while recognizing their strengths, is crucial to helping children and their families reach full potential. We must think of children with disabilities as equal and treasured members of their communities. Reducing limitations, barriers owing to stigma, and negative health outcomes are all key to supporting children with disabilities.

The prevention of unnecessary illness, suffering, or limitations comes in many forms. Advocating for the health and nutrition of women of childbearing years through nutritional support, and access to clean water, handwashing facilities and sanitation, and routine medical care are first steps. Many studies find that women with higher education levels and better money management skills have healthier pregnancies and infants, again arguing for the importance of education for all, and especially girls and young women.

Protecting children from violence and neglect can come through education in positive parenting and safe discipline; financial support; promotion of gender equality; programs to reduce use of alcohol, drugs, and weapons; and community organizations that promote cultural change through advocating for children of all abilities.

During early childhood, much can be done to help children reach their developmental potential (see sections on Parent Support, Caregiver Training, Center-Based Therapies, and Early Childhood Education). Recent work has addressed pairing nutrition support with developmental stimulation.[64,71,72] The UNICEF/World Health Organization Care for Child Development guidelines provide simple techniques that health care workers, field workers and others can use to support parents in providing responsive developmental stimulation and play for their child.[79]

INTERNATIONAL CHILD DEVELOPMENT CLINIC IN THE UNITED STATES

When children come to the United States from areas characterized by malnutrition and enteric disease, along with limited resources, physicians need to be aware of the importance of early childhood in promoting developmental thriving.

Growth

Young children with malnutrition, enteric disease, or disability are at high risk for growth failure. Careful and frequent measurements of weight, length, height, and head circumference upon arrival and at frequent intervals are important to assess risk factors, monitor growth, and ensure a child is making progress.

Developmental Stimulation

Children who hear a lot of words and receive reciprocal interactions from a responsive caregiver are given a good foundation. Providing information to families on resources in the community for high-quality child care and early childhood opportunities is key for helping a child reach his or her full potential. Intervention programs such as Incredible Years,[80,81] which teach caregivers about responsive interactions, are helpful in providing parents with skills and resources to use at home to promote development.

Inclusion in the School System

Children with disabilities around the world benefit from inclusion in educational systems. If children arrive in the United States from refugee or displacement situations, transition into the school system with an individualized education program (a legal requirement to receive special education services) may experience delays as the child's skills are assessed, as the family begins to learn another language, and as a plan to support social, emotional, and behavioral development in school is created. Multidisciplinary teams (pediatricians, social work, teachers, speech/language pathologists, developmental psychologists, nutritionists, occupational and physical therapists, physical medicine and rehabilitation, orthotists, and many others, along with a child's family) working together can seek a child's welfare in a new setting.

Community Resources

Participation in extracurricular activities such as story time at the library, swimming, and art or music classes can help to facilitate a child's transition to a new community. Local community groups that go out of their way to make new families feel welcomed are invaluable in helping children with disabilities, special health care needs, or developmental challenges feel connected to other children to learn language, culture and resources.

STRENGTHS-BASED PERSPECTIVES

When children face developmental challenges or health concerns, they and their families often experience significant stressors. However, these challenges may also give families unique opportunities to develop skill and networks, and to discover individual, family, and community strengths as they gather together in support. In Pakistan, researchers found that mothers caring for a child with a disability developed significant skills and gained unique community perspectives in navigating the world of care for their child.[82] There were many stressors, anxieties, and stigma for women, but also opportunities for empowerment. The study also notes the importance of interventions that seek to empower and strengthen caregivers. People with differing abilities have unique experiences, and can thus offer valuable strengths and perspectives to their communities.

LOOKING FORWARD

We sincerely believe there is reason for optimism. Around the world, children of all ability levels are increasingly included in health, education, and social systems. Care for children with unique health care needs is improving and interdisciplinary teams are working together to care for all children. Multiple programs have taken many forms in a variety of countries with local success. There is, however, a huge gap in understanding how to extend the reach of these programs, and in measuring the local and national impacts that programs have on communities and society as a whole. Further research is needed to optimize medical and educational approaches for children with disabilities, and sociologic research is needed to document the positive impact these programs have within and outside the child's family. The measure of a society can be estimated by how it treats its most vulnerable members. Disability care provides an opportunity to support and develop families and communities while contributing to early childhood thriving.

REFERENCES

1. Engle PL, Fernald LCH, Alderman H, et al. Child Development 2 Strategies for reducing inequalities and improving developmental outcomes for young children in low-income and middle-income countries. Lancet 2011;378(9799):1339–53.
2. Doyle O, Harmon CP, Heckman JJ, et al. Investing in early human development: timing and economic efficiency. Econ Hum Biol 2009;7(1):1–6.
3. Gertler P, Heckman J, Pinto R, et al. Labor market returns to an early childhood stimulation intervention in Jamaica. Science 2014;344(6187):998–1001.
4. Grantham-McGregor S, Cheung YB, Cueto S, et al. Child development in developing countries 1-Developmental potential in the first 5 years for children in developing countries. Lancet 2007;369(9555):60–70.
5. UNICEF. Child Disability. Child info: monitoring the situation of children and women 2009. Available at: http://www.childinfo.org/disability_challenge.html. Accessed May 1, 2011.
6. UNICEF. Children with disabilities. New York: UNICEF; 2013.
7. UNICEF. Promoting the rights of children with disabilities. Florence (Italy): UNICEF; 2007.
8. Robson C, Evans P. Educating children with disabilities in developing countries: the role of data sets. UNICEF. Huddersfield (UK): OECD; 2005. p. 55. Available at: http://www.childinfo.org/disability_references.html(World Bank).
9. Blackman JA. Early intervention: a global perspective. Infants Young Child 2002; 15(2):11–9.
10. Yousafzai AK, Pagedar S, Wirz S, et al. Beliefs about feeding practices and nutrition for children with disabilities among families in Dharavi, Mumbai. Int J Rehabil Res 2003;26(1):33–41.
11. Leeb RT, Bitsko RH, Merrick MT, et al. Does childhood disability increase risk for child abuse and neglect? J Ment Health Res Intellect Disabil 2012;5(1):4–31.
12. Kairys SW, Alexander RC, Block RW, et al. Assessment of maltreatment of children with disabilities. Pediatrics 2001;108(2):508–12.
13. Shah S, Tsitsou L, Woodin S. Hidden voices: disabled women's experiences of violence and support over the life course. Violence Against Women 2016; 22(10):1189–210.
14. Groce N. Violence against disabled children. UN secretary general's report on violence against children: findings and recommendations. New York: UNICEF; 2005.

15. International Labour Organization (ILO). Strategies for skills acquisition and work for people with disabilities: a report submitted to the International Labour Organization. Geneva (Switzerland): International Labour Organization; 2006.
16. World Health Organization (WHO). Early childhood development and disability: discussion paper. In: UNICEF, editor. Geneva (Switzerland): World Health Organization; 2012. p. 1–37.
17. Hurst R. The international disability rights movement and the ICF. Disabil Rehabil 2003;25(11–2):572–6.
18. Simeonsson RJ, Leonardi M, Lollar D, et al. Applying the International Classification of Functioning, Disability and Health (ICF) to measure childhood disability. Disabil Rehabil 2003;25(11–2):602–10.
19. Ustun TB, Chatterji S, Bickenbach J, et al. The International Classification of Functioning, Disability and Health: a new tool for understanding disability and health. Disabil Rehabil 2003;25(11–2):565–71.
20. World Health Organization (WHO). Towards a common language for functioning, disability and health: ICF. Geneva (Switzerland): World Health Organization; 2002.
21. Lake A. Early childhood development-global action is overdue. Lancet 2011; 378(9799):1277–8.
22. Veltman JA, Brunner HG. Applications of next-generation sequencing De novo mutations in human genetic disease. Nat Rev Genet 2012;13(8):565–75.
23. Crowe S, Utley M, Costello A, et al. How many births in sub-Saharan Africa and South Asia will not be attended by a skilled birth attendant between 2011 and 2015? BMC Pregnancy Childbirth 2012;12:9.
24. Saigal S, Doyle LW. Preterm birth 3: an overview of mortality and sequelae of preterm birth from infancy to adulthood. Lancet 2008;371(9608):261–9.
25. Dean JM, Shi ZJ, Fleiss B, et al. A critical review of models of perinatal infection. Dev Neurosci 2015;37(4–5):289–304.
26. Martinez-Morga M, Martinez S. Brain development and plasticity. Rev Neurol 2016;62:S3–8.
27. Oria RB, Murray-Kolb LE, Scharf RJ, et al. Early-life enteric infections: relation between chronic systemic inflammation and poor cognition in children. Nutr Rev 2016;74(6):374–86.
28. Guerrant RL, Deboer MD, Moore SR, et al. The impoverished gut-a triple burden of diarrhoea, stunting and chronic disease. Nat Rev Gastroenterol Hepatol 2013; 10(4):220–9.
29. Olson CL, Acosta LP, Hochberg NS, et al. Anemia of inflammation is related to cognitive impairment among children in Leyte, the Philippines. PLoS Negl Trop Dis 2009;3(10):e533.
30. Exhenry C, Nadal D. Vertical human immunodeficiency virus-1 infection: involvement of the central nervous system and treatment. Eur J Pediatr 1996;155(10): 839–50.
31. Alarcon A, Martinez-Biarge M, Cabanas F, et al. A prognostic neonatal neuroimaging scale for symptomatic congenital cytomegalovirus infection. Neonatology 2016;110(4):277–85.
32. Torgerson PR, Devleesschauwer B, Praet N, et al. World Health Organization estimates of the global and regional disease burden of 11 foodborne parasitic diseases, 2010: a data synthesis. PLoS Med 2015;12(12):e1001920.
33. Carabin H, Ndimubanzi PC, Budke CM, et al. Clinical manifestations associated with neurocysticercosis: a systematic review. PLoS Negl Trop Dis 2011;5(5): e1152.

34. Drake LJ, Bundy DAP. Multiple helminth infections in children: impact and control. Parasitology 2001;122:S73–81.

35. Brooker S. Estimating the global distribution and disease burden of intestinal nematode infections: adding up the numbers - a review. Int J Parasitol 2010; 40(10):1137–44.

36. Nokes C, Granthammcgregor SM, Sawyer AW, et al. Parasitic helminth infection and cognitive function in school-children. Proc Biol Sci 1992;247(1319):77–81.

37. Simeon DT, Granthammcgregor SM, Wong MS. Trichuris-trichiura infection and cognition in children - results of a randomized clinical-trial. Parasitology 1995; 110:457–64.

38. Levav M, Mirsky AF, Schantz PM, et al. Parasitic infection in malnourished school-children - effects on behavior and EEG. Parasitology 1995;110:103–11.

39. Sakti H, Nokes C, Hertanto WS, et al. Evidence for an association between hook-worm infection and cognitive function in Indonesian school children. Trop Med Int Health 1999;4(5):322–34.

40. Jukes MCH, Nokes CA, Alcock KJ, et al. Heavy schistosomiasis associated with poor short-term memory and slower reaction times in Tanzanian schoolchildren. Trop Med Int Health 2002;7(2):104–17.

41. Niehaus MD, Moore SR, Patrick PD, et al. Early childhood diarrhea is associated with diminished cognitive function 4 to 7 years later in children in a northeast Bra-zilian shantytown. Am J Trop Med Hyg 2002;66(5):590–3.

42. Jardim-Botelho A, Raff S, Rodrigues Rde A, et al. Hookworm, Ascaris lumbri-coides infection and polyparasitism associated with poor cognitive performance in Brazilian schoolchildren. Trop Med Int Health 2008;13(8):994–1004.

43. Shang Y, Tang L-H. Intelligence level and characteristics of cognitive structure in school-age children infected with soil-transmitted helminths. Zhongguo Ji Sheng Chong Xue Yu Ji Sheng Chong Bing Za Zhi 2010;28(6):423–6.

44. Guerrant RL, Oria RB, Moore SR, et al. Malnutrition as an enteric infectious dis-ease with long-term effects on child development. Nutr Rev 2008;66(9):487–505.

45. Black RE, Allen LH, Bhutta ZA, et al. Maternal and child undernutrition 1-: maternal and child undernutrition: global and regional exposures and health con-sequences. Lancet 2008;371(9608):243–60.

46. Congdon EL, Westerlund A, Algarin CR, et al. Iron deficiency in infancy is asso-ciated with altered neural correlates of recognition memory at 10 years. J Pediatr 2012;160(6):1027–33.

47. Chen P, Soares AM, Lima AAM, et al. Association of vitamin A and zinc status with altered intestinal permeability: analyses of cohort data from northeastern Brazil. J Health Popul Nutr 2003;21(4):309–15.

48. Bhutta ZA. Early nutrition and adult outcomes: pieces of the puzzle. Lancet 2013; 382(9891):486–7.

49. Georgieff MK. Nutrition and the developing brain: nutrient priorities and measure-ment. Am J Clin Nutr 2007;85(2):614S–20S.

50. Prado EL, Dewey KG. Nutrition and brain development in early life. Nutr Rev 2014;72(4):267–84.

51. Aboud FE, Yousafzai AK. Global health and development in early childhood. Annu Rev Psychol 2015;66:433–57.

52. Gowani S, Yousafzai AK, Armstrong R, et al. Cost effectiveness of responsive stimulation and nutrition interventions on early child development outcomes in Pakistan. Ann N Y Acad Sci 2014;1308:149–61.

53. Engle PL, Black MM, Behrman JR, et al. Child development in developing countries 3-Strategies to avoid the loss of developmental potential in more than 200 million children in the developing world. Lancet 2007;369(9557):229–42.
54. Meaney MJ. Epigenetics and the biological definition of gene x environment interactions. Child Dev 2010;81(1):41–79.
55. Shonkoff JP, Garner AS, Committee on Psychosocial Aspects of Child and Family Health, Committee on Early Childhood, Adoption, and Dependent Care, Section on Developmental and Behavioral Pediatrics. The lifelong effects of early childhood adversity and toxic stress. Pediatrics 2012;129(1):E232–46.
56. Pine DS, Costello J, Masten A. Trauma, proximity, and developmental psychopathology: the effects of war and terrorism on children. Neuropsychopharmacology 2005;30(10):1781–92.
57. Rice C. Prevalence of autism spectrum disorders. 2006. Available at: http://www.cdc.gov/mmwr/preview/mmwrhtml/ss5810a1.htm. Accessed December 1, 2016.
58. Walker SP, Wachs TD, Grantham-McGregor S, et al. Child development 1 inequality in early childhood: risk and protective factors for early child development. Lancet 2011;378(9799):1325–38.
59. Walker SP, Chang SM, Vera-Hernandez M, et al. Early childhood stimulation benefits adult competence and reduces violent behavior. Pediatrics 2011;127(5):849–57.
60. Currie J. Early childhood education programs. J Econ Perspect 2001;15(2):213–38.
61. Olusanya BO. Priorities for early childhood development in low-income countries. J Dev Behav Pediatr 2011;32(6):476–81.
62. Scharf RJ, Scharf GJ, Stroustrup A. Developmental milestones. Pediatr Rev 2016;37(1):25–37.
63. Madans JH, Loeb ME, Altman BM. Measuring disability and monitoring the UN convention on the rights of persons with disabilities: the work of the Washington Group on Disability Statistics. BMC Public Health 2011;11(Suppl 4):S4.
64. Yousafzai AK, Rasheed MA, Rizvi A, et al. Effect of integrated responsive stimulation and nutrition interventions in the Lady Health Worker programme in Pakistan on child development, growth, and health outcomes: a cluster-randomised factorial effectiveness trial. Lancet 2014;384(9950):1282–93.
65. Yousafzai AK, Rasheed MA, Rizvi A, et al. Parenting skills and emotional availability: an RCT. Pediatrics 2015;135(5):e1247–57.
66. Tofail F, Hamadani JD, Mehrin F, et al. Psychosocial stimulation benefits development in nonanemic children but not in anemic, iron-deficient children. J Nutr 2013;143(6):885–93.
67. Nahar B, Hossain MI, Hamadani JD, et al. Effects of psychosocial stimulation on improving home environment and child-rearing practices: results from a community-based trial among severely malnourished children in Bangladesh. BMC Public Health 2012;12:622.
68. Hamadani JD, Nahar B, Huda SN, et al. Integrating early child development programs into health and nutrition services in Bangladesh: benefits and challenges. Ann N Y Acad Sci 2014;1308:192–203.
69. Frongillo EA, Tofail F, Hamadani JD, et al. Measures and indicators for assessing impact of interventions integrating nutrition, health, and early childhood development. Ann N Y Acad Sci 2014;1308:68–88.
70. Yousafzai AK, Lynch P, Gladstone M. Moving beyond prevalence studies: screening and interventions for children with disabilities in low-income and middle-income countries. Arch Dis Child 2014;99(9):840–8.

71. Yousafzai AK, Aboud F. Review of implementation processes for integrated nutrition and psychosocial stimulation interventions. Ann N Y Acad Sci 2014;1308: 33–45.

72. Nahar B, Hossain MI, Hamadani JD, et al. Effects of a community-based approach of food and psychosocial stimulation on growth and development of severely malnourished children in Bangladesh: a randomised trial. Eur J Clin Nutr 2012;66(6):701–9.

73. Lo S, Das P, Horton R. A good start in life will ensure a sustainable future for all. Lancet 2017;389(10064):8–9.

74. Huebner G, Boothby N, Aber JL, et al. Beyond survival: the case for investing in young children globally. Natl Acad Med 2016;2016:1–32.

75. Karoly L, Kilburn M, Cannon J. Early childhood interventions: proven results, future promise. Santa Monica (CA): Rand Corporation; 2005.

76. Hallahan D, Kauffman J, Pullen P. 13th edition. Exceptional learners: an introduction to special education, vol. 13. Upper Saddle River (NJ): Pearson; 2015.

77. Benedict RE. Disparities in use of and unmet need for therapeutic and supportive services among school-age children with functional limitations: A comparison across settings. Health Serv Res 2006;41(1):103–24.

78. Chomba JM, Mukuria SG, Kariuki PW, et al. Education for students with intellectual disabilities in Kenya: challenges and prospects. Disabil Stud Q 2015;34: 1–14.

79. UNICEF. Care for child development: improving the care of young children. In: World Health Organization (WHO), editor. Malta: World Health Organization; 2012. p. 157.

80. Menting ATA, de Castro BO, Matthys W. Effectiveness of the Incredible Years parent training to modify disruptive and prosocial child behavior: a meta-analytic review. Clin Psychol Rev 2013;33(8):901–13.

81. O'Neill D, McGilloway S, Donnelly M, et al. A cost-effectiveness analysis of the incredible years parenting programme in reducing childhood health inequalities. Eur J Health Econ 2013;14(1):85–94.

82. Yousafzai AK, Farrukh Z, Khan K. A source of strength and empowerment? An exploration of the influence of disabled children on the lives of their mothers in Karachi, Pakistan. Disabil Rehabil 2011;33(12):989–98.

Neonatal and Perinatal Infections

Amira M. Khan, MBBS, DCH[a], Shaun K. Morris, MD, MPH[b],
Zulfiqar A. Bhutta, MBBS, FRCPCH, PhD[a,c],*

KEYWORDS

- Neonatal sepsis • Neonatal morbidity • Neonatal mortality • Maternal health
- Maternal infection • Younger-than-5 mortality • Antimicrobial resistance

KEY POINTS

- Globally, 2.6 million neonates die each year, with preterm birth, infections, and intrapartum-related conditions being the leading causes.
- Maternal, environmental, and infant factors are closely linked to neonatal health and influence acquisition of infection in the perinatal and neonatal period.
- Evidence-based preventive and therapeutic interventions have been identified that address risk factors and underlying causes of neonatal infections.
- The emergence of new infections, such as Zika, and increasing antimicrobial resistance present challenges that must be addressed to achieve substantial reductions in neonatal mortality.

BURDEN AND EPIDEMIOLOGY

Significant progress has been made toward reducing child mortality in low- and middle-income countries (LMIC). Younger-than-5 deaths have decreased from 12.7 million in 1990 to 5.8 million in 2015, of which 2.6 million were neonates.[1] In spite of a notable reduction in younger-than-5 mortality, the decrease in neonatal mortality has been unsatisfactory. Forty-five percent of younger-than-5 mortality now occurs in the first month of life.[2] In addition to 2.6 million newborn deaths, there are an

Disclosure Statement: The authors disclosure *no relationship* with a commercial company that has a direct financial interest in the subject matter or materials discussed in the article. There are no other conflicts of interest.
[a] Peter Gilgan Centre for Research and Learning (PGCRL), Centre for Global Child Health, The Hospital for Sick Children, 686 Bay Street, 11th Floor, Suite 11.9805, Toronto, Ontario M5G 0A4, Canada; [b] Division of Infectious Diseases, Department of Pediatrics, The Hospital for Sick Children, University of Toronto, 555 University Avenue, Toronto, Ontario M5G1X8, Canada; [c] Centre for Excellence in Women and Child Health, Aga Khan University, Stadium Road, Karachi 74800, Pakistan
* Corresponding author. Peter Gilgan Centre for Research and Learning (PGCRL), 686 Bay Street, 11th Floor, Suite 11.9805, Toronto, Ontario M5G 0A4, Canada.
E-mail address: Zulfiqar.bhutta@sickkids.ca

estimated additional 2.6 million still births, of which an estimated 12% are attributable to fetal infections.[3]

In 2015, the world transitioned from Millennium Development Goals to Sustainable Development Goals (SDGs). Along with intrapartum causes and preterm birth complications, infections are a major direct cause of neonatal deaths.[4] Preventing and managing neonatal infections are crucial to achieve subgoal 3.2 of SDGs, which aims to end preventable deaths of newborns and children younger than 5 years by 2030.

This article addresses neonatal infections that are primarily acquired in the perinatal period (late pregnancy, intrapartum, and postnatal period) (**Table 1**) and manifest clinically in the perinatal and neonatal period. Maternal infections acquired by the neonate early in pregnancy, such as rubella, syphilis, and toxoplasmosis, are not considered.

Conventionally, the perinatal period begins at 22 completed weeks of gestation and ends 7 days after birth. The neonatal period represents the first 28 days of life. The relative lack of structural barriers and an immature immune system put neonates at greater risk of infection and mortality. Preterm birth (36%), infections (23%), and intrapartum-related conditions, such as birth asphyxia (23%), are responsible for the greatest number of neonatal deaths[4] (**Fig. 1**). However, in the late neonatal period (>7 days), 48% of deaths are attributable to infections, the leading cause of death in this period[4] (see **Fig. 1**).

RISK FACTORS FOR NEONATAL AND PERINATAL INFECTIONS
Maternal Health and Infections

Poor maternal health and inadequate access to health care are determinants for neonatal outcomes.

Maternal infections
Infections during pregnancy are associated with spontaneous abortion, stillbirth, preterm delivery, and low birth weight (LBW).[5] Moreover, some infections are transmitted to the fetus, resulting in neonatal morbidity or fetal loss. Transmission can occur hematogenously from mother to baby or as an ascending infection via the uterine cervix. Early onset sepsis (EOS) and most infections in the perinatal period are associated with maternal factors. A neonate's immature immune system depends on maternal

Table 1
Key maternal infections acquired by neonates and period of transmission

	Early Pregnancy	Midpregnancy	Late Pregnancy	Intrapartum	Postnatal
Rubella	+	—	—	—	—
Toxoplasmosis	+	+	—	—	—
Syphilis	—	+	+	—	—
Cytomegalovirus	+	+	+	+	+
Zika virus	++	+	+	—	—
Chickenpox	—	—	+	+	+
Herpes simplex virus	—	—	—	+	—
HIV	—	—	+	++	+
Hepatitis B	—	—	—	+	—
Group B streptococcus	—	—	—	+	—

Abbreviation: HIV, human immunodeficiency virus.

Neonatal Period (0–28 d)

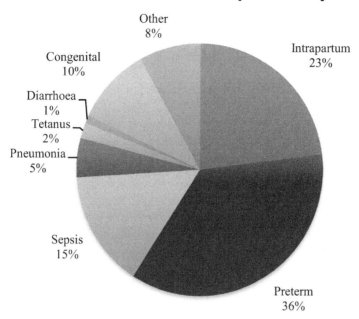

Other
8%

Intrapartum
23%

Congenital
10%

Diarrhoea
1%

Tetanus
2%

Pneumonia
5%

Sepsis
15%

Preterm
36%

Fig. 1. Causes of death in the neonatal period globally. (*Adapted from* Lawn J, Blencowe H, Oza S, et al. Every newborn: progress, priorities, and potential beyond survival. Lancet 2014;384(9938):189–205.)

antibodies that cross transplacentally. However, maternal infections occurring close to term may not generate sufficient immune protection to pass to the fetus.

Cytomegalovirus (CMV), rubella virus, varicella-zoster virus, hepatitis B and C, and Zika virus can transmit to the fetus through the blood. Important organisms acquired by the ascending route are group B streptococcus (GBS), herpes simplex virus (HSV), and *Escherichia coli*.[6] Chances of acquiring certain infections intrapartum increase with vaginal deliveries, and clinicians may opt for cesarean deliveries in such cases.

Premature rupture of membranes
Premature rupture of membranes (PROM) is when the amniotic sac ruptures more than 1 hour before the onset of labor. Ruptured membranes increase the risk of maternal infection, preterm birth, and EOS. Some estimates show that nearly 10%[6] of neonates develop infection following PROM, whereas others report lower (4%) or higher (33%) rates.[7,8] Risk is directly proportional to the time membranes rupture before delivery: the earlier the membranes rupture, the higher the risk of infection.

Organisms most commonly associated with EOS secondary to PROM include GBS. Studies in low-income settings report predominantly gram-negative organisms.[7] Gram-positive species, such as GBS and *Staphylococcus aureus*, though detected, were not as common as in developed settings.

Intra-amniotic infection
Aside from other causes, a mother can develop fever during labor due to chorioamnionitis or intra-amniotic infection (IAI). IAI is associated with adverse pregnancy and

neonatal outcomes, including stillbirth, preterm birth, and infections. Risk of neonatal septicemia in these cases is estimated at 5% to 15%. Neonatal outcomes are influenced by not only causative organisms but also birth weight and timing of antibiotic therapy.[6]

OTHER RISK FACTORS FOR ACQUIRING INFECTION
Environmental Factors

Late-onset neonatal infections are commonly associated with nosocomial or community-related environment factors.

Hospital-acquired infections

Hospitals, especially nurseries and intensive care units, are high-risk environments for acquiring infections. Infants are in frequent contact with health care workers, leading to spread of pathogenic organisms, especially multidrug-resistant types. With increasing facility-based deliveries in LMIC, the risk of hospital-acquired infections has also increased. Some studies from high-income countries (HIC) report that more than 20% of critically ill newborns who survive greater than 2 days acquire a nosocomial infection.[6] Major pathways for nosocomial spread of organisms in neonate are summarized in **Box 1**.

Community-acquired infections

Because of social and economic factors, many births, especially in rural areas of LMIC, take place at home. Risk of community-acquired infections in such home-delivered infants is higher. Other factors, such as lack of skilled birth attendants, unhygienic delivery practices, and unsterile cord cutting, further increase the risk of

---

Box 1
Common pathways for the nosocomial spread of sepsis in a neonate

Excessive vaginal examinations of mother

Lack of aseptic delivery

Inadequate hand hygiene and glove use

Failures in sterilization/disinfection or handling/storage of multiuser equipment, instruments, and supplies leading to contamination

Inadequate environmental cleaning and disinfection

Overuse of invasive devices

Reuse of disposable supplies without safe disinfection/sterilization procedures

Failures in isolation procedures/inadequate isolation facilities for babies infected with antibiotic-resistant or highly transmissible pathogens

Unhygienic bathing and skin care

Absence of mother-baby cohorting

Inappropriate and prolonged use of antibiotics

Lack of knowledge, training, and competency regarding infection control practice

Overcrowded and understaffed labor and delivery rooms

Adapted from Khan AM, Bhutta ZA. Childhood infectious diseases: overview. In: Quah SR, Cockerham WC, editors. The international encyclopedia of public health. 2nd edition. vol. 1. Oxford (United Kingdom): Academic Press; 2017. p. 517–38.

infections. In other settings, newborns discharged from the hospital can also acquire infections from household or community contact.

Infant Factors

Compared with other infants, those who have bacterial sepsis frequently possess distinctive risk factors, such as preterm birth, LBW, PROM, maternal IAI, and birth asphyxia.

The 20 million LBW babies born globally each year[9] are either preterm or small for gestational age (or both). Vulnerability to hypothermia, immature immune systems, and an underdeveloped skin barrier predispose them to infections.[10] Preterm birth is considered the chief risk factor for acquiring neonatal infections immediately before, during, or after delivery.[6] Preterm birth complications are now the number one killer of children younger than 5 years.[4]

Evidence indicates a low Apgar score at birth is associated with increased risk of infection-attributable neonatal mortality.[11] Fetal hypoxia and hypothermia can impair immune mechanisms as well as predispose to birth asphyxia, a risk factor for infections.[6]

PERINATAL VIRAL INFECTIONS

These viral infections are largely acquired from the mother in the perinatal period and manifest soon after birth.

Cytomegalovirus

CMV is the most common perinatal viral infection. Primary CMV infection in pregnant women can cause fetal infection in 40% of the cases. Ten percent to 15% are symptomatic, whereas the rest have subclinical congenital infection.[12] Moreover, perinatal infection can also occur by exposure to the virus in the maternal genital tract during delivery, through breastfeeding, or blood transfusions.

Symptomatic congenital CMV at birth occurs in 10% of infected infants and can present with jaundice, hepatosplenomegaly, and microcephaly. Complications in infants include sensorineural hearing loss (35%), neurologic deficits (66%), and death (4%).[13] Twenty-five percent of neonates with asymptomatic congenital CMV will have sequelae in the first 2 years of life.[6] Infants with perinatal CMV can develop a sepsis-like syndrome accompanied with hepatosplenomegaly.

Diagnosis of maternal CMV is through serologic tests for CMV antibodies. Amniocentesis is the best option for prenatal diagnosis of fetal congenital CMV infection.[12] Postnatal diagnosis of congenital CMV is recommended through virus isolation.

Antenatal treatment of maternal CMV with antiviral agents is not recommended except for research purposes. However, antiviral drugs can be used in symptomatic congenital CMV and have been shown to improve long-term hearing and neurologic outcomes.[13] Vaccine development remains a research priority.

Zika Virus

Zika virus generally causes a mild disease and can even be asymptomatic in pregnant women and adults. However, it can also cause a dengue-like constellation of symptoms, including rash, myalgias, fever, and conjunctivitis. In 2015, reports of association of Zika with increased incidence of Guillain-Barre syndrome and other neurologic conditions led to worldwide alarm. Further evidence suggested that infants born to Zika-infected women can have microcephaly and central nervous system abnormalities. In September 2016, the World Health Organization (WHO) concluded that Zika infection during pregnancy increases risk of congenital brain abnormalities, particularly with infection acquired in the first trimester.[14] Termed *congenital Zika syndrome* (CZS), it manifests with brain defects, craniofacial disproportion, limb contractures, and ocular and hearing abnormalities.[15] Infections in the third trimester are mostly associated with brain malformations but with normal-sized heads.[16]

Zika is transmitted by bite of the *Aedes aegypti* mosquito and less commonly through sexual contact and blood transfusion. Prevention includes control of mosquito breeding sites and protection against bites. Public health officials in pandemic regions continue to advise women to delay pregnancies until the virus is controlled. There is currently no vaccine for Zika. Treatment is supportive based on symptomatic and fluid management. Similarly, there is no specific treatment of infants with CZS other than supportive care.

Varicella

The 3 main forms of varicella associated with the perinatal and neonatal period are summarized in **Table 2**.

Varicella zoster immunoglobulin is indicated in infants whose mothers manifest the infection between 5 days before and 2 days after delivery. These neonates would not be protected by maternal antibodies.[6]

Introduction of the varicella vaccine has reduced the incidence of varicella zoster virus (VZV) infection among pregnant women, especially in HIC. Coverage of vaccine in LMIC remains low, however incidence of VZV is also low for unclear reasons.

Table 2
Varicella in the neonate in perinatal and neonatal period

	Transplacentally Acquired[a]		Postnatally Acquired
Acquisition by Infant	**Maternal Rash in Early or Midpregnancy**	**Maternal Rash, 5 d Before Delivery to 2 d After Birth**	**Postnatal Infant Chickenpox**
Clinical form in infant	Congenital varicella syndrome	Congenital/neonatal chickenpox	Chickenpox
Signs and symptoms in infant	Rare form with congenital lesions such as • Cicatricial skin lesions • Ophthalmic defects (chorioretinitis, microphthalmia) • Neurologic abnormalities • Hypoplastic limbs *Prematurity, LBW, and death are also possible complications of the syndrome*	Most severe form with • Signs of infection • Rash • Complications, such as hepatitis, pneumonia, or encephalitis *Can be associated with significant mortality*	Generally mild form with signs of infection and rash
Manifestation	First 10 d of life	First 10 d of life	10–28 d after birth

[a] Mother infected during pregnancy.

Herpes Simplex Virus

Eighty-five percent of cases of neonatal herpes are acquired by intrapartum virus exposure in the maternal genital tract. Five percent of neonates acquire disease in utero, whereas 10% acquire postnatally.[17] Disseminated herpes is the most severe form, with multisystem involvement.

Viral culture and polymerase chain reaction (PCR) for HSV DNA are used to diagnose neonatal herpes. Parenteral therapy with antiviral agents and long-term antiviral suppressive therapy are part of the treatment regimen.[18]

Human Immunodeficiency Virus

Mother-to-child perinatal transmission of human immunodeficiency virus (HIV) can occur in utero, most commonly intrapartum or postnatally through breastfeeding. Although a public health challenge, intensified services and global use of efficacious drugs has resulted in decreased rates of transmission. An estimated 1.4 million children were prevented from being infected between 2000 and 2014.[19]

HIV-positive infants could remain asymptomatic during the neonatal period or present with nonspecific symptoms. Suggested average age for onset of clinical signs of perinatally acquired HIV has been between 5 and 6 months.[20] Growth delay, oral thrush, lymphadenopathy, and hepatosplenomegaly are frequent, early findings. Importantly, these children are more susceptible to bacterial and opportunistic infections.

All HIV-exposed infants should receive antiretroviral (ARV) drugs to reduce the chance of perinatal transmission. If possible, prophylaxis should be initiated within 6 to 12 hours of delivery.

Children infected perinatally could present for the first time in adolescence. Conversely, some may have had multiple treatment regimens by adolescence and have a resistant strain, presenting a management challenge.[19]

Hepatitis B

Globally, hepatitis B virus (HBV) chronically infects more than 240 million individuals[21] and causes nearly 1 million deaths annually.[22] Most cases are a consequence of maternal-to-fetal transmission with the most frequent route being intrapartum. Early detection of HBV in mothers can inform prophylactic interventions postnatally.

An infant who has acquired HBV perinatally has a 90% risk of becoming a chronic carrier and a subsequent 15% to 20% chance of dying of chronic liver conditions in adulthood.[23] However, intervening postnatally with hepatitis B immunoglobulin and birth-dose vaccination provides the susceptible infant an 85% to 95% chance of being protected. Conversely, researchers have noted that mothers with a high viral load may pass on HBV to infants, underscoring the importance of peripartum use of antiviral drugs. Further studies are needed to assess appropriate timing of these drugs and their long-term safety in pregnancy.[21] Breastfeeding is not considered a risk factor for transmission and is recommended with accompanying prophylaxis.

Most infected newborns will remain asymptomatic until the first or second decade of life. Rarely, infants will manifest acute hepatitis with associated symptoms.[6] Diagnosis of HBV in neonates is generally made by detecting HBsAg or through PCR. Management is supportive, and treatment regimens available are for children older than 2 years.

BACTERIAL INFECTIONS
Neonatal Sepsis

Sepsis is a significant cause of newborn morbidity and mortality, particularly in preterm and LBW infants. Neonatal sepsis and meningitis are responsible for an estimated 420,000 deaths annually, accounting for 16% of neonatal mortality.[24]

Traditionally, neonatal sepsis is defined by systemic signs and blood stream infection identified in the first 4 weeks of life. Sepsis is classified as EOS or late-onset sepsis (LOS). There is a lack of consensus in the literature as to what age limits define both, though the most commonly used cutoff is less than 7 days (EOS) versus more than 7 days (LOS).

Neonates usually have nonspecific signs of infection, such as lethargy and irritability. Sepsis can be diagnosed both clinically and microbiologically. Some possible signs and symptoms of serious infection in newborns are shown in **Box 2**.

The organisms most commonly causing sepsis in developing and developed countries are given in **Table 3**.

Promptly identifying and treating neonates with infections is critical. Integrated management of childhood illness (IMCI) has been widely implemented, especially in LMIC. Modifications of IMCI to include the neonatal period and expansion to community settings have now been prioritized as a public health strategy.

Box 2
Possible symptoms and signs of sepsis in a neonate

Sepsis

Grunting

Not feeding well

Drowsiness or unconscious

Lethargy

Reduced movements

Fast breathing (60 breaths per minute or more)

Severe chest in-drawing

Increased body temperature (>38°C)

Hypothermia (<35.5°C)

Cyanosis

Convulsions

Signs of bacterial infection (in addition to the aforementioned signs)

Severe jaundice

Severe abdominal distension

Many or severe skin pustules

Umbilical redness

Pus draining from umbilicus

Bulging fontanelle

Joint swelling and tenderness

Adapted from Pocket book of hospital care for children. 2nd edition. Geneva (Switzerland): World Health Organization; 2013.

Table 3
Organisms most commonly causing sepsis in developing and developed countries

Neonatal Sepsis	
Developing Countries	Developed Countries
Gram-negative organisms (more common) 　*Klebsiella* 　*E coli* 　*Pseudomonas* 　*Salmonella*	Gram-negative organisms 　*E coli* (more common)
Gram-positive organisms (less common) 　*Staphylococcus aureus* 　*Streptococcus pneumoniae* 　*Streptococcus pyogenes*	Gram-positive organisms 　GBS (more common) 　CONS (NICU settings mostly) 　*Staphylococcus aureus*

Abbreviations: CONS, coagulase-negative staphylococci; NICU, neonatal intensive care unit.

Adapted from Khan AM, Bhutta ZA. Childhood infectious diseases: overview. In: Quah SR, Cockerham WC, editors. The International encyclopedia of public health. 2nd edition, vol. 1. Oxford (United Kingdom): Academic Press; 2017. p. 517–38.

Recent studies have established effectiveness of simpler treatment regimens that have achieved reductions in neonatal mortality with the use of oral cotrimoxazole and injectable gentamicin by community health workers. The African Neonatal Sepsis Trial (AFRINEST) demonstrated that simplified antibiotic regimens using combinations of injectable gentamicin, oral amoxicillin, and in some cases injectable procaine benzylpenicillin (given at home or at primary health care level) in possible serious bacterial infections (PSBI) were as effective as parenteral WHO-recommended regimens.[25] These strategies could be valuable where referral is a challenge.[26]

Facility-based treatment regimens for neonatal sepsis often use a combination of ampicillin and gentamicin with or without vancomycin. If at risk of *Staphylococcus aureus* infection, cloxacillin with gentamicin is recommended as an option, although rates of methicillin-resistant *Staphylococcus aureus* are rapidly increasing in many settings. The WHO recommends treating neonatal meningitis with ampicillin or a third-generation cephalosporin in combination with gentamicin, for at least 3 weeks.[27] (However, in some settings gentamicin is limited to 2 weeks because of ototoxicity.) **Table 4** shows the commonly used antibiotic treatment options for sepsis in neonates.

Possible Serious Bacterial Infection

As per the WHO's recommendations, serious bacterial infections[28] in neonates should be referred for hospital treatment with a 7-day course of benzylpenicillin with

Table 4
Commonly used antimicrobials for neonatal sepsis

	Antimicrobial Choice	
Likely Cause	Developed Countries	Developing Countries
Developed countries 　*Streptococcus* (group B) 　*E coli*	Ampicillin or penicillin plus 　gentamicin Or	Ampicillin or penicillin plus 　aminoglycoside Or
Developing countries 　*Klebsiella* 　*Pseudomonas* 　*Salmonella*	Third-generation 　cephalosporin	Cotrimoxazole plus gentamicin

gentamicin or ampicillin with gentamicin. However, considering the lack of access and compliance in many low-resource settings, the WHO now recommends that PSBI in neonates be treated at first-level care facilities by a trained health worker.[29] For this purpose, the diagnosis of PSBI is recommended based on the presence of one or more easily identifiable clinical signs.[29] Recommended treatment regimens include intramuscular gentamicin with oral amoxicillin.

GROUP B STREPTOCOCCAL INFECTIONS

GBS is the leading organism causing neonatal sepsis and meningitis and is well-documented in high-income regions. GBS burden in LMIC is poorly recognized. However, certain reviews have associated Africa with a GBS incidence 3 times higher than the Americas.[30] Current global incidence is estimated at 0.53 per 1000 livebirths, which is most likely an underestimate, as many cases in LMIC are fatal before diagnosis.[30]

Risk of infection with GBS is greatest in the first 90 days of life.[31] Colonization of the maternal genital tract, especially in the intrapartum phase, puts the neonate at risk of infection. Based on the age of onset, GBS infection can be early onset (0–6 days) or late onset (7–89 days). Early-onset disease (EOD) is largely a result of vertical transmission from the mother, whereas late-onset disease (LOD) can be from the mother or horizontal transmission from environmental sources. EOD usually manifests with nonspecific signs of bacteremia (80%–85%), pneumonia, or meningitis. LOD, with a lower fatality rate than EOD, can present with similar clinical features. More recently, the terminology late-late-onset infection has been applied to GBS disease occurring in infants older than 89 days, most of whom are preterm, which contributes to this late manifestation of GBS.[6]

GBS can be isolated from blood, cerebrospinal fluid, or focal site of infection. Penicillin G is the treatment of choice. However, in most scenarios, before confirmatory microbiology and transition to definitive therapy, initial therapy is started with ampicillin and an aminoglycoside. Fourteen- to 21-day parenteral therapy is advised for both meningitis and septic arthritis.

Most HICs implement universal GBS screening of women at 35 to 37 weeks of gestation through a rectovaginal swab followed by intrapartum antibiotic prophylaxis (IAP) in those with positive cultures. GBS bacteriuria or previous delivery of an infant with invasive GBS always requires IAP. Reliable prophylaxis consists of penicillin G or ampicillin given at least 4 hours before delivery. Widespread application of IAP has been instrumental in decreasing GBS burden in HIC. However, applying IAP in LMIC might prove to be challenging. GBS vaccine development trials are at various stages.[30]

NEONATAL TETANUS

Neonatal tetanus is usually acquired through the umbilical stump following unclean cutting of the cord. Approximately 85% untreated neonates die of the disease. It is completely preventable by immunization of mothers with at least 2 doses of tetanus toxoid. Although the disease cannot be eradicated, widespread maternal vaccination efforts for its elimination have led to a significant decrease in disease incidence and consequent fatalities.

EVIDENCE-BASED INTERVENTIONS FOR PREVENTION OF NEONATAL INFECTIONS

Well recognized in literature, out of all causes of death, severe infections are likely simplest to intervene, prevent, and treat.[32] The 2014 Lancet Every Newborn series concluded that scaling up of available interventions across the continuum of care (preconception to the postnatal period and beyond) could reduce neonatal infections by 84%[33] and prevent nearly 2 million deaths by 2025.

Antenatal Interventions

- Improved maternal nutrition, balanced protein energy and micronutrient supplementation in pregnancy, and early detection and management of intrauterine growth restriction have all been shown to reduce LBW and, indirectly, the risk of neonatal infections.
- Screening and management of maternal infections during pregnancy, such as HIV, syphilis, herpes, and hepatitis B, are central to preventing prenatal transmission.
- It is well established that tetanus toxoid vaccination of pregnant mothers (or women of childbearing age) has led to a significant reduction in neonatal tetanus and consequent mortality.[34] Rubella and varicella vaccination have reduced the incidence of the diseases in pregnant women. Influenza vaccine is recommended in pregnant women to reduce the incidence of disease and its complications in mothers and neonates. However, there is less consistent evidence to demonstrate positive effects of pneumococcal and *Haemophilus influenzae* type B.[33]

Intrapartum Interventions

- Optimal handwashing, clean birth practices, and sterile cord cutting can reduce the risk of neonatal sepsis and mortality. According to the *Lancet* Every Newborn series, handwashing with soap and water by birth attendants and caregivers could reduce the risk of neonatal tetanus by 42% and omphalitis by 31%.[33] Use of clean delivery kits has been proposed to promote safe delivery and reduce neonatal morbidity and mortality.[35]
- IAP against known GBS colonization can reduce the incidence of early infection in neonates.[33]
- Women with a history of PROM should be given prophylactic antibiotics. Evidence from LMIC indicates antibiotics for preterm PROM can help avert 4% of neonatal deaths due to prematurity and 8% of deaths due to postnatal infections.[36]

Postnatal Interventions

- Immediate postdelivery drying, thermal protection, delayed bathing, and kangaroo mother care for LBW infants help avert hypothermia. Systematic reviews have concluded that thermal care practices can prevent up to 10% of neonatal deaths caused by infections.[33]
- Percutaneous entry of organisms through the umbilical cord is an underlying cause of omphalitis and sepsis. The WHO currently recommends dry cord care for newborns in health facilities (lower neonatal mortality settings) and the application of chlorhexidine (CHX), a broad-spectrum topical antiseptic, to the cord stump for neonates born at home in high neonatal mortality settings. Evidence from Asia has supported the effectiveness of CHX[37,38]; however, recent studies from Africa[39,40] have indicated the role of CHX in moderate neonatal mortality settings is limited and further research is recommended.
- Innovations in neonatal skin care include topical emollient therapy, which has been shown to reduce risk of hospital-acquired infections and mortality by 50% and 27%, respectively.[41]

- Optimal feeding practices, that is, early initiation of breastfeeding, exclusive breastfeeding until 6 months of age, and continued breastfeeding until 2 years of age, contribute to prevention of infections. Breast milk possesses a variety of immune and nonimmune components that provide resistance to infection. Estimates indicate scaling up breastfeeding to a global level could prevent nearly 823,000 younger-than-5 deaths.[42]
- The WHO also recommends prophylactic antibiotics for neonates if certain risk factors exist, such as PROM (>18 hours before delivery), maternal fever (>38°C during labor), and/or foul-smelling amniotic fluid (usual recommended duration would be 48 hours until cultures are negative).

NEONATAL INFECTION AND ANTIMICROBIAL RESISTANCE

Antimicrobial resistance (AMR) is a global health challenge. Annually, an estimated 214,000 neonatal sepsis deaths are attributable to resistant organisms.[43] Most of these occur in LMIC where data on etiologic organisms is scarce and indiscriminate use of antimicrobials is high. Resistance to first-line antibiotic regimens (ampicillin/penicillin and gentamicin) is increasing globally.[32]

A recent prospective cohort study on neonatal sepsis from India[44] reported an 'alarming degree' of AMR with nearly 82% of *Acinetobacter* spp and 54% of *Klebsiella* spp demonstrating multidrug resistance. With increasing AMR and a growing number of facility-based births in LMICs, recognition of causative organisms, infection control measures, and appropriate use of antibiotics in community and health care facilities have never been more critical. The Etiology of Neonatal Infection in South Asia study (ANISA) initiated in 2010 and a proposed identical study in sub-Saharan Africa should provide crucial data on AMR patterns in organisms causing neonatal infections.[32]

REFERENCES

1. GBD 2015 Child Mortality Collaborators. Global, regional, national, and selected subnational levels of stillbirths, neonatal, infant, and under-5 mortality, 1980–2015: a systematic analysis for the Global Burden of Disease Study 2015. Lancet 2016;388(10053):1725–74.
2. World Health Organization. Children: reducing mortality. World Health Organization; 2016. Available at: http://www.who.int/mediacentre/factsheets/fs178/en/. Accessed October 20, 2016.
3. Khan AM, Bhutta ZA. Childhood infectious diseases: overview. In: Quah SR, Cockerham WC, editors. The international encyclopedia of public health, vol. 1, 2nd edition. Oxford (United Kingdom): Academic Press; 2017. p. 517–38.
4. Lawn J, Blencowe H, Oza S, et al. Every newborn: progress, priorities, and potential beyond survival. Lancet 2014;384(9938):189–205.
5. Velu PP, Gravett CA, Roberts TK, et al. Epidemiology and aetiology of maternal bacterial and viral infections in low- and middle-income countries. J Glob Health 2011;1(2):171–88.
6. Remington J, Klein J. Infectious diseases of the fetus and newborn infant. 1st edition. Philadelphia: Saunders/Elsevier; 2011.
7. Alam M, Saleem A, Shaikh A, et al. Neonatal sepsis following prolonged rupture of membranes in a tertiary care hospital in Karachi, Pakistan. J Infect Dev Ctries 2014;8(1):67–73.
8. Hossain MM, Afroza S, Shirin M, et al. Bacterial aetiology of neonatal sepsis in a tertiary care hospital in Bangladesh. Bangladesh J Child Health 2004;28:81–5.

9. Global nutrition report: from promise to impact: ending malnutrition by 2030. Washington, DC: International Food Policy Research Institute; 2016. Available at: http://globalnutritionreport.org/the-report/. Accessed October 29, 2016.
10. Schrag S, Cutland C, Zell E, et al. Risk factors for neonatal sepsis and perinatal death among infants enrolled in the prevention of perinatal sepsis trial, Soweto, South Africa. Pediatr Infect Dis J 2012;31(8):821–6.
11. Iliodromiti S, Mackay D, Smith G, et al. Apgar score and the risk of cause-specific infant mortality: a population-based cohort study. Lancet 2014;384(9956): 1749–55.
12. Society for Maternal-Fetal Medicine (SMFM), Hughes BL, Gyamfi-Bannerman C. Diagnosis and antenatal management of congenital cytomegalovirus infection. Am J Obstet Gynecol 2016;214(6):B5–11.
13. Kimberlin D, Jester P, Sanchez P. Valganciclovir for symptomatic congenital cytomegalovirus disease. N Engl J Med 2015;372:933–43.
14. World Health Organization. Zika causality statement. World Health Organization; 2016. Available at: http://www.who.int/emergencies/zika-virus/causality/en/. Accessed November 02, 2016.
15. World Health Organization. The history of Zika. World Health Organization; 2016. Available at: http://who.int/emergencies/zika-virus/history/en/. Accessed November 29, 2016.
16. França G, Schuler-Faccini L, Oliveira W, et al. Congenital Zika virus syndrome in Brazil: a case series of the first 1501 livebirths with complete investigation. Lancet 2016;388(10047):891–7.
17. Pinninti S, Kimberlin D. Preventing herpes simplex virus in the newborn. Clin Perinatol 2014;41(4):945–55.
18. Kimberlin D, Whitley R, Wan W, et al. Oral acyclovir suppression and neurodevelopment after neonatal herpes. N Engl J Med 2011;365(14):1284–92.
19. World Health Organization. Global health sector response to HIV, 2000-2015: focus on innovations in Africa: progress report. Geneva (Switzerland): World Health Organization; 2016. Available at: http://www.who.int/hiv/pub/progressreports/2015-progress-report/en/. Accessed November 11, 2016.
20. Galli L, Martino M, Tovo P, et al. Onset of clinical signs in children with HIV-1 perinatal infection. Italian register for HIV infection in children. AIDS 1995;9(5): 455–61.
21. Gentile I, Borgia G. Vertical transmission of hepatitis B virus: challenges and solutions. Int J Womens Health 2014;6:605.
22. Nayagam S, Thursz M, Sicuri E, et al. Requirements for global elimination of hepatitis B: a modelling study. Lancet Infect Dis 2016;16(12):1399–408.
23. Nguyet-Cam VL, Gotsch PB, Langan RC. Caring for pregnant women and newborns with hepatitis B or C. Am Fam Physician 2010;82(10):1225–9.
24. Laxminarayan R, Bhutta Z. Antimicrobial resistance—a threat to neonate survival. Lancet Glob Health 2016;4(10):e676–7.
25. Tshefu A, Lokangaka A, Ngaima S, et al. Simplified antibiotic regimens compared with injectable procaine benzylpenicillin plus gentamicin for treatment of neonates and young infants with clinical signs of possible serious bacterial infection when referral is not possible: a randomised, open-label, equivalence trial. Lancet 2015;385(9979):1767–76.
26. Nair H, Campbell H. Community management of neonatal infections. Lancet 2015;385(9979):1706–9.
27. World Health Organization. Pocket book of hospital care for children. 2nd edition. Geneva (Switzerland): World Health Organization; 2013.

28. Hibberd P, Qazi S. Population-based novel molecular diagnostics to move the neonatal sepsis agenda forward. Pediatr Infect Dis J 2016;35:S1–2.

29. World Health Organization. Guideline: managing possible serious bacterial infection in young infants when referral is not feasible. Geneva (Switzerland): World Health Organization; 2015. Available at: http://apps.who.int/iris/bitstream/10665/181426/1/9789241509268_eng.pdf. Accessed November 15, 2016.

30. Edmond K, Kortsalioudaki C, Scott S, et al. Group B streptococcal disease in infants aged younger than 3 months: systematic review and meta-analysis. Lancet 2012;379(9815):547–56.

31. Kobayashi M, Vekemans J, Baker C, et al. Group B streptococcus vaccine development: present status and future considerations, with emphasis on perspectives for low and middle income countries. F1000Res 2016;5:2355.

32. Saha S, Arifeen S, Schrag S. Aetiology of neonatal infection in South Asia (ANISA): An initiative to identify appropriate program priorities to save newborns. Pediatr Infect Dis J 2016;35:S6–8.

33. Bhutta Z, Das J, Bahl R, et al. Can available interventions end preventable deaths in mothers, newborn babies, and stillbirths, and at what cost? Lancet 2014; 384(9940):347–70.

34. Blencowe H, Lawn J, Vandelaer J, et al. Tetanus toxoid immunization to reduce mortality from neonatal tetanus. Int J Epidemiol 2010;39(Suppl 1):i102–9.

35. Turab A, Pell L, Bassani D, et al. The community-based delivery of an innovative neonatal kit to save newborn lives in rural Pakistan: design of a cluster randomized trial. BMC Pregnancy Childbirth 2014;14(1):315.

36. Cousens S, Blencowe H, Gravett M, et al. Antibiotics for pre-term pre-labour rupture of membranes: prevention of neonatal deaths due to complications of pre-term birth and infection. Int J Epidemiol 2010;39(Suppl 1):i134–43.

37. Mullany L, Darmstadt G, Khatry S, et al. Topical applications of chlorhexidine to the umbilical cord for prevention of omphalitis and neonatal mortality in southern Nepal: a community-based, cluster-randomised trial. Lancet 2006;367(9514):910–8.

38. Soofi S, Cousens S, Imdad A, et al. Topical application of chlorhexidine to neonatal umbilical cords for prevention of omphalitis and neonatal mortality in a rural district of Pakistan: a community-based, cluster-randomised trial. Lancet 2012;379(9820):1029–36.

39. Sazawal S, Dhingra U, Ali S, et al. Efficacy of chlorhexidine application to umbilical cord on neonatal mortality in Pemba, Tanzania: a community-based randomised controlled trial. Lancet Glob Health 2016;4(11):e837–44.

40. Semrau K, Herlihy J, Grogan C, et al. Effectiveness of 4% chlorhexidine umbilical cord care on neonatal mortality in Southern Province, Zambia (ZamCAT): a cluster-randomised controlled trial. Lancet Glob Health 2016;4(11):e827–36.

41. Salam R, Das J, Darmstadt G, et al. Emollient therapy for preterm newborn infants – evidence from the developing world. BMC Public Health 2013;13(Suppl 3):S31.

42. Victora C, Bahl R, Barros A, et al. Breastfeeding in the 21st century: epidemiology, mechanisms, and lifelong effect. Lancet 2016;387(10017):475–90.

43. Laxminarayan R, Matsoso P, Pant S, et al. Access to effective antimicrobials: a worldwide challenge. Lancet 2016;387(10014):168–75.

44. Investigators of the Delhi Neonatal Infection Study (DeNIS) Collaboration. Characterisation and antimicrobial resistance of sepsis pathogens in neonates born in tertiary care centres in Delhi, India: a cohort study. Lancet Glob Health 2016; 4(10):e752–60.

The Burden and Etiology of Diarrheal Illness in Developing Countries

 CrossMark

Karen L. Kotloff, MD

KEYWORDS

- Diarrhea • Rotavirus • *Shigella* • *Cryptosporidium* • ETEC • Gastroenteritis
- Developing countries • Burden

KEY POINTS

- Diarrheal disease contributes to one in eight deaths among children younger than 5 years, most of whom reside in developing countries.
- Four pathogens are responsible for most illnesses: rotavirus, *Cryptosporidium*, *Shigella*, and ETEC.
- A single episode of moderate-to-severe diarrhea has a significant impact on mortality and linear growth among survivors during the ensuing 2 to 3 months.
- The interventions available to prevent and treat diarrheal disease in developing countries are rotavirus vaccine, oral rehydration solutions (ORS), zinc, sanitation, hygiene, and targeted antibiotic treatment of dysentery and suspected cholera.

INTRODUCTION

Diarrheal disease is characterized by the onset of loose stools with or without vomiting, which may be associated with systemic manifestations, such as fever and abdominal cramps. The term acute gastroenteritis (AGE) is often used synonymously with diarrheal disease, although it is better suited to viral etiologies, such as rotavirus and norovirus, in which vomiting is a prominent symptom. Manifestations are shaped by the pathogen, the host, and the epidemiologic setting, which lead to a range of acute, subacute, and chronic intestinal and extraintestinal complications and outcomes.

Dr K.L. Kotloff receives funds from Merck, Sharp, and Dohme for a project entitled, "Surveillance study to monitor effectiveness and safety of the vaccine vial monitor compatible formulation of RotaTeq in routine use in a developing world setting (EP08011.027)" and to study the impact of vaccine introduction on rotavirus diarrhea in Mali, West Africa.
Division of Infectious Disease and Tropical Pediatrics, Center for Vaccine Development, Institute for Global Health, University of Maryland School of Medicine, 685 West Baltimore Street, HSF 480, Baltimore, MD 21201, USA
E-mail address: kkotloff@som.umaryland.edu

Pediatr Clin N Am 64 (2017) 799–814
http://dx.doi.org/10.1016/j.pcl.2017.03.006
pediatric.theclinics.com

DISEASE BURDEN

In 2015 an estimated 2.3 billion illnesses and 1.3 million deaths resulted from diarrheal disease worldwide.[1] Children younger than 5 years accounted for 40% of the diarrheal deaths even though they represent less than 10% of the world's population.[2] One in eight deaths in this age group, or a total of approximately 499,000 annually, are attributed to diarrheal disease,[1,2] 90% of which occurs in Sub-Saharan Africa and South Asia. The risk of growth faltering, ill health, and cognitive impairment increases among survivors.[3]

PATHOGENS

Table 1 describes the major viral, bacterial, and protozoal pathogens causing diarrheal disease in children.

Viral

Rotavirus is the most common cause of pediatric diarrhea. In the prevaccine era, greater than 90% of circulating human rotavirus strains globally belonged to the one of five common genotypes: G1P[8], G2P[4], G3P[8], G4P[8], and G9P[8]. In developing countries, there is greater genetic diversity and emergence of new and unusual strains.[4,5] The two genera of *Calicivirus* that cause diarrheal disease in humans are norovirus and sapovirus, each of which is further divided into genogroups and genotypes. Genetic drift among *Calicivirus* caused by point mutations and recombination events is common, resulting in emergence of antigenic variants. Since the 1990s, GII.4 norovirus has caused most infections worldwide. Among the more than 50 serotypes of adenovirus, types 40 and 41 are most often associated with diarrhea. Astroviruses that cause disease in humans belong to the *Mamastrovirus* genera (types 1–8).

Bacterial

The major bacterial enteropathogens are *Shigella*, nontyphoidal *Salmonella* (NTS), *Campylobacter*, and *Yersinia*. Four species of *Shigella* cause human disease: *S flexneri* (the major cause of shigellosis in low-resource countries), *S sonnei* (the second most common cause of shigellosis in low-income countries and the major cause in industrialized and transitional countries), and less commonly *S boydii* and *S dysenteriae*. *Salmonella* are classically divided into the human-restricted typhoidal *Salmonella* (*S typhi* and *S paratyphi* A and B), which cause enteric fever, and NTS, which contains most other serovars causing human diarrheal disease. *Salmonella typhimurium* and *Salmonella enteritidis* are the most common human NTS serovars globally. Two species of *Campylobacter* affect humans: *C jejuni* (90%–95% of infections) and *C coli*. Only 2 of the 11 species of *Yersinia* cause diarrhea in humans (*Y enterocolitica* and *Y pseudotuberculosis*). Five pathotypes of *Escherichia coli* infect humans: enterotoxigenic (ETEC), enteropathogenic, Shiga toxin-producing (also known as enterohemorrhagic) (STEC), enteroinvasive, and enteroaggregative. Pathogenic *E coli* are identified according to genotypic or phenotypic features that indicate virulence factors that they produce. There are greater than 200 serogroups of *Vibrio cholerae* but only two (O1 or O139) have been associated with epidemic cholera and cause nearly all sporadic cases. The O1 serogroup is further classified by serotype (eg, Ogawa and Inaba) and biotype (El Tor or classical). The seventh pandemic, which began in 1961 and is ongoing, is caused by *V cholerae* O1 El Tor. El Tor variants have emerged with genetic and phenotypic characteristics of classical biotype and seem more virulent.

Clostridium difficile that produce toxin are pathogenic for humans. Since 2000, a hypervirulent strain, North American Pulsed Field Type 1, polymerase chain reaction (PCR) ribotype 027 (NAP1/B1/027), has produced outbreaks of disease worldwide.[6]

Table 1
Pathogens causing diarrheal disease among children in developing countries

Agent	Clinically Relevant Species or Phenotypic, Antigenic, Serologic, or Genetic Types	
Viruses		
Rotavirus	Genotypes G1P[8], G2P[4], G3P[8], G4P[8], and G9P[8] are the predominant strains worldwide, although in low-income countries there is considerable diversity	
Calicivirus	Genera: *Norovirus, Sapovirus* Genogroups: *Norovirus*, GI and GII; *Sapovirus*, GI, GII, GIV, GV Genotypes: Many	
Enteric adenovirus	Enteric serotypes 40 and 41	
Astrovirus	Serotypes 1–8	
Bacteria		
Shigella (genus)	Species and number of serotypes:	• *S flexneri* (major species causing endemic diarrhea in developing countries), 15 serotypes and subtypes • *S sonnei* (second most common species causing endemic diarrhea in low-income countries) and major cause in middle and high income countries, 1 serotype • *S boydii* (uncommon), 20 serotypes • *S dysenteriae* (uncommon), 15 serotypes; *S dysenteriae* type 1 can cause pandemics
Salmonella (genus)	Species and subspecies: Serotypes:	*S enterica* • Those mainly causing enteric fever: *S* typhi, *S paratyphi* A, B, and C • Those mainly causing invasive disease in developing countries and diarrhea in middle- and high-income countries (nontyphoidal *Salmonella*): *S typhimurium, S enteritidis*
Campylobacter (genus)	Species:	*C jejuni* (90–95%) and *C coli*
Yersinia (genus)	Species:	*Y enterocolitica* and *Y pseudotuberculosis*
Enterotoxigenic *Escherichia coli*	*E coli* with genetic or phenotypic evidence of heat-labile toxin, and/or heat-stable toxin Colonization factor antigens (CFA/I, CFA/II, or CFA/IV)	
Shiga toxin–producing *E coli*[a]	*E coli* detected on sorbitol-MacConkey agar (presumed O157:H7) confirmed serologically, or producing Shiga toxin 1 and/or 2 (by immunoassay or polymerase chain reaction) Shiga toxin–producing serogroups other than O157 occur in 30%–50% of episodes in United States: O26, O111, O103, O121, O45, O145, and recently O104:H4 (detected at reference laboratories)	

(continued on next page)

Table 1 (continued)	
Agent	Clinically Relevant Species or Phenotypic, Antigenic, Serologic, or Genetic Types
Enteropathogenic E coli	E coli bearing eae and bfpA (present in typical but not atypical strains), and absent Shiga toxins 1 and 2
Enteroaggregative E coli	E coli with characteristic adherence pattern to cultured HEp-2 cells or genetic elements associated with virulence (eg, aggR regulon, aatA and aaiC)
Enteroinvasive E coli	E coli virulence genes: ipaH (genes encoding proteins capable of immune modulation)
Vibrio (genus)	Species: V cholerae Serogroup (98% of diarrheagenic strains are O type 1 or 139) Biotypes of O1: El Tor and classical (hybrid "altered El Tor" strains have emerged Serotypes of O1: Ogawa, Inaba, and Hikojima
Clostridium difficile[a]	Classified using several molecular methods (eg, toxinotyping, ribotyping, and pulse-field typing) Hypervirulent strain NAP1/B1/027 has caused outbreaks in North America and Europe since 2000
Other[a]	C perfringens Bacillus cereus (two forms: preformed emetic toxin and enterotoxin-producing) Staphylococcus aureus toxin A-E
Protozoa	
Cryptosporidium (genus)	Species: C hominus (most common), C parvum
Cyclospora (genus)	Species: C cavetanesis[a]
Entamoeba (genus)	Species: E histolytica
Giardia (genus)	Species: G intestinalis[a]

[a] Rare cause of diarrhea or unknown burden in developing countries.

Other bacterial pathogens are common causes of foodborne illness because of their ability to produce emetic and/or enterotoxins. These include *Bacillus cereus, Clostridium perfringens*, and *Staphylococcus aureus*. The burden of these pathogens has not been well-documented in developing countries and they are not discussed in detail.

Protozoal

Cryptosporidium is an oocyst-forming coccidian protozoa. At least 13 of the more than 60 species have been found to cause human disease, but *C hominus*, and to a lesser extent anthroponotic strains of *C parvum*, account for most (~90%) human infections.[7] *Cyclospora cayetanesis* is another coccidian protozoa. The genus *Entamoeba* includes six species that colonize humans; *Entamoeba histolytica* is thought to be the sole pathogen causing intestinal illness. *Giardia intestinalis* (formerly *Giardia lamblia* and *Giardia duodenalis*) is a flagellate protozoan that infects the small intestine and biliary tract.

RECENT DEVELOPMENTS IN ELUCIDATING THE CAUSE AND OUTCOMES OF DIARRHEAL DISEASES IN DEVELOPING COUNTRIES
Etiology of Diarrhea in Developing Countries

Two important studies conducted during the previous decade have advanced the understanding of the burden of diarrheal disease among young children living in developing countries. The GEMS (Global Enteric Multicentre Study) was a large, 3-year, population-based case-control study of acute, medically attended moderate-to-severe diarrhea (MSD) among children younger than 5 years living in Sub-Saharan Africa and South Asia.[3,8] Three age strata were included: 0 to 11 months, 12 to 23 months, and 24 to 59 months. The second was the MAL-ED (Malnutrition and Enteric Disease) Study of the cause, risk factors, and interactions of enteric infections and malnutrition and the consequences for child health. MAL-ED was a longitudinal community-based study with evaluation and sampling of newborn cohorts during health and acute diarrheal illnesses in eight low- and middle-income countries across Africa, Asia, and South America.[9,10] Children were followed until their second birthday.

Four major differences in the study design between GEMS and MAL-ED are notable. Similarities in study design are also worthy of mention as they allow comparisons of the findings to be made. First, GEMS used a case definition to enroll more severely ill children with blood in stool, evidence of dehydration (sunken eyes or decreased skin turgor), hospitalization, or administration of intravenous fluids. MAL-ED recruited milder cases from the community, with fewer than one-third meeting GEMS enrollment criteria. Together these studies capture the severe and less severe diarrheal diseases, which may have different etiologies. Second, GEMS sites were generally less developed; four of the seven GEMS sites and no MAL-ED sites were located in countries with the 35 highest under-5 mortality rates in 2010, so exposures and host vulnerability might differ. Third, GEMS was a case-control study in which children were visited a second time 2 to 3 months after enrollment to detect adverse outcomes. Although MAL-ED detected fewer adverse outcomes presumably because milder illnesses were captured, the longitudinal design was better suited to assess the sequence of events to determine causality and to measure disease burden over time (incidence). Both studies measured the proportion of diarrheal disease that was attributable to a broad array of pathogens, adjusting for asymptomatic detection of pathogens in controls. The end point, designated attributable fraction (AF), thus represented the proportion of cases significantly associated with diarrhea that could be prevented if an effective intervention were implemented. Finally, GEMS was conducted before introduction of rotavirus vaccine at any site, whereas three MAL-ED sites introduced vaccine before study initiation.

Across sites, most attributable cases in GEMS were caused by four pathogens (rotavirus, *Cryptosporidium*, *Shigella*, and ETEC producing heat-stable toxin [ST] alone or with labile-toxin [LT], herein termed ST-ETEC), and to a lesser extent, adenovirus 40/41.[3] Reanalysis of GEMS data using quantitative PCR (qPCR) substantially increased the AF of pathogens compared with estimates based on culture or immunoassay for key agents, such as *Shigella* and *C jejuni/coli* (two-fold), ST-ETEC (1.5-fold), and adenovirus 40/41 (five-fold).[11]

The public health importance of rotavirus in developing countries is a resounding message in GEMS. Rotavirus was the leading pathogen at every site during the first year of life, and at seven sites during the second year of life. The incidence of rotavirus among infants was more than two times higher than that seen for any other pathogen. GEMS data can be used to predict the public health impact of rotavirus vaccine introduction in developing countries. For example, a vaccine with 60% efficacy would prevent 4.2 episodes of rotavirus MSD per 100 child-years in the first year of life alone. In a low-resource African setting, such as Mali, with a birth cohort of 758,000 in 2016, this means that approximately 31,500 cases of life threatening rotavirus infection during the first year of life would be averted annually.

An unexpected observation in GEMS was the high prevalence of *Cryptosporidum* among episodes of MSD. *Cryptosporidium* ranked second among infants at all sites regardless of human immunodeficiency virus prevalence, and third among children 12 to 23 months of age. Although recognized as a cause of diarrhea and malnutrition in Sub-Saharan Africa, the importance of this pathogen in Asia had not previously been appreciated. Moreover, children with *Cryptosporidium* in the 12-to-23-month age group had a significantly higher risk of death during the ensuing 2 to 3 months, consistent with observations of excess mortality associated with this pathogen among infants and toddlers from Guinea-Bissau 15 years earlier.[12]

GEMS also illustrated the strong contribution of *Shigella* to the MSD burden at every study site. In contrast to rotavirus and *Cryptosporidium*, whose incidence declined with age, the incidence of *Shigella* increased with age, becoming the second most common pathogen identified among children 12 to 23 months, and the leading pathogen at 24 to 59 months of age. The qPCR analysis demonstrated not only that *Shigella* was the major pathogen associated with dysentery, which was expected (AF, 63.8%), but also the second most common agent associated with watery diarrhea (12.9%). The qPCR used in this analysis was not able to distinguish *Shigella* from enteroinvasive; however, further analysis suggested that most of these strains are *Shigella* (C. Stine and J. Nataro, unpublished data).

Several pathogens were important only in Asia (*Aeromonas*) or in Asia plus Mozambique (*C jejuni/coli* and *V cholerae* O1). Historically, an association between *Aeromonas* and diarrhea has been observed inconsistently, raising the possibility that only certain species or pathotypes were capable of causing diarrhea, or that *Aeromonas* was a cotraveler with pathogens acquired by the same route. Although coinfections involving *Aeromonas* were common in GEMS, particularly with *Shigella*, the association with diarrhea persisted when the analysis controlled for the presence of other pathogens and when *Aeromonas* was the only pathogen identified in a diarrheal episode.[13] In accordance with other reports, 26% of episodes were dysenteric.[14] These provocative data deserve further investigation.

Pathogens significantly associated with MSD at only one or two sites included (1) norovirus GII and *E histolytica* among infants; (2) norovirus GII, NTS, typical enteropathogenic (EPEC), and enteroaggregative *E. coli* among children aged 12 to 23 months; and (3) norovirus GII, NTS, and sapovirus in the 24-to-59-month age group. The paucity of NTS as a cause of diarrhea in developing countries deserves special mention. During the past several decades, distinct clones of NTS that have arisen in Sub-Saharan Africa are a frequent cause of often-fatal bloodstream infection in young children (particularly those with coincident malaria or malnutrition) and in adults infected with human immunodeficiency virus. In contrast to most NTS elsewhere, these strains do not seem to arise from zoonotic reservoirs and seldom cause diarrheal disease. A common feature involves high levels of genetic degradation (a characteristic of *S typhi*), rather than acquisition of new virulence factors.[15]

At least three pathogens are notable for their absence as a cause of MSD. First, STEC, a zoonotic infection that causes sporadic cases and outbreaks of diarrhea and hemorrhagic colitis linked to hemolytic uremic syndrome in high-income countries, was not found in any site. Second, ETEC strains producing LT only were not associated with diarrhea. This may be because LT-only ETEC produce less severe disease.[16] Third, *Yersinia*, generally found in cool climates, has occasionally been reported to occur in developing countries[17] but was not detected in either GEMS or MAL-ED.

Interestingly, *Giardia* was not associated with MSD but instead was found significantly more often in control subjects than in cases 12 to 59 months of age at most sites. This interesting finding has been observed by others[18] and suggests the hypothesis that in developing countries *Giardia* may actually interfere with the pathogenic mechanisms of other enteric pathogens. Along the same lines, one wonders whether

Giardia is a factor associated with suboptimal colonization and immune responses to live enteric vaccines that is commonly seen in developing countries.

In MAL-ED no pathogen exhibited a high AF in all individual sites. When an AF for all sites combined was calculated, the most common agents associated with diarrhea, in descending order, were norovirus GII, rotavirus, *Campylobacter*, astrovirus, and *Cryptosporidium* during infancy and *Campylobacter*, norovirus GII, rotavirus, astrovirus, and *Shigella* during the second year of life.[10] Rotavirus had the highest AF for sites without vaccine introduction and the fifth highest AF fraction for sites with vaccine introduction. During infancy, the AF in sites without vaccine introduction ranged from 3.2% to 9.6% compared with 16.3% to 27.8% in GEMS. These differences may reflect the observed trend for rotavirus to be identified with increasing frequency as the severity of illness increases; the clinical venue where cases are identified (community vs health center or hospital) is thought to be a proxy for disease severity.[19]

At first glance, it seems that norovirus GII played a leading role in MAL-ED, which is at odds with the GEMS results.[20] However, close examination reveals that norovirus GII has the highest AF during infancy in MAL-ED and the second highest during the second year of life for all sites combined. When sites were examined individually, however, norovirus GII was associated with diarrhea at only three sites during infancy and three sites during the second year of life. Two sites where norovirus GII predominated had introduced rotavirus vaccine, thus increasing the relative proportion of norovirus disease. In GEMS, norovirus GII was significantly associated with MSD in The Gambia (all age groups) and India (12–23 months old). The lack of association of norovirus with diarrhea at some sites in GEMS and MAL-ED was caused by high rates of asymptomatic carriage[21]; considerable geographic diversity in the prevalence of norovirus GII also contributed. Factors that might influence this diversity include geographic differences in the prevalence of genetic factors that mediate virus binding, which are less common in certain African and Latin American populations.[22,23] Temporal variations in the prevalence and severity of disease are seen when strains mutate in the hypervariable regions of the capsid genes resulting in emergence of new strains. GEMS and MAL-ED may have underestimated the burden of norovirus by excluding children who present with vomiting alone. Finally, GEMS may have captured less norovirus diarrhea because it produces a less severe illness.

As with norovirus, *Campylobacter* was identified in most children in MAL-ED by 1 year of age.[24] Despite high prevalence and high AFs for diarrhea when all sites were combined, infection was associated with diarrhea at only a few sites. Both norovirus and *Campylobacter* were associated with subsequent linear growth faltering in MAL-ED.

Outcomes of Moderate-To-Severe Diarrhea

An observation in both GEMS and MAL-ED was the geographic heterogeneity of pathogens. Nonetheless, both studies found rotavirus, *Shigella*, *Cryptosporidium*, and ST-ETEC to be associated with diarrhea in multiple sites. The widespread prevalence and high incidence of these four pathogens suggest that they should be prioritized for development and implementation of interventions to reduce the diarrheal disease burden.

EPIDEMIOLOGIC PATTERNS

Insufficient access to adequate hygiene, sanitation, and clean drinking water are the major risk factors for the heavy burden of diarrheal diseases in developing countries. Intrinsic properties of organisms that promote transmission include a low infectious dose, which enables person-to-person spread usually by the fecal-oral route without a food or water vehicle (eg, norovirus, *Shigella*, and *Cryptosporidium*). Other properties that promote transmission are bioavailability as conferred by a high level and/or prolonged fecal shedding, extended infectivity in the environment, and/or a large environmental or animal reservoir (eg, *Cryptosporidium*, *Giardia*, *Campylobacter*, *S typhi*), resistance to disinfection (eg, norovirus and *Cryptosporidium*), and the ability to circumvent immune surveillance (eg, the frequent antigenic changes of norovirus resulting from recombinational events). Organisms with higher infectious dose (eg, ETEC, *V cholerae*, *S typhi*, NTS) generally require a contaminated food or water vehicle. Exposure to animals or animal products may be important in some settings (eg, NTS in the United States) but not others (eg, NTS in developing countries, where source of transmission is unclear).[25] The more complex the pathogenesis, the longer the incubation period. At one end is AGE resulting from preformed toxin, such as *B cereus* and *S aureus* (12–24 hours), followed by most other viral and bacterial pathogens that generally require epithelial attachment or invasion sometimes followed by elaboration of toxins (1–5 days), and then protozoa that require excystation and phased development (1–4 weeks).

Host characteristics are also important. Most pathogens show an age predilection. The incidence of rotavirus and *Salmonella* are highest in infancy; in unvaccinated populations, nearly all infants experience at least one rotavirus infection by 24 months of age. Endemic shigellosis peaks in 1 to 4 year olds, whereas *Campylobacter* and *Cryptosporidium* show a bimodal distribution with the greatest number of reported cases in infants and young children and in young adults. Pandemic *V cholerae* and *S dysenteriae* type 1 emerge in immunologically naive populations and produce high attack rates and mortality in all age groups, and often affect displaced persons in emergency settings. Some agents (eg, NTS, *Shigella*, *Campylobacter*, *Yersinia*, and *Cryptosporidium*) are more frequent and more severe when the host is immunocompromised or malnourished.

CLINICAL EVALUATION

Diarrhea is usually defined as the passage of three or more loose or liquid stools per day (or more frequent passage than is normal for the individual). Frequent passage of formed stools is not diarrhea, nor is the passing of loose, "pasty" stools by breastfed babies. Mothers generally know when their children have diarrhea.

Clinical Symptoms According to Etiology

The clinical history is used to categorize a diarrheal episode into one of three clinical syndromes that have different (albeit overlapping) etiologies, outcomes, and treatments: (1) acute (nonbloody) diarrhea, (2) bloody diarrhea or frank dysentery (the frequent passage of scant stools containing blood with or without mucus, often accompanied by fever, lower abdominal cramps, and rectal tenesmus), and (3) persistent diarrhea (lasting more than 14 days). Profuse watery diarrhea is a subset of acute watery diarrhea that should raise suspicion for cholera.

Although there is considerable overlap, high fever greater than 40°C, overt fecal blood, abdominal pain, no vomiting before diarrhea onset, and high stool frequency (>10 per day) are more common with bacterial pathogens. High fever and overt fecal blood are often absent in bacterial enteritis, but when present, there is a high probability of a bacterial cause. Viral illnesses often begin with vomiting followed by frequent passage of watery nonbloody stools, associated with fever in about half the cases. Recovery with complete resolution of symptoms generally occurs within 7 days. Although disaccharide malabsorption is found in 10% to 20% of viral episodes, it is rarely clinically significant. A protozoal cause should be suspected when there is a prolonged diarrheal illness characterized by episodes of sometimes-explosive diarrhea with nausea, abdominal cramps, and abdominal bloating. The stools are usually watery, but can be greasy and foul smelling because of concomitant malabsorption of fats, which is more likely to occur if the parasite load is high. Occasionally diarrhea may alternate with constipation. Although infection with *E histolytica* causes the typical syndrome of protozoal diarrhea (known as intestinal amebiasis), a range of other syndromes may occur, including amebic dysentery and hepatic amebiasis. Amebic dysentery is characterized by bloody or mucoid diarrhea, which may be profuse and lead to dehydration or electrolyte imbalances or prolonged. Hepatic amebiasis is limited to abscess formation in the liver, which may occur with or without intestinal disease.

Defining Dehydration Severity

Classification of the severity of dehydration is used to guide rehydration therapy. The World Health Organization (WHO) guidelines simply use none, some, and severe dehydration (**Table 2**). Vital signs, weight, and length should be measured. The child's

Table 2
Classification of dehydration

Type of Dehydration	Signs	Fluids and Food Management
No dehydration	Signs of some or severe dehydration are absent	• Extra fluids at home • Continued breastfeeding • Normal diet of foods

Some dehydration	Two of the following signs:
	• Restless, irritable
	• Sunken eyes
	• Drinks eagerly, thirsty
	• Skin pinch goes back slowly
		• ORS for 4 h at the health center
		  ○ Continued breastfeeding
		  ○ Teach mother how to prepare ORS at home
		• After 4 h
		  ○ If still some dehydration
		    ■ Repeat ORS
		    ■ Refeed with age-appropriate, unrestricted diet[a]
		  ○ If rehydrated, follow steps for no hydration
		  ○ If severe dehydration develops at any time follow steps below

Severe dehydration	Two of the following signs: • Lethargic or unconscious • Sunken eyes • Not able to drink or drinking poorly • Skin pinch goes back very slowly	• Rapid intravenous rehydration • Switch to guidelines for some dehydration when improved

Abbreviation: ORS, oralrehydration.
    All children with diarrhea should be treated with zinc for 10–14 days. The daily oral dose is 10 mg for infants ≤6 months and 20 mg for older infants.
    [a] Recommended foods are those containing complex carbohydrates, fresh fruits, lean meats, yogurt, and vegetables.
    Specific guidelines for administration of ORS and intravenous rehydration can be found in World Health Organization. Handbook: IMCI integrated management of childhood illness. 2005. Available at: http://www.who.int/maternal_child_adolescent/documents/9241546441/en/. Accessed March 22, 2012; and World Health Organization. Pocket book of hospital care for children: guideline for the management of common illnesses with limited resources. 2005. Available at: http://whqlibdoc. who.int/publications/2005/9241546700.pdf. Accessed December 11, 2013.

nutritional status should be carefully evaluated and addressed as part of the management plan. The presence of lethargy, level of consciousness, and restlessness or irritability that interferes with feeding should be documented. The child should be offered fluid to see whether he or she is thirsty or drinks poorly. Hyperpnea (deep, rapid breathing) suggests acidosis secondary to dehydration, whereas respiratory distress (tachypnea, grunting, nasal flaring, head bobbing, and retractions) suggests pneumonia. Skin turgor is assessed by pinching a small skin fold on the lateral abdominal wall at the level of the umbilicus. If the fold does not promptly return to normal after release, the recoil time is quantified as delayed slightly or greater than or equal to 2 seconds. Note that excess subcutaneous tissue and hypernatremia may result in a false-negative test and malnutrition can prolong the recoil time.

Other signs of dehydration that have been found to be valuable include capillary refill time and hyperpnea,[26] recognizing that these have not been incorporated into the WHO algorithm. Capillary refill time is assessed by applying moderate pressure for 5 seconds to the nailbed of the child's distal fingertip, with the child's arm above heart level, until blanching occurs. When dehydration is present, the time elapsed until normal color is restored after release usually exceeds 3 seconds. Sunken fontanelle, dry mucus membranes, decreased urination, and crying without tears can also be seen in dehydrated infants and children.

Most episodes of dehydration are isonatremic. Serum electrolyte measurements, if available, should be reserved for children with severe dehydration, or children with some dehydration with suspected electrolyte abnormalities, such as when there is a history of frequent watery stools yet the skin pinch feels doughy without delayed recoil, suggesting hypernatremia, or inappropriate rehydration fluids have been administered at home. A blood culture should be obtained, if possible, for infants and children with fever and/or blood in the stool who are younger than 3 months, are immunocompromised, and have hemolytic anemia or other risk factors for bacteremia. A complete blood count, peripheral smear, serum electrolytes, and renal function tests are indicated when hemolytic uremic syndrome is suspected.

COMPLICATIONS

The major complications of diarrhea from any cause (**Table 3**) are dehydration and electrolyte abnormalities. At the extreme is cholera gravis, manifesting as rice water stools, vomiting, and leg cramps, which can lead to hypovolemic shock and death within hours. Bacterial diarrheal has been associated with a variety of intestinal and extraintestinal complications. The complications included in this category generally represent either end-organ damage that results directly from the infectious process and its extension to other sites, unusual manifestations of infection, or postinfectious immune-mediated events. Shigella is likely the major culprit with its ability to cause toxic megacolon, intestinal perforation, rectal prolapse, bacteremia (usually in immunocompromised or malnourished children), seizures, or encephalopathy. Hemolytic uremic syndrome can result from S dysenteriae type 1 and STEC.

Immune-mediated complications that are thought to result from immunologic cross-reactivity between bacterial antigens and host tissues are more often seen in adults than children. These include reactive arthritis following infection with the classical bacterial enteropathogens believed to be rare in developing countries at least in part because of the low prevalence of the HLA B27 haplotype,[27] and Guillain-Barré syndrome following Campylobacter infection.[28]

Table 3
Intestinal and extraintestinal complications of enteric infections

Complications, by Site and Time Frame	Major Causes
Intestinal complications	
Toxic megacolon	*Shigella, Clostridium difficile, Entamoeba histolytica*
Intestinal perforation	*Shigella, Yersinia, C difficile, E histolytica*
Rectal prolapse	*Shigella*, STEC, *C difficile*
Persistent diarrhea	All causes
Recurrent diarrhea (usually immunocompromised persons)	*Salmonella, Shigella, Yersinia, Campylobacter, C difficile*
Extraintestinal complications	
Dehydration and metabolic disturbances, malnutrition, micronutrient deficiency	All causes
Bacteremia with distant infectious foci	*Salmonella, Shigella, Yersinia, Campylobacter, C difficile*
Pseudoappendicitis (older children and adolescents)	*Yersinia* (rarely *Campylobacter*)
Exudative pharyngitis, cervical lymphadenopathy	*Yersinia*
Postinfectious complications	
Reactive arthritis[a]	NTS, *Shigella, Yersinia, Campylobacter*
Glomerulonephritis, myocarditis, pericarditis	*Campylobacter*
Guillain-Barré or Miller Fisher syndrome	*Campylobacter*
Hemolytic uremic syndrome	STEC, *Shigella dysenteriae* type 1
Seizure or encephalopathy	*Shigella*
Erythema nodosum or other rash	*Yersinia, Campylobacter, Salmonella*

Abbreviation: STEC, Shiga-toxin producing *E. coli*.
   [a] Arthritis can be seen alone or as part of a constellation of arthritis, conjunctivitis, uveitis, and urethritis and is rare in developing countries.

DIFFERENTIAL DIAGNOSIS

The infectious causes of watery and bloody diarrhea, and the noninfectious causes that should be considered in the differential diagnosis, are shown in **Table 4**. One entity that should be considered in particular when children younger than 3 years of age present with bloody stools is intussusception. The typical presentation of intussusception is the sudden onset of intermittent abdominal pain accompanied by crying and drawing legs up to abdomen, sometimes followed by vomiting. The stools often have the appearance of "currant jelly." Pain may become constant and severe over time. Initially the child is normal between episodes. A sausage-shaped mass may be palpable in the right side of the abdomen. Vigilance for intussusception is important because delay in diagnosis increases mortality, which can exceed 25% in developing country settings.

TREATMENT
Rehydration and Refeeding

The reader should refer to guidelines published by WHO for the management of diarrheal disease in children living in developing countries. The *Integrated Management of Childhood Illness* describes methods for prevention and management of diarrheal

Table 4
Infectious and noninfectious etiologies of diarrheal syndromes in infants and children

Clinical Presentation	Major Causes
Watery diarrhea	
Infections	Viruses (rotavirus, adenovirus 40/41, calicivirus, astrovirus)
	Bacteria (ETEC, EPEC, STEC, EAEC, EIEC, *Vibrio cholerae*, *Shigella*, NTS, *Campylobacter*, *Yersinia*, *Clostridium difficile*)
	Protozoa (*Cryptosporidium*)
Noninfectious causes	Metabolic (hyperthyroidism), food intolerance, medications (especially antibiotics), celiac disease
Bloody diarrhea/bloody stools	
Infections	Bacteria (*Salmonella*, *Shigella*, *Yersinia*, *Campylobacter*, *C difficile*, *Aeromonas*, STEC, EIEC)
	Protozoa (*Entamoeba histolytica*)
	Necrotizing enterocolitis (newborns)
Noninfectious causes	Inflammatory bowel disease
	Meckel diverticulum, intestinal polyps (usually painless rectal bleeding)
	Intussusception (intermittent crampy pain with "currant jelly" stools)
Chronic or relapsing diarrhea	
Infections	Intestinal protozoa, 10%–20% of all infectious diarrhea
Noninfectious causes	Cystic fibrosis, celiac disease, milk protein intolerance, congenital or acquired disaccharidase deficiency
Vomiting with or without abdominal pain	
Infections	Viruses (norovirus, rotavirus, adenovirus 40/41), astrovirus
Noninfectious causes	Pyloric stenosis, intestinal obstruction, pancreatitis, appendicitis, and cholecystitis

Abbreviations: EAEC, enteroaggregative; EIEC, enteroinvasive; EPEC, enteropathogenic; ETEC, enterotoxigenic; STEC, Shiga-toxin producing *E. coli*.

diseases at home and at outpatient facilities with limited diagnostic tools and medications.[29] Guidelines for inpatient management of children who reach a referral center are found in the *Pocketbook of Hospital Care for Children*.[30] A brief summary of the general principles of rehydration is provided in **Table 2**. Two situations require special attention. Children with severe acute malnutrition and those with persistent diarrhea and signs of dehydration require prompt hospitalization and treatment according to the guidelines that are outlined in the WHO guidelines. Specific feeding regimens are recommended for children with persistent diarrhea with or without associated dehydration.[30]

Zinc and Ancillary Treatments

WHO recommends that all children with diarrhea should be treated with zinc for 10 to 14 days. The daily oral dose is 10 mg for infants less than or equal to 6 months and 20 mg for older infants. Zinc replacement reduces the duration and severity of the episode and lowers the risk of diarrhea in the following 2 to 3 months. The following agents are *not* recommended for use in children: antimotility agents (eg, loperamide, or difenoxylate and atropine), antisecretory agents (eg, bismuth subsalicylate), and agents designed to adsorb toxins and water (kaolin and pectin).

Antibiotics

Judicious use of antibiotics is recommended for specific indications (**Table 5**). For acute diarrheal diseases, these indications are limited to dysentery and suspected

Table 5	
Antibiotic treatment of diarrhea	
Syndrome/Indication	**Management**
Dysentery	
Local susceptibility known	Follow local guidelines
Local susceptibility unknown	
First line	Ciprofloxacin, 15 mg/kg PO twice a day for 3 d
Second line (severely ill)	Ceftriaxone, 50–80 mg/kg/d IV or IM for 3 d

Not improved after 2 full days of antibiotics	• Stop first-line treatment
	• Look for other conditions
	• Choose one of the following
	  ○ An antibiotic known to be effective against *Shigella* in the area; OR
	  ○ Azithromycin, 20 mg/kg PO for 3 d or; OR
	  ○ Cefixime, 8 mg/kg/d PO for 3 d

Not improved after 2 more days of antibiotics	• Stop the previous antibiotic • Look for other conditions • Metronidazole, 10 mg/kg PO 3 times a day for 5 d if amebiasis is possible
Cholera: if child is 2 y or older, has severe dehydration, and there is cholera in the area	
Local susceptibility known	Follow local guidelines
Local susceptibility unknown	Choose one of the following • Erythromycin estolate, 12.5 mg/kg PO 4 times a day for 3 d; OR • Ciprofloxacin, 15 mg/kg PO twice a day for 3 d; OR • Azithromycin, 20 mg/kg PO for 3 d

Abbreviations: IM, intramuscularly; IV, intravenously.

Adapted from Pocket book of hospital care for children: guideline for the management of common illnesses with limited resources. 2005. Available at: http://whqlibdoc.who.int/publications/2005/9241546700.pdf. Accessed December 11, 2013.

cholera (see **Table 4**). Use outside of these indications is discouraged for several reasons. For one, most episodes of diarrhea are viral and thus self-limited. Second, the increasing prevalence of antibiotic resistance has prompted restrictions in promiscuous use of these drugs. Third, antibiotics may actually worsen outcome in some circumstances, such as in STEC infection antibiotics may increase the risk of hemolytic uremic syndrome, and in NTS they may prolong excretion and increase relapses.

PREVENTION

There are four strategies that are readily implemented by the clinician for prevention of diarrhea and its complications: (1) vaccination, (2) ORS, (3) zinc, and (4) hygiene (particularly handwashing). We are on the cusp of a dramatic shift in the epidemiology of pediatric diarrheal diseases since rotavirus vaccines became available and were recommended for routine immunization of all infants by WHO and the national regulatory authorities of numerous high- and middle-income countries. Three live oral vaccines are now licensed: the three-dose pentavalent G1, G2, G3, G4, P[8] human-bovine vaccine (RotaTeq); the two-dose monovalent human G1P[8] vaccine (ROTARIX); and the three-dose monovalent human-bovine 116E G6P[11] vaccine (Rotavax). In high- and middle-income countries, vaccine introduction has resulted in substantial reductions in rotavirus-associated and all-cause hospitalizations for diarrheal disease in vaccinated infants (direct protection) and unvaccinated individuals (indirect, or herd protection)[31]; in addition, substantial declines in less severe disease are demonstrated by reductions in office visits for rotavirus diarrhea.[32] Reductions in all-cause diarrhea deaths have been observed in Mexico and Brazil.[33,34] That norovirus has become the most common enteropathogen identified in US children hospitalized with AGE since the introduction of rotavirus vaccine provides a powerful illustration of the impact that rotavirus vaccines will have on the global epidemiology of pediatric diarrheal disease in the decades to come.

Programmatic uptake is lagging in low-resource settings where most severe disease and death occurs; however, Gavi, the Vaccine Alliance, a global health partnership that promotes vaccine access for the world's poorest countries, has supported introduction of rotavirus vaccine into approximately 40 countries. Lower point estimates of vaccine efficacy observed in clinical trials and in vaccine effectiveness during "real life" programmatic use in these settings (51%–64%) demonstrate smaller reductions in disease incidence compared with that seen in wealthier countries (85%–98%)[35,36]; however, with broad coverage, the life-saving potential is predicted to be substantial. The cause of hyporesponsiveness to oral vaccines in less-developed countries is unknown. Several avenues under investigation include small intestinal bacterial overgrowth, intestinal microbiome composition, genetic factors mediating pathogen attachment, coinfection with intestinal helminths or *Helicobacter pylori*, environmental enteropathy often accompanied by undernutrition, and micronutrient deficiency. Recent data on rotavirus vaccine suggest that improved efficacy may result from delaying the first dose to 8 to 10 weeks of age, which presumably minimizes interference of maternal antibody.[37] Investigators at the University of Maryland School of Medicine are assessing the impact of vaccine introduction on the incidence and cause of diarrhea in Sub-Saharan Africa. There is renewed interest in developing other vaccines against other enteric infections, including *Shigella* and ETEC, because the burden of disease has been better defined.

SUMMARY

Diarrheal diseases continue to cause substantial morbidity and mortality in developing countries. Four pathogens (rotavirus, *Shigella*, ST-ETEC, *Cryptosporidium*) contribute to most of the burden of diarrhea in developing countries. Efforts are needed to improve uptake of existing interventions (rotavirus vaccine, zinc, ORS) and to develop new methods that target the major causes of disease.

REFERENCES

1. GBD 2015 Disease and Injury Incidence and Prevalence Collaborators. Global, regional, and national incidence, prevalence, and years lived with disability for 310 diseases and injuries, 1990-2015: a systematic analysis for the Global Burden of Disease Study 2015. Lancet 2016;388:1545–602.
2. GBD 2015 Mortality and Causes of Death Collaborators. Global, regional, and national life expectancy, all-cause mortality, and cause-specific mortality for 249 causes of death, 1980-2015: a systematic analysis for the Global Burden of Disease Study 2015. Lancet 2016;388:1459–544.
3. Kotloff KL, Nataro JP, Blackwelder WC, et al. Burden and aetiology of diarrhoeal disease in infants and young children in developing countries (the Global Enteric Multicenter Study, GEMS): a prospective, case-control study. Lancet 2013;382:209–22.
4. Todd S, Page NA, Duncan Steele A, et al. Rotavirus strain types circulating in Africa: review of studies published during 1997-2006. J Infect Dis 2010;202(Suppl): S34–42.

5. Miles MG, Lewis KD, Kang G, et al. A systematic review of rotavirus strain diversity in India, Bangladesh, and Pakistan. Vaccine 2012;30(Suppl 1):A131–9.

6. Warny M, Pepin J, Fang A, et al. Toxin production by an emerging strain of *Clostridium difficile* associated with outbreaks of severe disease in North America and Europe. Lancet 2005;366:1079–84.

7. Sow SO, Muhsen K, Nasrin D, et al. The burden of cryptosporidium diarrheal disease among children < 24 months of age in moderate/high mortality regions of sub-saharan Africa and south Asia, utilizing data from the global enteric multicenter study (GEMS). PLoS Negl Trop Dis 2016;10:e0004729.

8. Kotloff KL, Blackwelder WC, Nasrin D, et al. The Global Enteric Multicenter Study (GEMS) of diarrheal disease in infants and young children in developing countries: epidemiologic and clinical methods of the case/control study. Clin Infect Dis 2012;55(Suppl 4):S232–45.

9. MAL-ED Network Investigators. The MAL-ED study: a multinational and multidisciplinary approach to understand the relationship between enteric pathogens, malnutrition, gut physiology, physical growth, cognitive development, and immune responses in infants and children up to 2 years of age in resource-poor environments. Clin Infect Dis 2014;59(Suppl 4):S193–206.

10. Platts-Mills JA, Babji S, Bodhidatta L, et al. Pathogen-specific burdens of community diarrhoea in developing countries: a multisite birth cohort study (MAL-ED). Lancet Glob Health 2015;3:e564–575.

11. Liu J, Platts-Mills JA, Juma J, et al. Use of quantitative molecular diagnostic methods to identify causes of diarrhoea in children: a reanalysis of the GEMS case-control study. Lancet 2016;388:1291–301.

12. Molbak K, Hojlyng N, Gottschau A, et al. Cryptosporidiosis in infancy and childhood mortality in Guinea Bissau, west Africa. BMJ 1993;307:417–20.

13. Qamar FN, Nisar MI, Quadri F, et al. *Aeromonas*-associated diarrhea in children under 5 years: the GEMS experience. Am J Trop Med Hyg 2016;95:774–80.

14. Soltan Dallal MM, Moezardalan K. *Aeromonas* spp associated with children's diarrhoea in Tehran: a case-control study. Ann Trop Paediatr 2004;24:45–51.

15. Feasey NA, Hadfield J, Keddy KH, et al. Distinct *Salmonella enteritidis* lineages associated with enterocolitis in high-income settings and invasive disease in low-income settings. Nat Genet 2016;48:1211–7.

16. Qadri F, Das SK, Faruque AS, et al. Prevalence of toxin types and colonization factors in enterotoxigenic *Escherichia coli* isolated during a 2-year period from diarrheal patients in Bangladesh. J Clin Microbiol 2000;38:27–31.

17. Okwori AE, Martinez PO, Fredriksson-Ahomaa M, et al. Pathogenic *Yersinia enterocolitica* 2/O:9 and *Yersinia pseudotuberculosis* 1/O:1 strains isolated from human and non-human sources in the Plateau State of Nigeria. Food Microbiol 2009;26:872–5.

18. Hollm-Delgado MG, Gilman RH, Bern C, et al. Lack of an adverse effect of *Giardia intestinalis* infection on the health of Peruvian children. Am J Epidemiol 2008; 168(6):647–55.

19. Tucker AW, Haddix AC, Bresee JS, et al. Cost-effectiveness analysis of a rotavirus immunization program for the United States. JAMA 1998;279:1371–6.

20. Lopman BA, Steele D, Kirkwood CD, et al. The vast and varied global burden of norovirus: prospects for prevention and control. PLoS Med 2016;13:e1001999.

21. Rouhani S, Penataro Yori P, Paredes Olortegui M, et al. Norovirus infection and acquired immunity in 8 countries: results from the MAL-ED study. Clin Infect Dis 2016;62:1210–7.

22. Corvelo TCO, Aguiar DCF, Sagica FES. The expression of ABH and Lewis antigens in Brazilian semi-isolated black communities. Genet Mol Biol 2002;25: 259–63.

23. Nordgren J, Nitiema LW, Ouermi D, et al. Host genetic factors affect susceptibility to norovirus infections in Burkina Faso. PLoS One 2013;8:e69557.

24. Amour C, Gratz J, Mduma E, et al. Epidemiology and Impact of campylobacter infection in children in 8 low-resource settings: results from the MAL-ED study. Clin Infect Dis 2016;63:1171–9.

25. Crump JA, Heyderman RS. A perspective on invasive salmonella disease in Africa. Clin Infect Dis 2015;61(Suppl 4):S235–40.

26. Steiner MJ, DeWalt DA, Byerley JS. Is this child dehydrated? JAMA 2004;291: 2746–54.

27. Gaston JS, Inman RD, Ryan ET, et al. Vaccination of children in low-resource countries against *Shigella* is unlikely to present an undue risk of reactive arthritis. Vaccine 2009;27:5432–4.

28. Islam Z, Gilbert M, Mohammad QD, et al. Guillain-Barre syndrome-related *Campylobacter jejuni* in Bangladesh: ganglioside mimicry and cross-reactive antibodies. PLoS One 2012;7:e43976.

29. World Health Organization. Handbook: IMCI integrated management of childhood illness. 2005. http://www.who.int/maternal_child_adolescent/documents/9241546441/en/. Accessed March 22, 2012.

30. World Health Organization. Pocket book of hospital care for children: guideline for the management of common illnesses with limited resources. 2005. Available at: http://whqlibdoc.who.int/publications/2005/9241546700.pdf. Accessed December 11, 2013.

31. Patel MM, Glass R, Desai R, et al. Fulfilling the promise of rotavirus vaccines: how far have we come since licensure? Lancet Infect Dis 2012;12:561–70.

32. Dennehy PH. Treatment and prevention of rotavirus infection in children. Curr Infect Dis Rep 2013;15:242–50.

33. do Carmo GM, Yen C, Cortes J, et al. Decline in diarrhea mortality and admissions after routine childhood rotavirus immunization in Brazil: a time-series analysis. PLoS Med 2011;8:e1001024.

34. Richardson V, Hernandez-Pichardo J, Quintanar-Solares M, et al. Effect of rotavirus vaccination on death from childhood diarrhea in Mexico. N Engl J Med 2010;362:299–305.

35. Zaman K, Dang DA, Victor JC, et al. Efficacy of pentavalent rotavirus vaccine against severe rotavirus gastroenteritis in infants in developing countries in Asia: a randomised, double-blind, placebo-controlled trial. Lancet 2010;376: 615–23.

36. Armah GE, Sow SO, Breiman RF, et al. Efficacy of pentavalent rotavirus vaccine against severe rotavirus gastroenteritis in infants in developing countries in sub-Saharan Africa: a randomised, double-blind, placebo-controlled trial. Lancet 2010;376:606–14.

37. Colgate ER, Haque R, Dickson DM, et al. Delayed dosing of oral rotavirus vaccine demonstrates decreased risk of rotavirus gastroenteritis associated with serum zinc: a randomized controlled trial. Clin Infect Dis 2016;63:634–41.

The Burden of Enteropathy and "Subclinical" Infections

Elizabeth T. Rogawski, PhD, MSPH[a,b,]*, Richard L. Guerrant, MD[b]

KEYWORDS

- Environmental enteropathy • Environmental enteric dysfunction • Enteric infections
- Growth faltering

KEY POINTS

- Environmental enteropathy in early childhood is associated with impaired vaccine responses, child growth faltering, cognitive impairment, and later life obesity, diabetes, and metabolic syndrome.
- It is challenging to define environmental enteropathy, which will be necessary for further research, prevention, and treatment.
- Enteric infections, even in the absence of overt diarrhea, are frequent in low-resource settings, contribute to environmental enteropathy, and may cause or aggravate growth faltering.
- New tools for detecting enteric pathogens, characterizing the microbiome, and assessing the transcriptome and metabolome may help to elucidate environmental enteropathy and identify potential interventions.

INTRODUCTION

As the cause of approximately 500,000 deaths in 2015[1] resulting from 1.7 billion episodes[2] globally, early childhood diarrhea has been a major focus of global health efforts to improve child health in low-resource settings. However, as we have witnessed substantial reductions in diarrhea-related mortality and learned how to provide

Disclosures: We declare no conflicts of interest. This work was supported by the Fogarty International Center, National Institutes of Health (D43-TW009359 to E.T. Rogawski).
[a] Department of Public Health Sciences, University of Virginia, PO Box 801379, Carter Harrison Research Building MR-6, 345 Crispell Drive, Room 2520, Charlottesville, VA 22908-1379, USA; [b] Division of Infectious Diseases and International Health, Department of Medicine, University of Virginia, PO Box 801379, Carter Harrison Research Building MR-6, 345 Crispell Drive, Room 2520, Charlottesville, VA 22908-1379, USA
* Corresponding author. Department of Public Health Sciences, University of Virginia, PO Box 801379, Carter Harrison Research Building MR-6, 345 Crispell Drive, Room 2520, Charlottesville, VA 22908-1379.
E-mail address: etr5m@virginia.edu

appropriate oral rehydration therapy, diarrhea has revealed itself to be only one, although particularly visible, consequence of exposure to enteropathogens in environments with poor sanitation and hygiene. A potentially more widespread and debilitating consequence for long-term development is environmental enteropathy (EE; also termed environmental enteric dysfunction), a chronic condition of the small intestine that is commonly considered a "subclinical" problem and often involves enteric infections without overt symptoms.[3] However, because it lacks definition as a "disease" and is challenging to diagnose, its magnitude and importance are only beginning to be appreciated.

Growing evidence for the diverse effects of EE on child development have revealed the "subclinical" designation to be a misnomer. There is a largely underrecognized range of potential impacts of common enteric infections and enteropathy that extend far beyond the typical assumption that they mainly cause diarrhea or other intestinal complaints like abdominal pain, nausea, or vomiting. Recognized examples of nonintestinal outcomes associated with enteric infections include associations of toxoplasmosis with birth defects and congenital brain damage ("TORCH" syndrome)[4] and of *Campylobacter* infections with Guillain-Barré syndrome.[5] However, as research studies include detection of wider arrays of bacterial, viral, and parasitic pathogens and longer term follow-up, potential effects of enteric infections and enteropathy on vaccine responses,[6,7] child growth,[8,9] cognitive development,[10,11] and even later life obesity, diabetes, and metabolic syndrome are increasingly being recognized.[12–15] Herein, we review the evolving challenges to defining EE and enteric infections, current evidence for the magnitude and determinants of its burden, new assessment tools, and relevant interventions.

HISTORICAL PERSPECTIVE

EE has its initial appreciation and origins in the mid-20th century as tropical sprue, a symptomatic disease first identified among military personnel and Peace Corps volunteers stationed in low-resource settings. Tropical sprue was characterized by chronic diarrhea, steatorrhea, weight loss, malabsorption, and abnormalities in intestinal morphology. In severe cases, it included manifestations of nutritional deficiencies, including night blindness and neurologic symptoms.[16] In 1966, a study found that 40% of volunteers stationed in Pakistan had signs of malabsorption and none of their jejunal biopsies showed normal fingerlike villous architecture with varying degrees of abnormality.[17] The condition was associated with residence in tropical countries, although the specific cause was unknown.

Further study of intestinal morphology by jejunal biopsy in asymptomatic individuals from Africa, Asia, and Latin America found common abnormalities of shorter and thickened villi, increased crypt depth, and inflammatory cellular infiltration, which did not necessarily result in overt symptoms.[18–24] Histologic abnormalities were often accompanied by excess fecal fat excretion and malabsorption of xylose and vitamin B_{12}.[21–23] Similar abnormalities were documented in malnourished children with Kwashiorkor and severe wasting.[25–27] Although the condition among expatriates reverted after returning to their home countries,[28] populations in endemic settings experienced the condition chronically.

CURRENT DEFINITIONS
Environmental Enteropathy

EE is thought (by most authors) to be the result of chronic exposure to enteropathogens, although the potentially synergistic and disruptive role of poor nutrition is increasingly being recognized. In addition to the histopathologic findings of villous blunting, the main components of EE are increased intestinal permeability (from impaired barrier function), mucosal inflammation, malabsorption, and systemic inflammation.[29–32] The condition is considered distinct from tropical sprue and overt symptoms of diarrhea.[29] Because it depends on exposure to unsanitary environments, it is common in both long-term residents and in travelers, and is reversible once the environment improves,[28] EE is thought to be environmentally derived and likely widespread in low-resource settings.[29]

However, the determination of a clear consensus definition for EE remains an elusive challenge. Because EE is without overt acute symptoms (although it may manifest in subacute weight loss and impaired growth or development over longer periods of time), the traditional gold standard for diagnosis has been intestinal biopsy to identify abnormalities in intestinal histology. Such an invasive diagnostic is infeasible in most research and many clinical settings and is also limited by potentially inadequate sampling, because the biopsied sample may not be representative of the whole intestine. However, the diagnosis of EE in the absence of these invasive procedures has proved challenging.

In response to the inability to regularly perform biopsies in healthy, "asymptomatic" individuals, recent research on EE has aimed to identify biomarkers to characterize EE that can be measured in stool, blood, or urine. At least 40 different biomarkers or metabolites have been investigated as potential indicators for EE that is clinically significant enough to result in growth faltering (**Table 1**).[6,29,33–39] These include markers of disrupted intestinal barrier or absorptive function (eg, lactulose and mannitol, rhamnose, or D-xylose absorption and excretion in the urine, alpha-1-antitrypsin in stool, tight junction components in plasma or intestinal tissue staining); translocation of microbes or their products (eg, lipopolysaccharide or anti-lipopolysaccharide antibody); intestinal inflammation (eg, myeloperoxidase, lactoferrin, calprotectin, or lipocalin in the stool); and systemic inflammation (eg, high sensitivity C-reactive protein or acid glycoprotein; serum amyloid A and other acute phase proteins). Other indicators include metabolites such as citrulline or tryptophan that may signal a healthy intestinal mucosa.

The biomarkers for these processes have varying specificity for EE-induced growth faltering. Lactulose absorption and excretion, like fecal alpha-1-antitripsin and plasma lipopolysaccharide markers, all reflect disrupted intestinal barrier dysfunction, which is a proximal component of EE. Conversely, markers of systemic inflammation have diverse causes and cannot specifically identify EE. Of course, measures of growth impairment alone, such as height-for-age z-score (HAZ) or stunting, have been included as markers in some studies, but they have poor specificity for EE because they may be due to nonintestinal causes. Like later impairments in cognitive development (especially in higher executive function or semantic fluency[40]), these measures are indicators of outcomes of EE and may occur too late in the disease process to be of timely diagnostic use to enable interventions. Tracking of growth trajectories may be useful to identify early decrements that could predict continuing growth deficits if EE conditions persist.

The identification of appropriate biomarkers for EE is challenged by their frequent comparison with nonspecific outcomes like linear growth rather than a true gold standard diagnostic. As noted, stunting is hypothesized to be an effect of EE and is highly multifactorial. The strongest predictor of stunting is birth size,[41] which is necessarily unrelated to the development of EE in early life in the child (although likely relevant to EE in the mother). Therefore, single anthropometric measurements have poor sensitivity and specificity as a standard against which to validate biomarkers. However,

Table 1
Potential biomarkers of environmental enteropathy

Function	Biomarker	Description	Sample Type
Intestinal absorptive function	Lactulose	Disaccharide, indicator of gut barrier disruption	Administered orally and measured in urine
	Mannitol	Monosaccharide, indicator of gut absorptive surface	Administered orally and measured in urine
	Lactulose:mannitol ratio (%L and %M)	Indicator of barrier disruption per surface area	Administered orally and measured in urine
	Rhamnose	Monosaccharide, indicator of absorptive surface	Administered orally and measured in urine
	D-Xylose	Monosaccharide, indicator of absorptive surface	Administered orally and measured in urine
	GMCSF antibody	Granulocyte macrophage colony stimulating factor autoantibody	Plasma
Intestinal barrier function	Alpha-1-antitrypsin	Plasma protease inhibitor, indicator of relatively severe gut barrier disruption	Stool
	Claudin-2	Tight junction peptide reflecting increased permeability	Intestinal tissue staining
	Claudin-15	A marker of "healthy" gut absorptive and barrier function	Urine
Translocation	LPS	Lipopolysaccharide	Plasma
	IgA and IgG anti-LPS	Antibody produced against lipopolysaccharide	Plasma
	IgA and IgG anti-FliC	Antibody produced against bacterial FliC (flagellin)	Plasma
	Zonulin	Tight junction peptide regulator of gut permeability (haptoglobin)	Plasma
	TJP1	Tight junction protein gene encoding for ZO-1	Intestinal biopsy, tissue DNA
Intestinal inflammation	MPO	Myeloperoxidase, a neutrophil granule component	Stool
	Calprotectin	Neutrophil marker	Plasma; stool
	Neopterin	Monocyte/macrophage marker of immune activation (GTP metabolite)	Stool
	Lactoferrin	Neutrophil granule component	Stool
	Lipocalin	Protein in neutrophils and epithelial cells	Stool
	Reg 1A	Regenerating islet-derived protein-α	
	Reg1β	Marker of epithelial repair	Stool
	I-FABP	Intestinal fatty acid binding protein	Plasma
	Fecal S100A12	Calcium (and zinc, copper)-binding protein regulator of inflammatory signaling	Stool

Category	Marker	Description	Sample
Systemic inflammation	AGP	Acid glycoprotein, a hepatic "acute phase reaction" product	Plasma
	IL-1β	Interleukin-1β, inflammatory cytokine produced by monocytes and macrophages	Plasma
	IL-4	Th2 cytokine	Plasma
	IL-5	Th2 and mast cell cytokine	Plasma
	IL-6	Proinflammatory or antiinflammatory T cell or macrophage cytokine or myokine	Plasma
	IL-7	Lymphokine stimulator of stem cell differentiation into B, T or NK lymphoid cells	Plasma
	IL-10	Antiinflammatory STAT3 inducer cytokine	Plasma
	TNFα	Proinflammatory cytokine	Plasma
	MIP1β	Macrophage inflammatory protein 1β (CCL4)	Plasma
	Ferritin	Iron-binding protein reflecting iron stores	Serum
	Hepcidin	Inflammation-driven inhibitor of iron exporter ferroportin, thus blocker of iron uptake or release into the circulation; hence anemia of chronic inflammation	Plasma
	C-reactive Protein (CRP)	An acute phase reactant (APR)	Plasma
	hsCRP	High sensitivity C-reactive protein (APR)	Plasma
	sCD14	Soluble CD14; shed by activated monocytes, binds LPS	Plasma
	EndoCAb	Antibody produced against bacterial lipopolysaccharide	Plasma
	Serum amyloid A	Acute phase reactant driver of inflammation	Plasma
	LBP	LPS binding protein	Plasma
Metabolites/growth markers	Tryptophan	Essential amino acid for protein synthesis and growth as well as the neurotransmitter, serotonin	Plasma
	Kynurenine	Tryptophan metabolite via IDO, potentially driven by inflammation	Plasma
	K:T ratio	Kynurenine:tryptophan ratio	Plasma
	Citrulline	Key amino acid for intestinal repair	Plasma
	IGFBP-3	IGF binding protein-3	Plasma
	IGF-1	Insulin-like growth factor 1	Plasma
	Activin	Growth regulation factor	Plasma

Abbreviations: GMCSF, granulocyte macrophage colony stimulating factor; GP, glycoprotein; Ig, immunoglobulin; LPS, lipopolysaccharide.
Data from Refs.[6,29,33]

growth trajectories, especially over the first 2 years of life (assessed as incremental changes in HAZ scores) may better reflect EE in early childhood. Validation against intestinal biopsy might be more specific, but is infeasible in many settings, as discussed.

In addition, the potential ubiquity of EE in low-resource settings makes it difficult to identify appropriate comparison groups. Because EE is acutely asymptomatic, it is unclear how to define "healthy" controls for a study in an environment conducive to EE and where the condition is expected to be common. Unlike the World Health Organization growth standards,[42] for example, there are no international reference standards for EE biomarkers based on a representative group of children from diverse areas. Distributions of EE biomarkers in healthy children in high-resource settings are also largely not available to be used as reference standards. Even if this information were available, external reference populations could be inappropriate because they would differ on many other characteristics that would confound comparisons. In multiple papers assessing EE among children in low-resource settings, the authors referenced comparison biomarker values based on small studies in healthy adults that were not assessing EE directly.[36,37,43,44] Clearly these reference values were suboptimal.

Beyond the uncertainties with biomarkers, the scientific community has not come to a consensus on what type of definitions are relevant for understanding EE. If EE is to be considered a disease, it will require a specific pathologic definition. Conversely, as a syndrome, EE could encompass multiple disease states. Arbitrary assemblages of morphologic or functional pathologies can have important acute or lasting consequences despite having multiple potential etiologies. Examples include pneumonia and diarrhea that are well-recognized as "disease" entities, even though they are composed of many component, more specific diagnoses, such as pneumococcal pneumonia or shigellosis. EE could be considered similarly as a set of functional pathophysiologic alterations, with varying degrees of morphologic pathology caused by diverse environmental determinants. However, distinguishing EE from similar pathologies as human immunodeficiency virus-associated enteropathy, for example, may be difficult. It is unclear whether and how similar presentations of enteropathy should be considered distinct when the conditions can be indistinguishable except for the underlying cause.

What needs to drive these definitions is the goal to identify EE as an entity for which its recognition and the development of effective interventions can improve long-term health outcomes that may range from growth to cognitive and even later life metabolic impairment. Both surveillance and clinical case definitions will be needed for future study of EE. A surveillance definition would be used to identify sentinel cases to inform population-level interventions, which would be relevant because EE seems to be widespread in low-resource settings. Because populations suffering from EE show a population shift in biomarker distributions, it may be difficult to make individual diagnoses, and population-level interventions may be most appropriate. In contrast, a clinical case definition will be needed for targeted treatment and other individual-level interventions.

Geographic differences in EE manifestations may also pose challenges. Variations in environmental exposures across low-resource settings likely result in different pathologies. Perhaps it is more important to describe an EE spectrum, where milder cases may not include systemic inflammation, for example, and more severe cases may be associated with villous blunting and poor growth outcomes. It may be necessary to distinguish between consequential EE, with observable poor outcomes, and inconsequential EE, in which a child may show abnormal histology or biomarker levels, but no related outcomes such as poor growth. In this conception, EE constitutes a risk factor for health outcomes, such as a significant decrease in HAZ in the formative early years of childhood or an impairment of normal cognitive development, especially in higher executive function. EE describes a state that is probabilistically associated with poor development (eg, growth, vaccine response, cognitive impairment), but is not a necessary or sufficient cause and may lead to no observable clinical outcomes in a significant proportion of cases.

As the field is quickly evolving, new biomarkers are being identified and refined to help enhance our understanding, if not the definition, of EE. In spite of the complex challenges in defining EE, improved clarity of this entity will help to develop appropriate surveillance and clinical case definitions against which to study risk factors, which will be vital to advancing our understanding and to testing, and ultimately investing in, potentially effective interventions.

Specific Enteric Infections

Overt diarrhea (defined as 3 or more unformed stools per day[45]), especially when prolonged or persistent, has predicted growth and even cognitive failure in many previous studies.[11,46–51] However, reduced diarrhea rates observed in more recent studies have made overt diarrhea less useful in predicting growth and developmental outcomes. Despite these reductions, "subclinical" pathogen detection in stools continues to be common in many impoverished settings and has been associated with poor outcomes.[8,9,52]

These infections are hypothesized to be a key contributor to EE, and asymptomatic carriage of known enteric pathogens may cause or aggravate linear growth faltering, even in the absence of recognized episodes of diarrhea.[8,9,53,54] For example, asymptomatic excretion of enteroaggregative *E. coli* (EAEC) has been associated with linear growth faltering.[53] The mechanism for the growth effect may be through subclinical gut inflammation, which has been associated with EAEC detection in MAL-ED (Etiology, Risk Factors, and Interactions of Enteric Infections and Malnutrition and the Consequences for Child Health and Development Project), a birth cohort study performed at 8 sites in South America, sub-Saharan Africa, and South Asia (Rogawski and colleagues, manuscript in preparation). Carriage of *Campylobacter* spp. has also been associated with both linear and ponderal growth faltering.[8,55] This association may be mediated through EE; *Campylobacter* detection was associated with increased markers of permeability (alpha-1-antitrypsin), intestinal inflammation (myeloperoxidase), and systemic inflammation (acid glycoprotein) in MAL-ED.[8] Similarly, persistent *Giardia* detection in the first 6 months of life has been associated with malabsorption[9] and reduced linear growth in two studies.[9,56] *Cryptosporidium parvum* excretion has also been associated with growth faltering, although it is unclear if this association is driven by prolonged excretion after a symptomatic infection.[57] These data suggest that a primary mechanism for the pathogenesis of EE may involve exposure to pathogens through poor hygiene practices and contaminated food and water, resulting in enteric infections.

Because these infections are commonly diagnosed in stool by culture or molecular methods, it is challenging to distinguish between colonization and infection. Many microorganisms can play both the roles of commensal and pathogenic organism and mere detection does not illuminate the multifactorial impact of the organism.[58] Some organisms, like *Clostridium difficile*, *Salmonella*, and likely many other enteric bacterial pathogens, may change from commensal to pathogenic within an individual over time, and pathogenicity is highly dependent on the presence of other microorganisms and a wide range of environmental and genetically determined host factors.[59]

Further, the distinction between commensal and pathogenic is often made among organisms within the same species, as is the case for *E coli*. Pathogenic *E coli* are generally identified by an array of virulence factors, the significance of some of which have yet to be fully elucidated.[60]

The identification, quantification, and attribution of pathogenic versus nonpathogenic organisms is complicated in endemic settings by differences in host resistance, normal microbiota, and acquired immunity. Organisms that are known causes of diarrhea outbreaks, such as waterborne *Giardia* outbreaks, are often not associated with diarrhea among children in endemic settings. *Giardia*, for example, was more commonly identified in nondiarrheal stools than diarrheal stools in both major studies of diarrhea etiology, MAL-ED and GEMS (Global Enteric Multicenter Study).[52,61] Even organisms that are statistically associated with diarrhea in these studies are commonly found in nondiarrheal stools and "healthy" controls. New methods to use quantitative polymerase chain reaction (PCR) to incorporate quantity of pathogen have helped to distinguish cases from controls, but they remain imperfect and quantities significantly associated with case status necessarily only apply at the population level. Detections above these quantities cannot conclusively identify etiology in individual cases. In contrast, detections of these pathogens are rare in high-resource settings, which makes it easier to confidently assign etiology.

Pathogenic organisms must be considered in the context of the gut microbiota, a highly complex "organ" of the body which impacts myriad processes from metabolism to cognition. However, microbiota-related studies rarely consider the presence of specific pathogenic organisms, and it is unknown what bilateral impact they may have. Although the microbiota has been shown to be altered in many diseases states, it is unclear which compositions constitute beneficial microbiota and which represent dysbiosis. Diversity parameters for the microbiota (either alpha diversity within a sample or beta diversity between samples)[62] can simplify the highly dimensional composition data, but high diversity is not uniformly positive. For example, while exclusive breastfeeding is recommended in early infancy, the predominant bacteria in the microbiota of breastfed infants are *Bifidobacterium* and *Lactobacillus*,[63,64] whereas infants fed with formula milk have a more complex microbiota.[63,65] Recently, measures of microbiota "maturity" have been developed to describe how malnourished children often have microbiota compositions that mirror the compositions of younger, healthy children.[66] However, the organisms identified as discriminating for immaturity differ across populations, limiting the generalizability of the index.[66,67] These discriminating organisms are not those classically considered as enteric pathogens, and it is unclear if they are harmful themselves or simply indicators for generalized dysbiosis.

Animal models can help to separate and elucidate the roles of specific pathogen infections versus the microbiota by experimentally controlling infections and the microbiota in specific diet and host contexts. For example, protozoal, bacterial, and viral infections in murine models have strikingly different effects in the context of specific nutrient deficiencies with normal microbiota. Protein deficiency greatly enhanced both the intensity of cryptosporidial infection as well as its impact on growth, documenting a bidirectional impact of worsened infection with protein malnutrition and conversely worsened growth with infection.[68,69] Cryptosporidial infection in the setting of protein deficiency also caused impaired turnover of infected epithelial cells.[70] Similar synergies with protein or zinc deficiency were seen with EAEC infections.[71–73] Conversely, murine rotavirus infections were less severe in undernourished conditions,[74] which may be because the intestinal villi were blunted and less efficiently provided the lactase needed to "uncoat" the virus as part of pathogenesis.

The microbiota also affect susceptibility to infection in mouse models. Early studies from the 1960s and 1970s showed the intestinal flora was antagonistic to *Salmonella, Shigella,* and *Vibrio cholerae* infection.[75] Several other recent studies have found that a normal microbiota in mice successfully prevents colonization by *Salmonella enterica* serovar Typhimurium. Conversely, mice with altered microbiotas owing to antibiotic administration are more susceptible to intestinal infection and disease due to *Salmonella* and other enterobacteria such as *E coli*.[76–78] One study showed a dose–response such that greater alterations to the microbiota led to higher colonization by *S enterica* serovar Typhimurium, with more severe inflammation and intestinal pathology.[77,79] Further, modification of the microbiota through the antibiotic treatment of mice increased susceptibility to infection by vancomycin-resistant *Enterococcus* and *C difficile*.[77]

In terms of the microbiota and susceptibility to viral infections, there are examples both where intestinal bacteria promote and are antagonistic to viral infection.[78,80,81] For example, *Bacteroides thetaiotaomicron* and *Lactobacillus casei* have been shown to prevent infection of the intestinal epithelial cells by rotavirus in vitro. Similarly, mice with depleted microbiotas through antibiotic treatment or development in germ-free conditions are more susceptible to influenza compared with normal mice.[78,80] On the other hand, the gastrointestinal microbiota has been shown to enhance replication and infection of other viruses.[80,82,83] Antibiotic-treated mice were less susceptible to poliovirus compared with mice with normal microbiota, resulting in a mortality rate among normal mice twice that among antibiotic-treated mice.[82] A similar study demonstrated that mouse mammary tumor virus, a retrovirus, was more efficiently transmitted in the presence of a rich microbiota, and correspondingly virus transmission to offspring was reduced in antibiotic-treated mice and germ-free mice.[83]

Clinical studies have supported laboratory based evidence of the importance of the microbiota. Prior antibiotic treatment has been associated with increased susceptibility to *E coli*, *Salmonella*, *Shigella*, and *Campylobacter* infections and with longer duration of infection compared with patients who did not receive antibiotics.[78,84,85] Antibiotic treatment also reduces the inoculum required to cause infection with *Salmonella*.[85] The clear association between the microbiota and susceptibility to infection has led some researchers to suggest that people with an altered microbiota are functionally immunocompromised and less resilient against new and opportunistic pathogens and recurrent infections.[77] The complex interactions in the gut between enteropathogens and the microbiota likely play a key role in development of EE.

MAGNITUDE OF BURDEN

Because a clear case definition with diagnostic cutoffs for EE biomarkers has not yet been developed to classify individuals with and without EE using noninvasive methods, no large-scale population-based surveillance has been completed to estimate the global burden of EE. Symptomatic diarrhea remains the main indicator for pediatric enteric disease. Only symptomatic diarrhea was included in the most recent Global Burden of Disease study, and the longer-term consequences remain controversial and poorly defined.[1] The inadequacy of definitions of EE has limited the ability to include its consequences in enteric disease-associated disability-adjusted life-year calculations, which would help to garner the attention needed for their amelioration.[86]

Smaller scale studies of histology are not necessarily globally representative, but provide evidence for the universality of EE in low-resource settings. In a study of 57 Indian children with chronic diarrhea, almost three-quarters showed abnormal histology of the jejunum and approximately two-thirds showed atrophy of villi.[87] In a cohort study of 200 adults in Zambia, all of the jejunal biopsies demonstrated some degree of enteropathy, with varying levels of abnormality in villous height and crypt depth.[88] Among 414 children presenting to a hospital in London with chronic diarrhea, almost one-half had mild (25%), moderate (10%), or severe (9%) enteropathy by proximal small intestinal mucosal biopsy.[89]

EE biomarkers are increasingly being measured in studies of enteric disease. In MAL-ED, a large multisite birth cohort study from 8 countries, a panel of potential EE biomarkers was measured across the first 2 years of life.[38] In a subset of children with biomarkers measured at 3 to 9 months of age, median alpha-1-antitrypsin, neopterin, and myeloperoxidase concentrations in stool were elevated compared with sparse but available data from healthy individuals in nontropical countries.[36] Specifically, in quarterly stools from 3 to 21 months of age from the complete MAL-ED cohort in the Bangladesh site, more than one-half of samples were higher than normal for alpha-1-antitrypsin and myeloperoxidase, and 95% were abnormal for neopterin.[37] Similarly, in PROVIDE (Exploration of the Biologic Basis for Underperformance of Oral Polio and Rotavirus Vaccines in Bangladesh), a study of EE and oral polio and rotavirus vaccine response in Bangladesh, fecal EE biomarkers measured at 12 weeks of age were abnormal in the majority of infants (82% abnormal for myeloperoxidase and alpha-1-antitrypsin, and 94% abnormal for calprotectin).[6] These results suggest that the majority of infants had enteric inflammation even in the first few months of life. The entire distribution of EE biomarkers in study populations from low-resource settings is likely shifted compared with populations in high-resource settings.

Nondiarrheal enteric infections are more straightforward to measure through detection of the enteropathogens in stool samples when diarrhea symptoms are not reported. The prevalence of such infections is high in low-resource settings, which has made it critical to assess the presence of pathogens in both diarrheal and nondiarrheal stools when attributing population-level diarrhea etiology. In GEMS, a large study of moderate-to-severe diarrhea in 7 sites in Africa and Asia, the prevalences of *Shigella*, *Cryptosporidium*, and heat-labile enterotoxigenic *Escherichia coli* by quantitative PCR were 27%, 21%, and 29% in enrolled controls without diarrhea in the second year of life.[90] In MAL-ED, the prevalences of *Campylobacter*, *Giardia,* and EAEC using conventional methods[91] in quarterly nondiarrheal stools from the same age period were 36%, 29%, and 26%, respectively.[8,9] Because the prevalences of *Giardia* and EAEC were similar in diarrheal and nondiarrheal stools, neither pathogen was statistically associated with diarrhea for any age group or at any site in MAL-ED.[52] *Giardia* carriage measured by repeated detections in nondiarrheal stools was common; 63% of the *Giardia* detections in diarrheal stools were preceded by *Giardia* detections in nondiarrheal stools in the prior 2 months, suggesting the *Giardia* detected during diarrhea may have been from previous infection.[9]

Even if the burden of EE may be difficult to define, the prevalence of risk factors for EE is high and widespread. The World Health Organization estimates that approximately 900 million people around the world do not have access to an improved drinking water source, including more than 40% of people in sub-Saharan Africa.[92] Even those with access to an improved water source may have poor quality water owing to recontamination and unsafe storage. Similarly, sanitation coverage and use is poor. The prevalence of open defecation globally was 18% in 2006 and is widely practiced in South Asia (48%) and sub-Saharan Africa (28%). Improved sanitation facilities that ensure hygienic separation between humans and their excreta are available to fewer than one-third of people in sub-Saharan Africa.[92]

Many challenges also remain to providing optimal nutrition both in utero and during early childhood. Globally each year, approximately 13 million infants are born with intrauterine growth restriction and about 20 million with low birth weight.[93] Breastfeeding in the first 6 months of life is not exclusive as recommended for 16% of infants, and 14% of children discontinue breastfeeding before 2 years of age.[94] Micronutrient deficiencies are also common; one-quarter of the global population has vitamin A deficiency,[94] including 190 million children (33.3%) under 5 years of age.[95] Overall, 16% of the global population has zinc deficiency, and 17% of women have iron deficiency,[94] with anemia affecting almost one-half of the preschool age population.[93] These risk factors are likely major contributors to EE. A global study of risk factors for stunting, an outcome associated with EE, identified fetal growth restriction and preterm birth as the leading risk factors for stunting prevalence, followed by environmental factors (unimproved water, unimproved sanitation, and biomass fuel use) and maternal and child nutrition. This analysis estimates that 22% of stunting cases were attributable to environmental factors and 14% were attributable to child nutrition.[41]

Challenges to Assessing Causality

The complex interplay between many of these factors, which are often associated, but related nonlinearly, make it challenging to assign causality in population-based studies. For example, the highly cited vicious cycle between malnutrition and illness posits that malnutrition can both be a cause and effect of enteric infections.[12] Even with longitudinal data to track children over time, it is difficult to model the complex system and determine temporality. Risk factors can confound the causal effect of other risk factors if the confounding factor is associated with both the risk factor of interest and the EE outcome. However, they could also be mediators, on the causal pathway between more distal risk factors and EE, or modifiers, which change the magnitude of association between risk factors and EE. We diagram the relationship between these different types of variables in **Fig. 1**A, and provide an example in the context of EE in **Fig. 1**B. These diagrams draw on the concepts of directed acyclic graphs,[96] which are useful to develop causal models, but are extended here to include modifiers and allow multiple variables at 1 node.

In observational studies, it may be difficult to disentangle highly correlated risk factors such as socioeconomic status and education. The distribution of risk factors associated with nutrition, WaSH (Water, Sanitation and Hygiene for All), and social factors vary across and often within countries, as was shown in the multisite MAL-ED study, where there were major variations in breastfeeding practices, water, sanitation, handwashing, animal ownership, and antibiotic use across sites.[8,9,97] These differences may limit the interpretation of cross-site comparisons. Alternatively, risk factors may be ubiquitous in some settings, such that it is impossible to compare outcomes between exposed and unexposed. For example, all participants had access to an improved water source (as defined by the World Health Organization[92]) in 5 of the 8 research sites in the MAL-ED study.[8]

Many of these risk factors are difficult to measure. Caregiver report, especially for behavioral factors such as handwashing behavior, is notoriously unreliable.[98,99] Improved measurement of risk factors alongside better models of their complex interactions will all be needed to identify appropriate targets and develop interventions for EE.

NEW ASSESSMENT TOOLS CREATE NEW PERSPECTIVES AND RECOGNITION OF IMPACT
Detection of Enteric Pathogens

The relatively recent focus on enteropathy and subclinical enteric infections has been spurred by technological advances that have made closer study of EE feasible. A widening array of protozoan, bacterial, and viral enteric pathogen assays are now

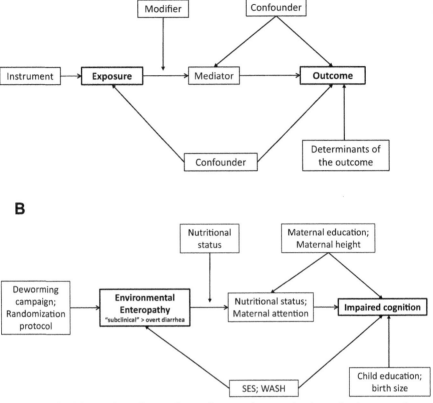

Fig. 1. Modified directed acyclic graphs to diagram the complex interplay between factors associated with environmental enteropathy and its effects. (*A*) Different types of variables that could affect exposure–outcome relationships. (*B*) Relationships between relevant variables in the context of environmental enteropathy. SES, socioeconomic status; WaSH, Water, Sanitation and Hygiene for All.

available to assess pathogen burden in stool samples, including those for *Cryptosporidium*, *Campylobacter*, and multiple types of diarrheagenic *E coli* based on increasingly appreciated virulence traits such as heat labile or heat stable enterotoxins, attaching and effacing traits, invasiveness (EIEC), shigatoxin, aggregative adherence (EAEC), and viral agents.[91,100]

Although traditional culture and microscopy methods are still commonly used to detect these pathogens, new molecular methods have been developed with superior sensitivity and specificity in many cases.[90,101] For example, culture assays for *Shigella* are known to have low sensitivity. In a reanalysis of stool samples from the GEMS case-control study, the use of quantitative PCR diagnostics increased *Shigella* attributable incidence approximately 2.5-fold in the second year of life from 2.7 cases per 100 child-years to 7.0 cases per 100 child-years.[90]

Molecular tools not only provide greater sensitivity than most traditional methods, they also enable quantification of the pathogen load, indicating the intensity of each pathogen infection.[90,101] The quantification cycle (Cq) in quantitative PCR, the cycle number at which fluorescence from target amplification exceeds the background fluorescence, can be used as an inverse metric of nucleic acid quantity. For many of the diarrhea-associated pathogens, higher pathogen quantities, as indicated by lower Cq values, are more strongly associated with stools from diarrhea cases compared with nondiarrheal stools from controls. For example, the association between diarrhea and Rotavirus detected at a Cq of 34 was near the null, while the magnitude of the odds ratio for diarrhea with Rotavirus detected at a Cq of 20 was greater than 10 in GEMS.[90] The difficulty of assigning diarrhea etiology has long been recognized given the frequent presence of enteropathogens in nondiarrheal stools. Quantification allows greater resolution to better discriminate causative organisms from potentially unrelated infections.

However, with the increased sensitivity of molecular tools, poor specificity may be a problem if quantity of pathogen is not taken into account. To limit false positives, a Cq cutoff (eg, at 35 cycles) is regularly set to classify amplifications beyond that cycle number as negative in the analysis. However, beyond the strength of statistical associations between pathogen quantity and diarrhea compared with nondiarrheal stools, the necessary or sufficient pathogen burdens to cause illness are unknown and likely vary across individuals and settings. Therefore, although these methods are especially useful for assigning etiology at the population level, they are less useful for determining causes of individual cases.

There are further limitations of these methods in standardization and comparability. Comprehensive platforms such as the TaqMan Array Card can detect more than 40 pathogens simultaneously and are standardized to allow comparison of Cq values across assays.[101] However, PCR Cq values are difficult to compare when measured by single reactions without a standardized platform. Cq values may differ by PCR machine as well as across experiments on the same machine, making cross-site comparisons of pathogen quantity unreliable. In addition, in many PCR programs, Cq values must be calculated or at least reviewed by a technician by eye, which can further increase variability. Assaying pathogen standards of known quantity to create quantification curves can improve comparability across platforms.[102]

Microbiome and Innovative Biomarker Assays

Because the majority of bacteria in the gastrointestinal microbiota cannot be cultured, early studies of the microbiota that relied on bacterial culture provided a skewed representation of microbiota composition. Newer molecular techniques, which most commonly amplify and characterize nucleic acids from the 16S rRNA conserved gene through high-throughput sequencing technologies, have allowed higher resolution for the complex and diverse communities of the microbiota.[103] These techniques are also rapidly becoming less expensive, which allows for larger sample sizes needed for group comparisons.

Similarly, as assays for current biomarkers are being refined, transcriptomics and metabolomics offer innovative methods to identify new types of biomarkers. In a recent study of Malawian children from 12 to 61 months of age, lactulose permeability as an indicator of EE was correlated with fecal messenger RNA copy number to identify transcripts with differential expression in EE. Twelve transcripts associated with EE and mapped to pathways related to cell adhesion and immune responses to viral, bacterial, and parasitic organisms. Transcripts associated with the maintenance of the mucous layer were underexpressed in children with EE.[104] These transcripts may prove to be useful targets as relevant EE biomarkers.

Metabolomics also has the potential to identify new biomarkers associated with EE. In a study of urinary metabolites in children enrolled in the case-control study component of MAL-ED in Northeast Brazil, an ^1H nuclear magnetic resonance spectroscopy-based metabolic profiling approach was used to identify metabolites associated with stunting (HAZ <−2) and catch-up growth (ΔHAZ between baseline and 2–5 months of follow-up). Undernutrition was associated with altered choline and tryptophan metabolism and increased proteolytic activity of the gut microbiome. The authors suggest that urinary N-methylnicotinamide and β-aminoisobutyric acid may be promising biomarkers for identifying children at risk for further growth shortfalls.[105]

INTERVENTIONS

As our understanding of the mechanisms of EE pathogenesis increases, we can begin to appreciate the optimal markers to help define and track potentially effective interventions. This understanding will likely best derive from linking field clinical studies with targeted animal model studies that dissect metabolic pathways that are seen in both affected children and in the models. Examples include disrupted choline and tryptophan metabolism in both children and murine models. Furthermore, field and laboratory model studies can identify hypotheses to be tested in other study designs and raise potential interventions worthy of testing. For example, the impairment of cell turnover noted with protein deficiency that greatly increases the intensity and severity of cryptosporidial infection noted above[70] raises the possibility that intestinal repair nutrients like glutamine or citrulline might reduce the impaired growth and development seen with this infection in clinical studies.

Multiple key interventions will likely be needed in combination to realize reductions in EE and its potentially devastating intermediate and long-term consequences. For example, behavioral or structural interventions that reduce exposure to enteric pathogens, such as interventions targeted to improve water, sanitation, and hygiene, will likely synergize with nutritional interventions, vaccines, and innovative interventions that directly target EE, such as those to repair intestinal injury. Because even many of the available enteric vaccines have shown reduced efficacy in low-resource settings where EE is common,[106] reducing the quantity of the pathogen ingested from contaminated food and water may improve vaccine impact. Likewise, key nutrients likely enhance protective host immune (and other) responses to pathogen disruption of intestinal function. Such protection could range from improved innate or acquired immunity to epithelial cell turnover, an important component of host defense.[70] Equally, very limited, carefully targeted, single-dose antimicrobials might enable catch-up growth responses to nutrition therapy to set a child's growth onto a new trajectory. Finally, an alert and healthy child will engage more parental and caregiver interactions to support the critical impact of cognitive stimulation on child development.

Further more, the potential to identify subtypes of EE may help to identify targeted interventions which will be most effective. For example, high levels of fecal myeloperoxidase, suggesting an invasive pathogen like Shigella, enteroinvasive E coli (EIEC), or Campylobacter infections might be promptly ameliorated by a single-dose antimicrobial treatment (such as azithromycin). Alternatively, disrupted intestinal absorptive or barrier function might suggest that interventions targeting injury repair, such as certain amino acids in an oral rehydration and repair therapy, could be helpful. Vaccines are available for only a few enteropathogens, including rotavirus, cholera, and polio, and are limited by suboptimal effectiveness in low-resource settings. The development of new vaccines, especially for Shigella, may be warranted given the recently appreciated burden of both moderate to severe watery diarrhea and dysentery associated with Shigella.[90]

Challenges remain with regional and cultural differences in the uptake, effectiveness, and adherence to selected interventions. Water, sanitation, and hygiene interventions have been particularly challenged by suboptimal coverage, even in the setting of randomized trials with intense community interaction and follow-up.[107,108] Appropriate water treatment processes, latrine designs, and sanitation and hygiene behaviors must be tailored to individual communities to maximize acceptability.[109] Intervention planning should also account for existing practices in the targeted community. For example, interventions involving targeted antimicrobial use may be severely limited by current widespread use even early in life[110] and concerns about antimicrobial resistance.

SUMMARY

The complexities inherent in defining and studying EE and subclinical infections have made it difficult to characterize burden as well as test potential interventions. Calls to update diarrhea disability-adjusted lie-years[86] have largely been unanswered because of the difficulty in quantifying nondiarrheal impact of enteric pathogen exposure and EE. A significant decrease in HAZ in the formative early years of childhood or an impairment of normal cognitive development remain to be counted, largely because we still desperately need better data on their causes and burden. The years lost to disability (YLD) due to early childhood EE in the form of growth and cognitive developmental deficits, as well as long-term metabolic effects, may exceed the rapidly decreasing years of life lost (YLL) due to diarrhea. Including these components into the disability-adjusted life-years will appropriately highlight the importance and value of diagnosis and effective interventions needed to improve these outcomes for impoverished children around the world.

Similar pathways and effects may also have relevance among the elderly, whose quality of life is also impaired by poor sanitation and physical and cognitive impairment. Although these are not addressed in this overview, they likely involve similar, largely unrecognized effects of EE, as shown by the surprising frequencies of evidence for intestinal inflammation and of *C difficile* infections that may be seen in more than 30% to 40% of "asymptomatic" nursing home residents.[111–113] Further expanding the potential disability-adjusted life-years impact of the often clinically unrecognized problem of EE in this population is also likely warranted.

Numerous research and translational gaps remain in the appreciation of EE and its causes, biomarkers, and consequences. Because EE can develop in the first few months of life, methods for early recognition are vitally needed to intervene before long-term consequences manifest. The appropriate targets of these interventions and mode of delivery for greatest impact are still unknown. Some of the most important long-term outcomes for growth or cognitive development require much longer follow-up than most current projects or funding mechanisms address. Focus on shorter term outcomes may miss critical aspects of EE or of its impact, and inappropriately discount the effectiveness of interventions. Innovative enteropathogen detection, biomarker, microbiota, and metabolomics methods noted have improved our ability to tackle questions about which pathogens have the greatest relevance, which host and microbial pathways are involved, and which biomarkers will be most relevant for diagnosis, health outcomes, and interventions. It is clear that we can no longer consider EE to be "subclinical." It does a disservice to the field by understating the potential long-term and multifaceted impact of EE among children in low-resource settings.

ACKNOWLEDGMENTS

The authors thank Dr Sean Moore and Dr James Platts-Mills for their helpful input.

REFERENCES

1. GBD 2015 Mortality and Causes of Death Collaborators. Global, regional, and national life expectancy, all-cause mortality, and cause-specific mortality for 249 causes of death, 1980-2015: a systematic analysis for the Global Burden of Disease Study 2015. Lancet 2016;388(10053):1459–544.
2. Walker CLF, Rudan I, Liu L, et al. Global burden of childhood pneumonia and diarrhoea. Lancet 2013;381(9875):1405–16.
3. Keusch GT, Denno DM, Black RE, et al. Environmental enteric dysfunction: pathogenesis, diagnosis, and clinical consequences. Clin Infect Dis 2014;59(Suppl 4):S207–12.
4. Neu N, Duchon J, Zachariah P. TORCH infections. Clin Perinatol 2015;42(1): 77–103, viii.
5. Loshaj-Shala A, Regazzoni L, Daci A, et al. Guillain Barré syndrome (GBS): new insights in the molecular mimicry between C. jejuni and human peripheral nerve (HPN) proteins. J Neuroimmunol 2015;289:168–76.
6. Naylor C, Lu M, Haque R, et al. Environmental enteropathy, oral vaccine failure and growth faltering in infants in Bangladesh. EBioMedicine 2015;2(11): 1759–66.
7. Gilmartin AA, Petri WA. Exploring the role of environmental enteropathy in malnutrition, infant development and oral vaccine response. Philos Trans R Soc Lond B Biol Sci 2015;370(1671). http://dx.doi.org/10.1098/rstb.2014.0143.
8. Amour C, Gratz J, Mduma E, et al. Epidemiology and impact of Campylobacter infection in children in eight low-resource settings: results from the MAL-ED study. Clin Infect Dis 2016. http://dx.doi.org/10.1093/cid/ciw542.
9. Rogawski ET, Bartelt LA, Platts-Mills JA, et al. Determinants and impact of Giardia infection in the first two years of life in the MAL-ED birth cohort. J Pediatric Infect Dis Soc 2016, in press.
10. Eppig C, Fincher CL, Thornhill R. Parasite prevalence and the worldwide distribution of cognitive ability. Proc Biol Sci 2010;277(1701):3801–8.
11. Pinkerton R, Oriá RB, Lima AAM, et al. Early childhood diarrhea predicts cognitive delays in later childhood independently of malnutrition. Am J Trop Med Hyg 2016. http://dx.doi.org/10.4269/ajtmh.16-0150.
12. Guerrant RL, DeBoer MD, Moore SR, et al. The impoverished gut–a triple burden of diarrhoea, stunting and chronic disease. Nat Rev Gastroenterol Hepatol 2013; 10(4):220–9.
13. Scharf RJ, Deboer MD, Guerrant RL. Recent advances in understanding the long-term sequelae of childhood infectious diarrhea. Curr Infect Dis Rep 2014;16(6):408.
14. DeBoer MD, Lima AAM, Oría RB, et al. Early childhood growth failure and the developmental origins of adult disease: do enteric infections and malnutrition increase risk for the metabolic syndrome? Nutr Rev 2012;70(11):642–53.
15. DeBoer MD, Chen D, Burt DR, et al. Early childhood diarrhea and cardiometabolic risk factors in adulthood: the Institute of Nutrition of Central America and Panama Nutritional Supplementation Longitudinal Study. Ann Epidemiol 2013; 23(6):314–20.
16. Batheja MJ, Leighton J, Azueta A, et al. The face of tropical sprue in 2010. Case Rep Gastroenterol 2010;4(2):168–72.
17. Lindenbaum J, Kent TH, Sprinz H. Malabsorption and jejunitis in American Peace Corps volunteers in Pakistan. Ann Intern Med 1966;65(6):1201–9.

18. Cook GC, Kajubi SK, Lee FD. Jejunal morphology of the African in Uganda. J Pathol 1969;98(3):157–69.
19. Sprinz H, Sribhibhadh R, Gangarosa EJ, et al. Biopsy of small bowel of Thai people. With special reference to recovery from Asiatic cholera and to an intestinal malabsorption syndrome. Am J Clin Pathol 1962;38:43–51.
20. Colwell EJ, Welsh JD, Legters LJ, et al. Jejunal morphological characteristics in South Vietnamese residents. JAMA 1968;206(10):2273–6.
21. Lindenbaum J, Alam AK, Kent TH. Subclinical small-intestinal disease in East Pakistan. Br Med J 1966;2(5530):1616–9.
22. García S. Malabsorption and malnutrition in Mexico. Am J Clin Nutr 1968;21(9): 1066–76.
23. England NW, O'Brien W. Appearances of the jejunal mucosa in acute tropical sprue in Singapore. Gut 1966;7(2):128–39.
24. Mathan VI, Baker SJ. An epidemic of tropical sprue in southern India. I. Clinical features. Ann Trop Med Parasitol 1970;64(4):439–51.
25. Amin K, Walia BN, Ghai OP. Small bowel functions and structure in malnourished children. Indian Pediatr 1969;6(2):67–72.
26. Cook GC, Lee FD. The jejunum after kwashiorkor. Lancet 1966;2(7476):1263–7.
27. Stanfield JP, Hutt MS, Tunnicliffe R. Intestinal biopsy in kwashiorkor. Lancet 1965;2(7411):519–23.
28. Lindenbaum J, Gerson CD, Kent TH. Recovery of small-intestinal structure and function after residence in the tropics. I. Studies in Peace Corps volunteers. Ann Intern Med 1971;74(2):218–22.
29. Korpe PS, Petri WA Jr. Environmental enteropathy: critical implications of a poorly understood condition. Trends Mol Med 2012;18(6):328–36.
30. Watanabe K, Petri WA. Environmental enteropathy: elusive but significant subclinical abnormalities in developing countries. EBioMedicine 2016;10:25–32.
31. Syed S, Ali A, Duggan C. Environmental enteric dysfunction in children. J Pediatr Gastroenterol Nutr 2016;63(1):6–14.
32. Keusch GT, Rosenberg IH, Denno DM, et al. Implications of acquired environmental enteric dysfunction for growth and stunting in infants and children living in low- and middle-income countries. Food Nutr Bull 2013;34(3):357–64.
33. Guerrant RL, Leite AM, Pinkerton R, et al. Biomarkers of Environmental Enteropathy, Inflammation, Stunting, and Impaired Growth in Children in Northeast Brazil. PLoS One 2016;11(9):e0158772.
34. Prata MM, Havt A, Bolick DT, et al. Comparisons between myeloperoxidase, lactoferrin, calprotectin and lipocalin-2, as fecal biomarkers of intestinal inflammation in malnourished children. J Transl Sci 2016;2(2):134–9.
35. Gosselin KB, Aboud S, McDonald CM, et al. Etiology of diarrhea, nutritional outcomes and novel intestinal biomarkers in Tanzanian infants: a preliminary study. J Pediatr Gastroenterol Nutr 2016. http://dx.doi.org/10.1097/MPG.000000000000 1323.
36. Kosek M, Haque R, Lima A, et al. Fecal markers of intestinal inflammation and permeability associated with the subsequent acquisition of linear growth deficits in infants. Am J Trop Med Hyg 2013;88(2):390–6.
37. Arndt MB, Richardson BA, Ahmed T, et al. Fecal markers of environmental enteropathy and subsequent growth in Bangladeshi children. Am J Trop Med Hyg 2016;95(3):694–701.
38. Kosek M, Guerrant RL, Kang G, et al. Assessment of environmental enteropathy in the MAL-ED cohort study: theoretical and analytic framework. Clin Infect Dis 2014;59(Suppl 4):S239–47.

39. Uddin MI, Islam S, Nishat NS, et al. Biomarkers of environmental enteropathy are positively associated with immune responses to an oral cholera vaccine in Bangladeshi children. PLoS Negl Trop Dis 2016;10(11):e0005039.

40. Oriá RB, Costa CMC, Lima AAM, et al. Semantic fluency: a sensitive marker for cognitive impairment in children with heavy diarrhea burdens? Med Hypotheses 2009;73(5):682–6.

41. Danaei G, Andrews KG, Sudfeld CR, et al. Risk factors for childhood stunting in 137 developing countries: a comparative risk assessment analysis at global, regional, and country levels. PLoS Med 2016;13(11):e1002164.

42. World Health Organization. WHO child growth standards: length/height-for-age, weight-for-age, weight-for-length, weight-for-height and body mass index-for-age, Methods and Development. 2006. Available at: http://www.who.int/childgrowth/standards/Technical_report.pdf?ua=1. Accessed May 9, 2016.

43. Saiki T. Myeloperoxidase concentrations in the stool as a new parameter of inflammatory bowel disease. Kurume Med J 1998;45(1):69–73.

44. Ledjeff E, Artner-Dworzak E, Witasek A, et al. Neopterin Concentrations in Colon Dialysate. Pteridines 2013;12(4):155–60.

45. World Health Organization. The treatment of diarrhoea: a manual for physicians and other senior health workers. 2005. Available at: http://www.who.int/maternal_child_adolescent/documents/9241593180/en/index.html.

46. Guerrant DI, Moore SR, Lima AA, et al. Association of early childhood diarrhea and cryptosporidiosis with impaired physical fitness and cognitive function four-seven years later in a poor urban community in northeast Brazil. Am J Trop Med Hyg 1999;61(5):707–13.

47. Lima AA, Moore SR, Barboza MS Jr, et al. Persistent diarrhea signals a critical period of increased diarrhea burdens and nutritional shortfalls: a prospective cohort study among children in northeastern Brazil. J Infect Dis 2000;181(5):1643–51.

48. Niehaus MD, Moore SR, Patrick PD, et al. Early childhood diarrhea is associated with diminished cognitive function 4 to 7 years later in children in a northeast Brazilian shantytown. Am J Trop Med Hyg 2002;66(5):590–3.

49. Checkley W, Epstein LD, Gilman RH, et al. Effects of acute diarrhea on linear growth in Peruvian children. Am J Epidemiol 2003;157(2):166–75.

50. Moore SR, Lima NL, Soares AM, et al. Prolonged episodes of acute diarrhea reduce growth and increase risk of persistent diarrhea in children. Gastroenterology 2010;139(4):1156–64.

51. Assis AMO, Barreto ML, Santos LMP, et al. Growth faltering in childhood related to diarrhea: a longitudinal community based study. Eur J Clin Nutr 2005;59(11):1317–23.

52. Platts-Mills JA, Babji S, Bodhidatta L, et al. Pathogen-specific burdens of community diarrhoea in developing countries: a multisite birth cohort study (MAL-ED). Lancet Glob Health 2015;3(9):e564–75.

53. Steiner TS, Lima AA, Nataro JP, et al. Enteroaggregative Escherichia coli produce intestinal inflammation and growth impairment and cause interleukin-8 release from intestinal epithelial cells. J Infect Dis 1998;177(1):88–96.

54. Acosta GJ, Vigo NI, Durand D, et al. Diarrheagenic Escherichia coli: prevalence and pathotype distribution in children from peruvian rural communities. Am J Trop Med Hyg 2016;95(3):574–9.

55. Lee G, Pan W, Peñataro Yori P, et al. Symptomatic and asymptomatic Campylobacter infections associated with reduced growth in Peruvian children. PLoS Negl Trop Dis 2013;7(1):e2036.

56. Donowitz JR, Alam M, Kabir M, et al. A prospective longitudinal cohort to investigate the effects of early life Giardiasis on growth and all cause diarrhea. Clin Infect Dis 2016;63(6):792–7.

57. Checkley W, Epstein LD, Gilman RH, et al. Effects of Cryptosporidium parvum infection in peruvian children: growth faltering and subsequent catch-up growth. Am J Epidemiol 1998;148(5):497–506.

58. Galdys AL, Nelson JS, Shutt KA, et al. Prevalence and duration of asymptomatic Clostridium difficile carriage among healthy subjects in Pittsburgh, Pennsylvania. J Clin Microbiol 2014;52(7):2406–9.

59. Levine MM, Robins-Browne RM. Factors that explain excretion of enteric pathogens by persons without diarrhea. Clin Infect Dis 2012;55(Suppl 4):S303–11.

60. Kaper JB, Nataro JP, Mobley HL. Pathogenic Escherichia coli. Nat Rev Microbiol 2004;2(2):123–40.

61. Kotloff KL, Nataro JP, Blackwelder WC, et al. Burden and aetiology of diarrhoeal disease in infants and young children in developing countries (the Global Enteric Multicenter Study, GEMS): a prospective, case-control study. Lancet 2013;382(9888):209–22.

62. Morgan XC, Huttenhower C. Chapter 12: human microbiome analysis. PLoS Comput Biol 2012;8(12):e1002808.

63. Hopkins MJ, Sharp R, Macfarlane GT. Variation in human intestinal microbiota with age. Dig Liver Dis 2002;34(Suppl 2):S12–8.

64. Di Mauro A, Neu J, Riezzo G, et al. Gastrointestinal function development and microbiota. Ital J Pediatr 2013;39:15.

65. Guarino A, Wudy A, Basile F, et al. Composition and roles of intestinal microbiota in children. J Matern Fetal Neonatal Med 2012;25(Suppl 1):63–6.

66. Subramanian S, Huq S, Yatsunenko T, et al. Persistent gut microbiota immaturity in malnourished Bangladeshi children. Nature 2014. http://dx.doi.org/10.1038/nature13421. Advance online publication.

67. Blanton LV, Charbonneau MR, Salih T, et al. Gut bacteria that prevent growth impairments transmitted by microbiota from malnourished children. Science 2016; 351(6275). http://dx.doi.org/10.1126/science.aad3311.

68. Coutinho BP, Oriá RB, Vieira CMG, et al. Cryptosporidium infection causes undernutrition and, conversely, weanling undernutrition intensifies infection. J Parasitol 2008;94(6):1225–32.

69. Costa LB, Noronha FJ, Roche JK, et al. Novel in vitro and in vivo models and potential new therapeutics to break the vicious cycle of Cryptosporidium infection and malnutrition. J Infect Dis 2012;205(9):1464–71.

70. Liu J, Bolick DT, Kolling GL, et al. Protein malnutrition impairs intestinal epithelial turnover: a potential mechanism of increased cryptosporidiosis in a murine model. Infect Immun 2016. http://dx.doi.org/10.1128/IAI.00705-16.

71. Roche JK, Cabel A, Sevilleja J, et al. Enteroaggregative Escherichia coli (EAEC) impairs growth while malnutrition worsens EAEC infection: a novel murine model of the infection malnutrition cycle. J Infect Dis 2010;202(4):506–14.

72. Bolick DT, Roche JK, Hontecillas R, et al. Enteroaggregative Escherichia coli strain in a novel weaned mouse model: exacerbation by malnutrition, biofilm as a virulence factor and treatment by nitazoxanide. J Med Microbiol 2013; 62(Pt 6):896–905.

73. Bolick DT, Kolling GL, Moore JH, et al. Zinc deficiency alters host response and pathogen virulence in a mouse model of enteroaggregative Escherichia coli-induced diarrhea. Gut Microbes 2014;5(5):618–27.

74. Preidis GA, Saulnier DM, Blutt SE, et al. Host response to probiotics determined by nutritional status of rotavirus-infected neonatal mice. J Pediatr Gastroenterol Nutr 2012;55(3):299–307.

75. Hentges DJ. Role of the intestinal microflora in host defense against infection. In: Hentges DJ, editor. Human intestinal microflora in health and disease. New York: Academic Press, Inc; 1983. p. 311–31.

76. Wardwell LH, Huttenhower C, Garrett WS. Current concepts of the intestinal microbiota and the pathogenesis of infection. Curr Infect Dis Rep 2011;13(1): 28–34.

77. Sekirov I, Finlay BB. The role of the intestinal microbiota in enteric infection. J Physiol 2009;587(Pt 17):4159–67.

78. Looft T, Allen HK. Collateral effects of antibiotics on mammalian gut microbiomes. Gut Microbes 2012;3(5):463–7.

79. Sekirov I, Tam NM, Jogova M, et al. Antibiotic-induced perturbations of the intestinal microbiota alter host susceptibility to enteric infection. Infect Immun 2008; 76(10):4726–36.

80. Moon C, Stappenbeck TS. Viral interactions with the host and microbiota in the intestine. Curr Opin Immunol 2012;24(4):405–10.

81. Grzybowski MM, Długońska H. Natural microbiota in viral and helminth infections. Addendum to: Personalized vaccination. II. The role of natural microbiota in a vaccine-induced immunity. Ann Parasitol 2012;58(3):157–60.

82. Kuss SK, Best GT, Etheredge CA, et al. Intestinal microbiota promote enteric virus replication and systemic pathogenesis. Science 2011;334(6053):249–52.

83. Kane M, Case LK, Kopaskie K, et al. Successful transmission of a retrovirus depends on the commensal microbiota. Science 2011;334(6053):245–9.

84. DuPont AW, DuPont HL. The intestinal microbiota and chronic disorders of the gut. Nat Rev Gastroenterol Hepatol 2011;8(9):523–31.

85. Finegold SM, Mathisen GE, George WL, et al. Changes in human intestinal flora related to the administration of antimicrobial agents. In: Human intestinal microflora in health and disease. New York: Academic Press, Inc; 1983. p. 355–446.

86. Guerrant RL, Kosek M, Lima AAM, et al. Updating the DALYs for diarrhoeal disease. Trends Parasitol 2002;18(5):191–3.

87. Mishra OP, Dhawan T, Singla PN, et al. Endoscopic and histopathological evaluation of preschool children with chronic diarrhoea. J Trop Pediatr 2001;47(2): 77–80.

88. Kelly P, Menzies I, Crane R, et al. Responses of small intestinal architecture and function over time to environmental factors in a tropical population. Am J Trop Med Hyg 2004;70(4):412–9.

89. Thomas AG, Phillips AD, Walker-Smith JA. The value of proximal small intestinal biopsy in the differential diagnosis of chronic diarrhoea. Arch Dis Child 1992; 67(6):741–3 [discussion: 743–4].

90. Liu J, Platts-Mills JA, Juma J, et al. Use of quantitative molecular diagnostic methods to identify causes of diarrhoea in children: a reanalysis of the GEMS case-control study. Lancet 2016;388(10051):1291–301.

91. Houpt E, Gratz J, Kosek M, et al. Microbiologic methods utilized in the MAL-ED cohort study. Clin Infect Dis 2014;59(Suppl 4):S225–32.

92. World Health Organization and United Nations Children's Fund Joint Monitoring Programme for Water Supply and Sanitation, (JMP). Progress on Drinking Water and Sanitation: Special Focus on Sanitation. New York; Geneva (Switzerland): UNICEF, WHO; 2008. Available at: http://www.wssinfo.org/fileadmin/user_upload/resources/1251794333-JMP_08_en.pdf. Accessed February 5, 2016.

93. World Health Organization. Comprehensive implementation plan on maternal, infant and young child nutrition. 2014. Available at: http://www.who.int/nutrition/publications/CIP_document/en/. Accessed November 29, 2016.

94. Forouzanfar MH, Afshin A, Alexander LT, et al. Global, regional, and national comparative risk assessment of 79 behavioural, environmental and occupational, and metabolic risks or clusters of risks, 1990–2015: a systematic analysis for the Global Burden of Disease Study 2015. Lancet 2016;388(10053): 1659–724.

95. World Health Organization. Essential nutrition actions: improving maternal, newborn, infant and young child health and nutrition. 2013. Available at: http://www.who.int/nutrition/publications/infantfeeding/essential_nutrition_actions/en/. Accessed November 29, 2016.

96. Greenland S, Pearl J, Robins JM. Causal diagrams for epidemiologic research. Epidemiology 1999;10(1):37–48.

97. Lang D, MAL-ED Network Investigators. Opportunities to assess factors contributing to the development of the intestinal microbiota in infants living in developing countries. Microb Ecol Health Dis 2015;26:28316.

98. Curtis V, Cousens S, Mertens T, et al. Structured observations of hygiene behaviours in Burkina Faso: validity, variability, and utility. Bull World Health Organ 1993;71(1):23–32.

99. Biran A, Rabie T, Schmidt W, et al. Comparing the performance of indicators of hand-washing practices in rural Indian households. Trop Med Int Health 2008; 13(2):278–85.

100. Panchalingam S, Antonio M, Hossain A, et al. Diagnostic microbiologic methods in the GEMS-1 case/control study. Clin Infect Dis 2012;55(Suppl 4):S294–302.

101. Liu J, Gratz J, Amour C, et al. A laboratory-developed TaqMan array card for simultaneous detection of 19 enteropathogens. J Clin Microbiol 2013;51(2): 472–80.

102. Rutledge RG, Côté C. Mathematics of quantitative kinetic PCR and the application of standard curves. Nucleic Acids Res 2003;31(16):e93.

103. Carroll IM, Threadgill DW, Threadgill DS. The gastrointestinal microbiome: a malleable, third genome of mammals. Mamm Genome 2009;20(7):395–403.

104. Yu J, Ordiz MI, Stauber J, et al. Environmental enteric dysfunction includes a broad spectrum of inflammatory responses and epithelial repair processes. Cell Mol Gastroenterol Hepatol 2016;2(2):158–74.e1.

105. Mayneris-Perxachs J, Lima AAM, Guerrant RL, et al. Urinary N-methylnicotinamide and β-aminoisobutyric acid predict catch-up growth in undernourished Brazilian children. Sci Rep 2016;6:19780.

106. Serazin AC, Shackelton LA, Wilson C, et al. Improving the performance of enteric vaccines in the developing world. Nat Immunol 2010;11(9):769–73.

107. Clasen T, Boisson S, Routray P, et al. Effectiveness of a rural sanitation programme on diarrhoea, soil-transmitted helminth infection, and child malnutrition in Odisha, India: a cluster-randomised trial. Lancet Glob Health 2014;2(11): e645–53.

108. Patil SR, Arnold BF, Salvatore AL, et al. The effect of India's total sanitation campaign on defecation behaviors and child health in rural Madhya Pradesh: a cluster randomized controlled trial. PLoS Med 2014;11(8):e1001709.

109. Luby S. Is targeting access to sanitation enough? Lancet Glob Health 2014; 2(11):e619–20.

110. Rogawski ET, Platts-Mills JA, Seidman JC, et al. Use of antibiotics in children younger than two years in eight countries: a prospective cohort study. Bull World Health Organ 2017;95:49–61.
111. Archbald-Pannone L, Sevilleja JE, Guerrant R. Diarrhea, clostridium difficile, and intestinal inflammation in residents of a long-term care facility. J Am Med Dir Assoc 2010;11(4):263–7.
112. Bentley DW. Clostridium difficile-associated disease in long-term care facilities. Infect Control Hosp Epidemiol 1990;11(8):434–8.
113. Rybolt AH, Bennett RG, Laughon BE, et al. Protein-losing enteropathy associated with Clostridium difficile infection. Lancet 1989;1(8651):1353–5.

Cryptosporidium and Giardia Infections in Children: A Review

Blandina T. Mmbaga, MD, MMed, PhD[a], Eric R. Houpt, MD[b],*

KEYWORDS

- *Cryptosporidium* • Diarrhea • Children

KEY POINTS

- Consider *Cryptosporidium* in any child, particularly younger than 2 years old, with severe acute watery diarrhea.
- Diagnosis of *Cryptosporidium* can be made by acid-fast microscopy, enzyme-linked immunosorbent assay (ELISA), or immunofluorescent antibody staining, or molecular diagnostics.
- Diarrhea due to *Cryptosporidium* is usually self-limited in 1 to 2 weeks but vigilance is needed in immunocompromised patients in whom the clinical course may be protracted and severe.
- Nitazoxanide is approved for treatment of *Cryptosporidium* in immunocompetent children older than the 1 year old.
- Inquire about possible sources of exposure, such as recreational water and close contacts, with similar symptoms because outbreaks occur and *Cryptosporidium* and *Giardia* are reportable disease in many jurisdictions and Consider giardiasis in cases of prolonged diarrhea, particularly in travelers.

CRYPTOSPORIDIUM

Cryptosporidium is an apicomplexan protozoan parasite that was first identified as a human pathogen in 1976 in a 3-year-old child with severe acute enterocolitis[1] (**Figs. 1** and **2**). Another publication later that year described an immunosuppressed adult with a similar presentation of severe diarrhea without clear cause.[2] In both instances, biopsy of intestinal tissue with electron microscopy was performed and lesions showed mucosal injury and tiny 2 to 4 μm organisms on the intestinal epithelial surface that

No Commercial or Financial Conflicts of Interest. No funding sources.
[a] Department of Pediatrics, Kilimanjaro Christian Medical Centre, Kilimanjaro Clinical Research Institute, Box 3010, Moshi, Tanzania 0255; [b] Division of Infectious Diseases and International Health, University of Virginia, 345 Crispell Drive, Charlottesville, VA 22908, USA
* Corresponding author.
E-mail address: erh6k@virginia.edu

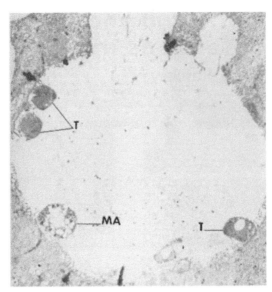

Fig. 1. The original photomicrograph of a rectal biopsy showing trophozoites (T) and macrogametes (MA) of *Cryptosporidium* attached to the epithelial surface. (*Data from* Nime FA, Burek JD, Page DL, et al. Acute enterocolitis in a human being infected with the protozoan *Cryptosporidium*. Gastroenterology 1976;70:592–8.)

were determined to be *Cryptosporidium* based on morphology. These are now known to be intracellular forms, such as trophozoites, schizonts, and gametes. When these forms produce oocysts that are excreted into the environment then transmission to other hosts can continue.

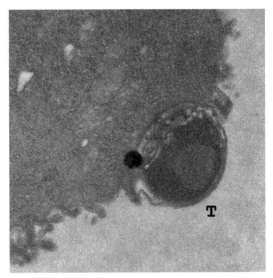

Fig. 2. High-power electron micrograph of *Cryptosporidium*. Trophozoite form (T) with an internal vacuole is present, after infection of HCT-8 intestinal epithelial cells. The dark black dot is artifact. (*Courtesy of* Christopher Huston, University of Vermont.)

Since that original description, cases of severe and fatal disease in patients with acquired immune deficiency syndrome (AIDS),[3] and the massive 1993 outbreak of waterborne *Cryptosporidium* affecting 403,000 persons in Milwaukee, Wisconsin,[4] have increased attention to the pathogen. Now *Cryptosporidium* is recognized as a leading cause of childhood diarrhea around the world, revealed largely by the large Global Enteric Multicenter Study (GEMS).[5] According to the Global Burden of Disease Study, it is now the second most implicated diarrheal pathogen after rotavirus, causing 60,400 deaths alone in 2015, or 12% of the total diarrhea mortality burden.[6] This article provides an overview of this enigmatic pathogen, focusing on pediatric disease, which merits investment to research better treatments and vaccines.

Cryptosporidium Epidemiology

The authors reviewed the recent literature on *Cryptosporidium* diarrhea in children, summarizing several studies published since 2000 involving children 15 years of age and younger who had diarrhea in Africa,[5,7–17] Asia,[5,17–23] and Latin America[17,24–26] (**Table 1**). Across diverse settings, the prevalence of diarrhea cases is 1% to 35% (median 18%), with variations in hospital versus community settings and diagnostic methodology. Many studies included control stools for comparison, whereby the rates of *Cryptosporidium* were virtually always lower (median 6%), confirming *Cryptosporidium*'s association with diarrhea. Most studies focused on *Cryptosporidium* alone or on a small number of pathogens. The largest studies were the multisite GEMS[5] and Malnutrition and Enteric Disease Study (MAL-ED)[17] studies, which tested case and control stools for dozens of enteropathogens and allowed an examination of the importance of *Cryptosporidium* relative to others. Because these are the most recent and comprehensive studies to date, they are explored in further detail.

The GEMS study was a case control study of children younger than 5 years old performed in 4 sites in Africa and 3 in Asia. Cases had moderate-to-severe diarrhea and controls were age, sex, and geographically matched. Enzyme-linked immunosorbent assay (ELISA) was used for *Cryptosporidium* diagnosis. This study found that *Cryptosporidium* was the second most attributable pathogen among infants (a metric that combines both prevalence and magnitude of diarrhea-association) after rotavirus in all 4 African sites (located in Gambia, Mali, Mozambique, and Kenya) plus India, and was also common in the other South Asian sites. In the second year of life, *Cryptosporidium* remained the second most important pathogen in Mali, Kenya, and India. Moreover, *Cryptosporidium* diarrhea was associated with a high risk of death in 90-day follow-up. After 2 years of age, *Cryptosporidium*'s importance declined dramatically. These *Cryptosporidium* burden estimates were reaffirmed in a reanalysis of the GEMS study that used quantitative polymerase chain reaction (PCR) for diagnosis.[27] Although the burden was similar, *Cryptosporidium*'s position in the enteropathogen hierarchy dropped slightly relative to other pathogens, particularly *Shigella*, which was better detected with the molecular diagnostics. That said, *Cryptosporidium* remained extremely important; for example, accounting for 17% of cases in Malian infants, second to only rotavirus at 23%. Note that the GEMS study was performed in 2007 to 2011 in regions before implementation of the rotavirus vaccine.

The MAL-ED study was conducted in 2009 to 2014 in similar settings in Africa, Asia, as well as South America, at which time a few sites had implemented rotavirus vaccine.[17] This was a community-based active surveillance study that captured milder diarrheal episodes. *Cryptosporidium* was also diagnosed by ELISA and was measured

Table 1
Prevalence of *Cryptosporidium* in diarrhea in children

Region (Reference)	Country	Age Included (y)	Setting	Diagnostic Method	Diarrhea Samples (N)	*Cryptosporidium* %	Comments
Asia							
Khan et al,[18] 2004	Bangladesh	0–5	H	Microscopy	1672	3	—
Haque et al,[19] 2009	Bangladesh	0–14 and adults	H & C	ELISA	3646	3	Rate in nondiarrhea 2% (n = 2575)
Bera et al,[20] 2014	India	0–5	H	ELISA	175	27	—
Mirzaei et al,[21] 2007	Iran	0–15	C	Microscopy	89	35	Rate in nondiarrhea 3% (n = 51)
Hawash et al,[22] 2014	Saudi Arabia	0–9	C	PCR	95	17	—
Wongstitwilairroong et al,[23] 2007	Thailand	0–5	C	ELISA	236	1	Rate in nondiarrhea 3% (n = 236)
Africa							
Wegayehu et al,[7] 2013	Ethiopia	0–14	C	Microscopy	0	NA	Rate in nondiarrhea 7% (n = 384)
Firdu et al,[8] 2014	Ethiopia	0–13	H	Microscopy	230	10	Rate in nondiarrhea 6% (n = 115)
Adjei et al,[9] 2004	Ghana	0–5	H	Microscopy	304	28	Rate in nondiarrhea 16% (n = 304)
Eibach et al,[10] 2015	Ghana	0–15	H	PCR	2232	5	Includes gastrointestinal symptoms
Moyo et al,[11] 2011	Tanzania	0–5	H	ImmunoCard	270	19	—

Reference	Location	Age	Setting	Method	N		Rate in nondiarrhea
Elfving,[12] 2014	Tanzania	0–5	H	PCR	165	30	Rate in nondiarrhea 11% (n = 165)
Desilva et al,[13] 2016	Tanzania	0–5	H	PCR	701	16	Rate in nondiarrhea 3% (n = 558) HIV+ 24% vs HIV− 4%
Tumwine et al,[14] 2005	Uganda	0–5	H	Microscopy	243	32	HIV+ 74% vs HIV− 6%
Tumwine et al,[15] 2003	Uganda	0–5	H	PCR	1779	25	Rate in nondiarrhea 9% (n = 667)
Amadi et al,[16] 2001	Zambia	0–5	H	Microscopy	200	26	HIV+ 29% vs HIV− 19%
Latin America							
Medeiros et al,[24] 2001	Brazil	0–10	H & C	Microscopy	1836	2	—
Carvalho-Costa et al,[25] 2007	Brazil	0–5	H	Microscopy	193	9	—
Laubach et al,[26] 2004	Guatemala	0–5	C	Microscopy	100	32	—
Worldwide multisite							
Kotloff et al,[5] 2013	Bangladesh, India, Pakistan, Gambia, Mali, Kenya, Mozambique	0–5	H & C	ELISA	9439		Attributable fraction = 5.3%–14.7% in year 1 of life
Platts-Mills et al,[17] 2015	Bangladesh, India, Nepal, Pakistan, Tanzania, South Africa, Brazil Peru	0–2	C	ELISA	7318		Attributable fraction = 2.0% in year 1 of life; 3.8% in year 2

Attributable fraction combines prevalence and odds ratio, according to the formula AF = prevalence (1−1/odds ratio).

Abbreviations: C, community; H, hospital; NA, not applicable; PCR, polymerase chain reaction.

to be the fourth most attributable diarrheal pathogen in the first year of life (overall ~2% of episodes) and sixth most in the second year of life (overall ~4% of episodes). Cryptosporidiosis was enriched among more severe episodes, consistent with the higher rates in the GEMS study. Taken together, these studies point to the clear importance of *Cryptosporidium* as a major cause of diarrhea in Africa and parts of Asia in children younger than 2 years, and this importance will likely increase as rotavirus vaccine is implemented.

Cryptosporidium is a risk factor for mortality in malnourished children with diarrhea.[16] Breastfeeding seems to confer some protection.[8,15,13] In high-income countries, disease has been linked to water-borne outbreaks.[28–30] In resource-limited settings, contaminated water has been associated with *Cryptosporidium* in some studies[26] but not others.[31] An increase during the rainy season has been repeatedly noted.[10,15,23,13,32] For instance, in the MAL-ED study, during the rainy season in Pakistan, more than half of diarrheal episodes could be attributed to *Cryptosporidium*. There does not seem to be a consistent gender predisposition to infection.[8,22,26]

CRYPTOSPORIDIUM SPECIES

Most early publications used the term *C parvum*; however, in 2002 biological and molecular data suggested many of these infections were in fact due to a different but structurally indistinguishable species termed *C hominis*.[33] These 2 species are quite similar at the DNA level (~96%)[34] compared with, for example, only approximately 70% among *Giardia* subtypes.[35] Several other species of *Cryptosporidium* have also been identified in humans, notably *C meleagridis* and many others.[14,36,37] *C viatorum* has recently been noted as a pathogen in returning travelers with diarrhea.[38] However, it is now appreciated that *C hominis* is the main cause globally in childhood diarrhea cases[10,14,13,36,37,39–41] **(Table 2)**. In the GEMS study, 78% of *Cryptosporidium* cases were *C hominis* and another 10% were *C parvum*, with the remainder undetermined.[39] These high rates have also been seen in several other studies.[10,13,36,37,41] Furthermore, even among *C parvum* infections, subtyping of these strains has shown that many are so-called anthroponotic subtypes,[10,39,42] suggesting human-human acquisition of these cases as well. Thus the zoonotic relevance of *Cryptosporidium* in childhood diarrhea in most settings seems to be modest or confined to certain areas, particularly parts of the United Kingdom. That said, close contact with animals at home has been a risk factor for *Cryptosporidium* in some studies.[7,8]

Table 2
Distribution of *Cryptosporidium hominis* and *Cryptosporidium parvum*

Reference, Year	Country	C Hominis %	C Parvum %
Sow et al,[39] 2016	Multisite	78	10
Tellevik et al,[13] 2015	Tanzania	85	8
Gatei et al,[37] 2006	Kenya	87	9
Gatei et al,[40] 2003	Multisite	75	22
Tumwine et al,[14] 2005	Uganda	73	18
Sarkar et al,[41] 2013	India	79	16
Eibach et al,[8] 2015	Ghana	58	42
Xiao et al,[36] 2001	Peru	79	9

Clinical differences between *Cryptosporidium* species has been reported in some studies but have often conflicted, such as more vomiting with *C parvum* in Ghana versus more vomiting with *C parvum* in Peru.[10,43] In general, these analyses have been complicated by confounders, the possibility of other enteropathogens not tested for, and intrinsically small sample sizes for other species given the predominance of *C hominis*.

CRYPTOSPORIDIUM AND THE HUMAN IMMUNODEFICIENCY VIRUS INFECTION IN CHILDREN

Cryptosporidiosis has long been associated with immunodeficiency. *Cryptosporidium* prevalence in human immunodeficiency virus (HIV) infection is typically higher in cross-sectional studies than in non-HIV infected individuals (see **Table 1**). Diarrhea severity is often worse and duration protracted in HIV and malnourished subsets. This likely reflects the importance of CD4+ cell-mediated immune responses in controlling the infection,[44] a phenomenon that may underlie the susceptibility of the youngest children.

CRYPTOSPORIDIUM CLINICAL PRESENTATION

Watery diarrhea is the chief clinical syndrome,[15,18,13,37] frequently severe and with dehydration,[13,37] usually not bloody, and sometimes with vomiting. Cryptosporidial diarrhea is often prolonged or persistent compared with other causes,[15,14,17,13] explaining about one-third of such cases. In 1 study, diarrhea with *Cryptosporidium* was less likely to occur with abdominal pain than did other entities.[19] Overall, however, no specific signs or symptoms implicate *Cryptosporidium* over other organisms that cause watery diarrhea such as rotavirus, enterotoxigenic *Escherichia coli* (ETEC), adenovirus, or even *Shigella* or *Campylobacter*, which are also important causes of watery diarrhea in children. Severity seems to correlate with parasite burden, at least in AIDS in which histopathologic disease correlates with parasite load.[45] In immunocompromised patients, infection can extend throughout the gastrointestinal tract and disseminate to other sites, including biliary tree and lung,[46] and present with right upper quadrant pain or pathologic conditions of the lung. In a study from Uganda, 12% of young children presenting with diarrhea had *Cryptosporidium* by microscopy, 25% of whom had *Cryptosporidium* detectable in respiratory specimens by PCR, and many had cough.[46]

In addition to diarrhea, asymptomatic intestinal infection with *Cryptosporidium* has been associated with poor childhood growth.[47] The impact and magnitude of this effect is a subject of active study because asymptomatic intestinal infection is much more common than diarrhea on a community level. Asymptomatic *Cryptosporidium* carriage can also occur in HIV patients, even with advanced AIDS, presumably reflecting sufficient immune responses other than CD4 cells, persistent low level infections after diarrhea, or incubating preclinical disease.[48]

CRYPTOSPORIDIUM LABORATORY DIAGNOSIS

Unfortunately, in resource poor settings, *Cryptosporidium* is not routinely tested for because it requires special stains, even though this technology is straightforward. The modified acid-fast stain uses Kinyoun carbol fuchsin, does not require heat, and stains oocysts. Several approved ELISA and immunofluorescent antibody tests are also commercially available. These target oocyst antigens and provide improved sensitivity versus microscopy. Molecular diagnostics are also increasingly available; for example, the FilmArray Gastrointestinal Panel (Biofire Diagnostics, Salt Lake City, UT, USA) and the xTAG Gastrointestinal Pathogen Panel (Luminex, Austin, TX, USA). These diagnostics detect more than a dozen enteropathogens, including Cryptosporidium, and are highly sensitive compared with microscopy or ELISA; however, they are costly.[49]

CRYPTOSPORIDIUM TREATMENT

Typical therapy for childhood diarrhea is supportive care with rehydration. Only in particularly severe or bloody episodes is laboratory diagnosis or antibiotic therapy pursued.[50] Similarly, most cases of Cryptosporidium diarrhea are self-limited and do not require specific therapy, although the course frequently lasts 2 weeks. Nitazoxanide is a broad spectrum antiparasitic approved by the US Food and Drug Administration for the treatment of Cryptosporidium.[51–53] The drug is well tolerated with mild side effects.[54] It has been shown to be effective in immunocompetent (HIV-negative) children and adults with Cryptosporidium[51,55,56] but is not efficacious in HIV-positive individuals. The effect size seems modest, however, with cessation of diarrhea occurring in only 56% of individuals in the Zambia study, with duration reduced by only 2 days in adults. Perhaps the most compelling result was the improvement in mortality within 8 days in HIV-negative children with cryptosporidial diarrhea (0% vs 18% in placebo, n = 25 and 22 per arm). This was a small study with an extremely high mortality rate, even among HIV-uninfected children (eg, several-fold higher than GEMS) and, as of yet, such an impressive mortality effect has not been redemonstrated. Nitazoxanide is also effective against other protozoal infections[57] and has been approved for treatment of Giardia.[54] Understanding these caveats, the authors recommend treatment with nitazoxanide if Cryptosporidium diarrhea is severe. It is available as oral suspension or tablets and is administered twice daily for 3 days. In children with solid organ transplant and cryptosporidial diarrhea, longer duration (>14 days) of nitazoxanide have been used.[58] Paromomycin is an alternative agent with mixed results[59,60] and is available only in capsule form in the United States. Additive azithromycin has also been attempted in extreme cases.[61] Immunotherapy, such as bovine anti-Cryptosporidium oocyst colostrum, has been tried without success. In HIV-infected individuals, highly active antiretroviral therapy and supportive care are the mainstays of treatment. In sum, better and more available treatments for Cryptosporidium are likely needed[49] but will need to be paired with more available diagnostics given the long list of pathogens that can present with severe watery diarrhea.

CRYPTOSPORIDIUM PREVENTION

Given the difficulty in treating Cryptosporidium, prevention is important. The infectious dose is low and the parasite is relatively resistant to chlorination. Municipal water utilities test drinking water sources for Cryptosporidium in the United States; however, outbreaks still occur, particularly during the summer recreational water season.[62] Surprisingly, in a longitudinal study in India, children who used bottled water did not have lower rates of Cryptosporidium,[41] which casts doubt on the importance of drinking water in transmission in highly endemic settings. Boiling, absolute 1 micron filters, or UV treatments are effective. Of course, careful food and water hygiene during travel is advised; however, Cryptosporidium is not commonly reported in travelers returning with diarrhea.[63] Vaccines are not currently available but several candidates are being explored.[49]

Cryptosporidium case vignettes

1. A child immigrated from a resource-limited setting and presents to a US pediatrician's office with diarrhea.
   - If severe with clinical signs of dehydration, the authors recommend diagnostic evaluation to include *Cryptosporidium* and treatment with nitazoxanide if positive.

2. A child traveled to such an endemic country and now is presenting with mild diarrheal symptoms.
   - Supportive care only. Even if the diagnosis is *Cryptosporidium*, the course should self-limit after about 2 weeks.

3. A child plans to visit an endemic country with her family.
   - *Cryptosporidium* is not a common cause of traveler's diarrhea but routine hygiene precautions are advised, such as washing hands before eating and avoiding tap water and food exposed to tap water. Boiled, UV treated, or bottled water may be consumed.

GIARDIA LAMBLIA

Giardia lamblia (also known as *Giardia duodenalis)* is a flagellated protozoan pathogen that is commonly found in nearly all human populations. The ability of *G lamblia* to cause diarrhea was established without question in the course of human volunteer studies in the 1980s.[64] Moreover, clinical experience in industrialized countries supports the causal association between the shedding of *Giardia* cysts and trophozoites, and diarrheal symptoms, with resolution of symptoms accompanying eradication of the organism.

GIARDIA EPIDEMIOLOGY

Despite the clear implication of *Giardia* as a diarrheal pathogen in industrialized countries, its role in diarrhea in developing countries is less certain. In GEMS, detection of *Giardia* by immunoassay was not associated with diarrhea at any site or in any age stratum.[5] This observation was confirmed using molecular detection methods.[27] Interestingly, some sites reported a protective epidemiologic association of *Giardia* against moderate to severe diarrhea, although a mechanism to account for this observation was not suggested.[5] Speculation regarding different roles for *Giardia* as an enteric pathogen in industrialized versus developing countries focuses on possible age-related susceptibility, protective effects of prior experience with the pathogen, heterogeneous virulence of individual isolates, or the possibility that low levels of exposure may induce colonization without symptomatology.

A more recent and possibly more important implication of *Giardia* in human disease has focused on childhood growth. Donowitz and colleagues[65] have recently conducted a prospective longitudinal birth cohort study in Bangladesh, in which stools were assayed for *Giardia* monthly and whenever diarrhea occurred. In this study, the presence of *Giardia* in the monthly surveillance stools within the first 6 months of life resulted in a decreased length-for-age Z score at 2 years of age by 0.4. Bartelt and colleagues[66] have developed a mouse model that recapitulates this effect. Persistent shedding of *Giardia* in the mice was associated with decreased growth in the absence of diarrhea. This effect was exacerbated by inducing a state of malnutrition in the mice. Intestinal histopathology of giardia-infected mice mirrored what had been described in humans. Thus the burden of *Giardia* infection in *Homo sapiens* is likely to reflect both diarrheal disease, possibly mostly in industrialized countries, and growth in developing countries. This requires further elucidation.

LABORATORY DIAGNOSIS

In direct microscopic examination of stool, the presence of trophozoites or cysts has long been the standard for detection of *Giardia* infection. A single smear from a diarrheal specimen has a sensitivity of 75% to 95% in the hands of an experienced technician. More recently, enzyme immunoassay has replaced microscopic examination in most clinical laboratories and many epidemiologic studies. The sensitivity and specificity is as good as or better than microscopic examination.[67,68] PCR has been available for decades.[69,70] Molecular detection, such as the panels described for *Cryptosporidium*, may be most valuable in industrialized countries where asymptomatic shedding is uncommon.

TREATMENT

Treatment of giardiasis has long been problematic because no therapy is 100% effective. This may be because some cases are falsely ascribed to *Giardia* or because particularly heavy infestations may be resistant to pharmacologic eradication. Metronidazole administered for 5 to 7 days produces cure rates of 80% to 95%. Tinidazole is similarly or slightly more effective after administration of just a single dose for children 3 years of age or older. Both of these drugs are only available as tablets and thus need to be crushed or made into preparations for children unable to swallow tablets. Nitazoxanide oral suspension given in a 3-day course can be used down to 1 year of age, and is as effective as metronidazole and tinidazole. Albendazole, mebendazole, and paromomycin are well-tolerated and may be effective. In cases of relapse, most experts recommend a repeat course of therapy in immunocompetent patients, possibly including 2 drugs[71] to cover drug resistance, and a more prolonged treatment regimen in immunocompromised patients. Patients should be warned after treatment that transient lactose-deficiency is common and to avoid or minimize lactose-containing foods for a few weeks. Postinfective irritable bowel syndrome and chronic fatigue syndrome have been clearly documented from an outbreak in Norway that primarily affected adults.[72]

SUMMARY

Given the importance of *Cryptosporidium* as a cause of severe watery diarrhea, in any child with severe diarrhea of unknown cause presenting for care, immunocompromised or not, the authors recommend testing for *Cryptosporidium* and treatment with nitazoxanide if the child is older than 1 year of age. Rehydration remains paramount, as well as investigation for underlying immunocompromisation. *Giardia* is a common infection worldwide but its burden of disease is controversial. In industrialized countries, it is typically found in cases of persistent diarrhea and should be treated in symptomatic patients; however, it can represent diagnostic, therapeutic, and post-therapeutic challenges.

REFERENCES

1. Nime FA, Burek JD, Page DL, et al. Acute enterocolitis in a human being infected with the protozoan *Cryptosporidium*. Gastroenterology 1976;70(4):592–8.
2. Meisel JL, Perera DR, Meligro C, et al. Overwhelming watery diarrhea associated with a cryptosporidium in an immunosuppressed patient. Gastroenterology 1976; 70(6):1156–60.
3. Wittner M, Goldfarb J, Vogl S, et al. Fatal cryptosporidiosis complicating Kaposi's sarcoma in an immunocompromised man. Am J Med Sci 1984;287(2):47–8.

4. Mac Kenzie WR, Hoxie NJ, Proctor ME, et al. A massive outbreak in Milwaukee of cryptosporidium infection transmitted through the public water supply. N Engl J Med 1994;331(3):161–7.
5. Kotloff KL, Nataro JP, Blackwelder WC, et al. Burden and aetiology of diarrhoeal disease in infants and young children in developing countries (the Global Enteric Multicenter Study, GEMS): a prospective, case-control study. Lancet 2013; 382(9888):209–22.
6. GBD 2015 Mortality and Causes of Death Collaborators. Global, regional, and national life expectancy, all-cause mortality, and cause-specific mortality for 249 causes of death, 1980-2015: a systematic analysis for the Global Burden of Disease Study 2015. Lancet 2016;388(10053):1459–544.
7. Wegayehu T, Adamu H, Petros B. Prevalence of *Giardia duodenalis* and *Cryptosporidium* species infections among children and cattle in North Shewa Zone, Ethiopia. BMC Infect Dis 2013;13(1):419.
8. Firdu T, Abunna F, Girma M. Intestinal protozoal parasites in diarrheal children and associated risk factors at Yirgalem Hospital, Ethiopia: a case-control study. Int Sch Res Notices 2014;1–8.
9. Adjei AA, Armah H, Rodrigues O, et al. *Cryptosporidium* spp., a frequent cause of diarrhea among children at the Korle-Bu Teaching Hospital, Accra, Ghana. Jpn J Infect Dis 2004;57(5):216–9.
10. Eibach D, Krumkamp R, Al-Emran HM, et al. Molecular Characterization of *Cryptosporidium* spp. among children in rural Ghana. PLoS Negl Trop Dis 2015;9(3): e0003551.
11. Moyo SJ, Gro N, Matee MI, et al. Age specific aetiological agents of diarrhoea in hospitalized children aged less than five years in Dar es Salaam, Tanzania. BMC Pediatr 2011;11(1):19.
12. Elfving K, Andersson M, Msellem MI, et al. Real-time PCR threshold cycle cutoffs help to identify agents causing acute childhood diarrhea in Zanzibar. J Clin Microbiol 2014;52(3):916–23.
13. Tellevik MG, Moyo SJ, Blomberg B, et al. Prevalence of *Cryptosporidium parvum/hominis*, *Entamoeba histolytica* and *Giardia lamblia* among Young Children with and without Diarrhea in Dar es Salaam, Tanzania. PLoS Negl Trop Dis 2015; 9(10):1–16.
14. Tumwine JK, Kekitiinwa A, Bakeera-Kitaka S, et al. Cryptosporidiosis and microsporidiosis in Ugandan children with persistent diarrhea with and without concurrent infection with the human immunodeficiency virus. Am J Trop Med Hyg 2005; 73(5):921–5.
15. Tumwine JK, Kekitiinwa A, Nabukeera N, et al. *Cryptosporidium parvum* in children with diarrhea in Mulago Hospital, Kampala, Uganda. Am J Trop Med Hyg 2003;68(6):710–5.
16. Amadi B, Kelly P, Mwiya M, et al. Intestinal and systemic infection, HIV, and mortality in Zambian children with persistent diarrhea and malnutrition. J Pediatr Gastroenterol Nutr 2001;32(5):550–4.
17. Platts-Mills JA, Babji S, Bodhidatta L, et al. Pathogen-specific burdens of community diarrhoea in developing countries: a multisite birth cohort study (MAL-ED). Lancet Glob Heal 2015;3(9):564–75.
18. Khan WA, Rogers KA, Karim MM, et al. Cryptosporidiosis among Bangladeshi children with diarrhea: a prospective matched case-control study of clinical feature, epidemiology and systemic, antibody response. Am J Trop Med Hyg 2004;71(4):412–9.

19. Haque R, Mondal D, Karim A, et al. Prospective case-control study of the association between common enteric protozoal parasites and diarrhea in Bangladesh. Clin Infect Dis 2009;48(9):1191–7.

20. Bera P, Das S, Saha R, et al. *Cryptosporidium* in children with diarrhea: a hospital-based study. Indian Pediatr 2014;51(11):906–8.

21. Mirzaei M. Prevalence of *Cryptosporidium* sp. infection in diarrheic and non-diarrheic humans in Iran. Korean J Parasitol 2007;45(2):133–7.

22. Hawash Y, Dorgham LS, Al-Hazmi AS, et al. Prevalence of *Cryptosporidium*-associated diarrhea in a high altitude-community of Saudi Arabia detected by conventional and molecular methods. Korean J Parasitol 2014;52(5):479–85.

23. Wongstitwilairroong B, Srijan A, Serichantalergs O, et al. Intestinal Parasitic infections among pre-school children in Sangkhlaburi, Thailand. Am J Trop Med Hyg 2007;76(2):345–50.

24. Medeiros MIC, Neme SN, da Silva P, et al. Etiology of acute diarrhea among children in Ribeirão Preto-SP, Brazil. Rev Inst Med Trop Sao Paulo 2001;43:21–4.

25. Carvalho-Costa FA, Gonçalves AQ, Lassance SL, et al. Detection of *Cryptosporidium* spp and other intestinal parasites in children with acute diarrhea and severe dehydration in Rio de Janeiro. Rev Soc Bras Med Trop 2007;40(3):346–8.

26. Laubach HE, Bentley CZ, Ginter EL, et al. A study of risk factors associated with the prevalence of *Cryptosporidium* in villages around Lake Atitlan, Guatemala. Braz J Infect Dis 2004;8:319–23.

27. Liu J, Platts-Mills JA, Juma J, et al. Use of quantitative molecular diagnostic methods to identify causes of diarrhoea in children: a reanalysis of the GEMS case-control study. Lancet 2016;388(10051):1291–301.

28. Desilva MB, Schafer S, Kendall Scott M, et al. Communitywide cryptosporidiosis outbreak associated with a surface water-supplied municipal water system—Baker City, Oregon, 2013. Epidemiol Infect 2016;144(2):274–84.

29. Alden NB, Ghosh TS, Vogt RL, et al. Cryptosporidiosis outbreaks associated with recreational water use—Five states, 2006. MMWR Morb Mortal Wkly Rep 2007; 56(29):729–32.

30. Widerström M, Schönning C, Lilja M, et al. Large Outbreak of *Cryptosporidium hominis* infection transmitted through the public water supply, Sweden. Emerg Infect Dis 2014;20(4):581–9.

31. Iqbal J, Munir MA, Khan MA. *Cryptosporidium* infection in young children with diarrhea in Rawalpindi, Pakistan. Am J Trop Med Hyg 1999;60(5):868–70.

32. Katsumata T, Hosea D, Wasito EB, et al. Cryptosporidiosis in Indonesia: a hospital-based study and a community-based survey. Am J Trop Med Hyg 1998;59(4): 628–32.

33. Morgan-Ryan UM, Fall A, Ward LA, et al. *Cryptosporidium hominis n. sp.* (*Apicomplexa: Cryptosporidiidae*) from *Homo sapiens*. J Eukaryot Microbiol 2002; 49(6):433–40.

34. Xu P, Widmer G, Wang Y, et al. The genome of *Cryptosporidium hominis*. Nature 2004;431(7012):1107–12.

35. Adam RD, Dahlstrom EW, Martens CA, et al. Genome sequencing of *Giardia lamblia* genotypes A2 and B isolates (DH and GS) and comparative analysis with the genomes of genotypes A1 and E (WB and Pig). Genome Biol Evol 2013;5(12): 2498–511.

36. Xiao L, Bern C, Limor J, et al. Identification of 5 types of *Cryptosporidium* parasites in children in Lima, Peru. J Infect Dis 2001;183(3):492–7.

37. Gatei W, Wamae CN, Mbae C, et al. Cryptosporidiosis: prevalence genotype analysis and symptoms associated with infection in children in Kenya. Am J Trop Med Hyg 2006;75(1):78–82.
38. Elwin K, Hadfield SJ, Robinson G, et al. *Cryptosporidium viatorum* n. sp. (*Apicomplexa*: *Cryptosporidiidae*) among travellers returning to Great Britain from the Indian subcontinent, 2007-2011. Int J Parasitol 2012;42(7):675–82.
39. Sow SO, Muhsen K, Nasrin D, et al. The Burden of *Cryptosporidium* Diarrheal Disease among Children < 24 Months of Age in Moderate/High Mortality Regions of Sub-Saharan Africa and South Asia, Utilizing Data from the Global Enteric Multicenter Study (GEMS). PLoS Negl Trop Dis 2016;10(5):e0004729.
40. Gatei W, Greensill J, Ashford RW, et al. Molecular analysis of the 18S rRNA gene of *Cryptosporidium* parasites from patients with or without human immunodeficiency virus infections living in Kenya, Malawi, Brazil, the United Kingdom, and Vietnam. J Clin Microbiol 2003;41(4):1458–62.
41. Sarkar R, Ajjampur SSR, Prabakaran AD, et al. Cryptosporidiosis among children in an endemic semiurban community in southern India: Does a protected drinking water source decrease infection? Clin Infect Dis 2013;57(3):398–406.
42. Xiao L, Ryan UM. Cryptosporidiosis: an update in molecular epidemiology. Curr Opin Infect Dis 2004;17(5):483–90.
43. Cama VA, Bern C, Roberts J, et al. *Cryptosporidium* species and subtypes and clinical manifestations in children, Peru. Emerg Infect Dis 2008;14(10):1567–74.
44. Griffiths JK, Theodos C, Paris M, et al. The gamma interferon gene knockout mouse: a highly sensitive model for evaluation of therapeutic agents against *Cryptosporidium parvum*. J Clin Microbiol 1998;36(9):2503–8.
45. Goodgame RW, Genta RM, White AC, et al. Intensity of infection in AIDS-associated cryptosporidiosis. J Infect Dis 1993;167(3):704–9.
46. Mor SM, Tumwine JK, Ndeezi G, et al. Respiratory cryptosporidiosis in HIV-seronegative children in Uganda: potential for respiratory transmission. Clin Infect Dis 2010;50(10):1366–72.
47. Checkley W, Gilman RH, Epstein LD, et al. Asymptomatic and symptomatic cryptosporidiosis: their acute effect on weight gain in Peruvian children. Am J Epidemiol 1997;145(2):156–63.
48. Houpt ER, Bushen OY, Sam NE, et al. Short report: asymptomatic *Cryptosporidium hominis* infection among human immunodeficiency virus-infected patients in Tanzania. Am J Trop Med Hyg 2005;73(3):520–2.
49. Checkley W, White AC, Jaganath D, et al. A review of the global burden, novel diagnostics, therapeutics, and vaccine targets for cryptosporidium. Lancet Infect Dis 2015;15(1):85–94.
50. WHO. The treatment of diarrhoea: a manual for physician and other health care workers 4th revision. WHO; 2005.
51. Rossignol JF. Nitazoxanide in the treatment of acquired immune deficiency syndrome-related cryptosporidiosis: results of the United States compassionate use program in 365 patients. Aliment Pharmacol Ther 2006;24(5):887–94.
52. Snelling WJ, Xiao L, Ortega-pierres G, et al. Review article cryptosporidiosis in developing countries. Asian Pac J Trop Biomed 2013;3(11):916–24.
53. White AC. Nitazoxanide: an important advance in anti-parasitic therapy. Am J Trop Med Hyg 2003;68(4):382–3.
54. Fox LM, Saravolatz LD. Nitazoxanide: a new thiazolide antiparasitic agent. Clin Infect Dis 2005;40(8):1173–80.

55. Rossignol JF, Ayoub A, Ayers MS. Treatment of diarrhea caused by *Cryptosporidium parvum*: a prospective randomized, double-blind, placebo-controlled study of Nitazoxanide. J Infect Dis 2001;184(1):103–6.

56. Amadi BC, Mwiya M, Musuku J, et al. Effect of nitazoxanide on morbidity and mortality in Zambian children with cryptosporidiosis: a randomised controlled trial. Lancet 2002;360(9343):1375–80.

57. Ali A, Abdelrahim M, Elmoslamy N, et al. Comparison between nitazoxanide and metronidazole in the treatment of protozoal diarrhea in Children. Med Sci Int Med J 2013;3(2):1.

58. Krause I, Amir J, Cleper R, et al. Cryptosporidiosis in children following solid organ transplantation. Pediatr Infect Dis J 2012;31(11):1135–8.

59. Hewitt RG, Yiannoutsos CT, Higgs ES, et al. Paromomycin: no more effective than placebo for treatment of cryptosporidiosis in patients with advanced human immunodeficiency virus infection. AIDS Clinical Trial Group. Clin Infect Dis 2000; 31(4):1084–92.

60. White AC, Chappell CL, Hayat CS, et al. Paromomycin for cryptosporidiosis in AIDS: a prospective, double-blind trial. J Infect Dis 1994;170(2):419–24.

61. Legrand F, Grenouillet F, Larosa F, et al. Diagnosis and treatment of digestive cryptosporidiosis in allogeneic haematopoietic stem cell transplant recipients: a prospective single centre study. Bone Marrow Transplant 2011;46(6):858–62.

62. Painter JE, Hlavsa MC, Collier SA, et al, Centers for Disease Control and Prevention. Cryptosporidiosis surveillance – United States, 2011-2012. MMWR Suppl 2015;64(3):1–14.

63. Harvey K, Esposito DH, Han P, et al. Surveillance for travel-related disease–GeoSentinel Surveillance System, United States, 1997-2011. MMWR Surveill Summ 2013;62:1–23.

64. Nash TE, Herrington DA, Losonky GA, et al. Experimental human infections with Giardia lamblia. J Infect Dis 1987;156(6):974–84.

65. Donowitz JR, Alam M, Kabir M, et al. A prospective longitudinal cohort to investigate the effects of early life giardiasis on growth and all cause diarrhea. Clin Infect Dis 2016;63(6):792–7.

66. Bartelt LA, Roche J, Kolling G, et al. Persistent G. lamblia impairs growth in a murine malnutrition model. J Clin Invest 2013;123(6):2672–84.

67. Josko D. Updates in immunoassays: parasitology. Clin Lab Sci 2012;25(3): 185–90.

68. Gaafar MR. Evaluation of enzyme immunoassay techniques for diagnosis of the most common intestinal protozoa in fecal samples. Int J Infect Dis 2011;15(8): e541-4.

69. Mahbubani MH, Bej AK, Perlin M, et al. Detection of *Giardia* cysts by using the polymerase chain reaction and distinguishing live from dead cysts. Appl Environ Microbiol 1991;57(12):3456–61.

70. Singh B. Molecular methods for diagnosis and epidemiological studies of parasitic infections. Int J Parasitol 1997;27(10):1135–45.

71. Nash TE. Unraveling how *Giardia* infections cause disease. J Clin Invest 2013; 123(6):2346–7.

72. Hanevik K, Wensaas K-A, Rortveit G, et al. Irritable bowel syndrome and chronic fatigue 6 years after giardia infection: a controlled prospective cohort study. Clin Infect Dis 2014;59(10):1394–400.

Malaria in Children

Lauren M. Cohee, MD, Miriam K. Laufer, MD, MPH*

KEYWORDS

- Malaria • *Plasmodium* • *Falciparum* • *Vivax*

KEY POINTS

- Malaria is a significant cause of morbidity and mortality in endemic areas.
- Travelers to endemic areas are at risk of malaria.
- Identifying patients who may have malaria and providing prompt evaluation and treatment are critical to limit disease and its complications.
- Malaria has the potential to be fatal. In cases where the index of suspicion is high, treatment can be started before testing results are available, so that there is no delay in therapy. If presumptive treatment is initiated, diagnostic specimens should still be obtained.
- Updated guidelines are available through the US Centers for Disease Control and Prevention and should be consulted whenever a physician is treating patients with suspected or confirmed malaria.

INTRODUCTION

Malaria causes substantial morbidity and mortality in many of the most resource-limited areas of the world. In addition, malaria is a threat to travelers to endemic areas and should be considered in the evaluation of any traveler returning from a malaria-endemic region presenting with fever. Malaria infection can rapidly develop into severe disease that can be fatal. Prompt, effective treatment is critical to limiting these complications. Understanding the species-specific epidemiology and drug-resistance patterns in the geographic area where infection was acquired guides treatment. This review contains an overview of the epidemiology and pathogenesis of malaria with a focus on components relevant to treating malaria in nonendemic areas. Guidance for treatment and management of malaria in returned travelers is provided.

CAUSE AND PATHOGENESIS

Malaria is caused by infection with *Plasmodium* parasites. Five species cause disease in humans: *Plasmodium falciparum*, *Plasmodium vivax*, *Plasmodium malariae*,

Disclosures: Neither author has any commercial or financial conflicts of interest.
Division of Malaria Research, Institute for Global Health, University of Maryland School of Medicine, HSF-II, Room 480, 685 West Baltimore Street, Baltimore, MD 21201, USA
* Corresponding author.
E-mail address: mlaufer@som.umaryland.edu

Plasmodium ovale, and *Plasmodium knowlesi*. Infection is spread by the bite of a female *Anopheles* mosquito and has obligatory human and mosquito stages of the life cycle. The species of *Anopheles* mosquitoes responsible for *Plasmodium* transmission has a broad geographic distribution. Typically, *Anopheles* bite from dusk to dawn. However, exact biting patterns vary based on specific species.

The life cycle of the 5 *Plasmodium* species is similar, apart from the dormant stages of *P vivax* and *P ovale*:

- Sporozoites are inoculated into humans by an *Anopheles* mosquito and immediately invade hepatocytes.
- Asexual replication takes place initially in the liver, leading to the release of thousands of merozoites per infected hepatocyte into the blood. This release occurs 1 to 2 weeks after the bite of the infectious mosquito.
- Blood stage infection causes clinical disease.
- Merozoites invade erythrocytes, undergo asexual reproduction, and then rupture out of the erythrocyte, allowing the daughter merozoites to continue the cycle of invasion and replication.
- Some blood stage parasites develop into male and female gametocytes, the stage that is responsible for transmission to the mosquito.
- For the infection to be transmitted, a female *Anopheles* mosquito must ingest erythrocytes containing male and female gametocytes.
- Sexual reproduction takes place in the mosquito midgut where the gametocytes mature into gametes, merge to form a zygote, and then develop into an ookinete.
- Ookinetes invade the mosquito stomach wall and develop into oocysts, which rupture and release sporozoites.
- Sporozoites migrate to the mosquito salivary gland and may infect another human during the mosquito's next blood meal.
- Of note, in *P vivax* and *P ovale*, dormant stages, called hypnozoites, may remain quiescent in the liver of the infected human for weeks to years from the initial infection, leading to onset of clinical symptoms or relapses of infections much later. Treatment specifically targeting these dormant stages is required to completely clear infections with *P vivax* and *P ovale*.

Malarial disease results from multiple complex parasite-host interactions during the asexual, blood stage of infection. Clinical manifestations of disease are related to parasite modification of the erythrocyte and parasite-induced inflammation.

Plasmodium pathogenesis can be divided into inflammation, anemia, and end-organ damage. Inflammation is caused by the downstream effects of parasite metabolism and erythrocyte rupture, and, in *P falciparum*, parasite sequestration. Splenic macrophages and monocytes release large amounts of proinflammatory cytokines in response to phagocytosis of hemozoin, a toxic metabolite from the parasite digestion of heme, and other erythrocyte remnants. Proinflammatory cytokines in turn give rise to (1) the systemic inflammatory response syndrome, (2) edema and inflammation in perivascular tissues in end organs due to disruption of endothelial basal lamina and extravasation,[1] and (3) increased expression of adhesion molecules and increased sequestration of parasitized erythrocytes.

The anemia caused by *Plasmodium* infection is multifactorial. Asexual reproduction in infected erythrocytes leads directly to hemolysis. Moreover, intraerythrocytic parasites decrease erythrocyte deformability, leading to increased hemolysis and splenic clearance, compounded by splenic sequestration in *P falciparum* infection. Hematopoiesis, which would normally compensate for hemolysis, is suppressed by tumor necrosis factor-alpha released during infection.

End organ damage due to *P falciparum* infection is mediated by cytoadherence of infected erythrocytes, also referred to as sequestration. Intraerythrocytic parasites produce proteins that are expressed on the surface of infected erythrocytes and lead to binding to a variety of cell types. Binding of parasitized erythrocytes in the microvasculature along with uninfected erythrocytes, inflammatory cells, and platelets leads to partial blood flow obstruction, breakdown of the endothelium, and inflammation that causes end organ damage. Sequestered erythrocytes can be found in any organ. Sequestration in the brain leads to the clinical syndrome of cerebral malaria described in later discussion. Sequestration in the placenta leads to the adverse birth outcomes associated with malaria during pregnancy. Sequestration also removes parasites from the circulation, preventing splenic clearance during one phase of parasite replication and permitting on-going infection.

EPIDEMIOLOGY

Although rarely encountered in the United States, malaria causes approximately 45% of the world's population to be at risk of infection.[2] *P falciparum* and *P vivax* are the most common causes of human malaria and have distinct geographic distributions, as in **Fig. 1**. *P malariae* is found in a similar distribution as *P falciparum*; *P ovale* is primarily found in West Africa, but cases have been reported in other sub-Saharan African countries. The limited cases of *P knowlesi*, a primarily nonhuman primate parasite, are reported in Southeast Asia.

Worldwide over the last 15 years, there has been a 60% decrease in the malaria death rate due to increased availability of preventive measures, such as bed nets, and effective new diagnostics and treatments. Since 2007 when the World Health Organization (WHO) endorsed a global commitment to eradicate malaria, 5 countries have been declared malaria free (United Arab Emirates, Morocco, Turkmenistan, Armenia, and Sri Lanka), and 26 more are poised for elimination by 2020.[3] Despite this progress, in 2015, it is estimated that there were still 214 million new cases of malaria and 438,000 deaths. The vast majority of morbidity and mortality occur in sub-Saharan Africa, where the heaviest burden of disease is shouldered by children less than 5 years of age. Further progress is threatened by the spread of drug and insecticide resistance, the need for new tools for malaria control in areas that have not reduced transmission with current interventions, and the continued demand for a global financial commitment to the goal of eradication.

In the United States, there has been a consistent increase the number of cases of malaria reported to the US Centers for Disease Control and Prevention (CDC) since 1973. In 2013, 1727 cases were reported. All infections in which origin was determined (99.6%) were acquired abroad. Most occurred in US residents, and 17% occurred in children (age <18 years). Severe malaria, infection associated with end organ damage, was more common in children less than 5 year old compared with older children and adults. However, none of the 10 deaths caused by malaria in the United States were among children.[4]

SUSCEPTIBILITY TO INFECTION

In nonendemic and low transmission areas, all individuals are at risk of infection. In highly endemic settings, primarily some areas in sub-Saharan Africa, multiple malaria infections lead to the development of partial immunity. As children in these areas have repeated exposure to malaria infection, they become less likely to experience clinical disease. By adulthood, individuals in high transmission settings may still become infected, but the parasite load is lower and there is very low risk of clinical disease.

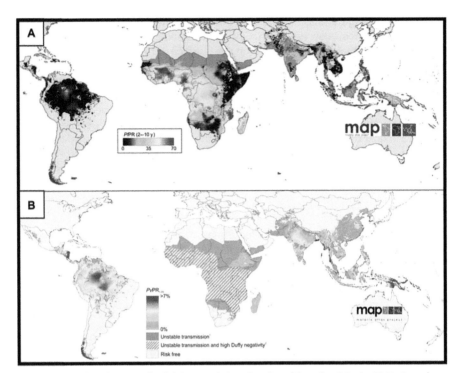

Fig. 1. Spatial distribution of *P falciparum* (*A*) and *P vivax* (*B*) endemicity in 2010. Prevalence rates are presented in different populations and different scales based on species. The *P falciparum* map (*A*) shows the prevalence rate in 2 to 10 year olds (PfPR) and ranges from 0% to 70%; see color scale on map. The *P vivax* map (*B*) shows the prevalence rate in 1 to 99 year olds (PvPR) and ranges from 0 to greater than 7%. Shaded areas have unstable transmission (<0.1%), and hatched areas have greater than 90% prevalence of Duffy antigen negativity. Duffy antigen is required for the invasion of *P vivax* into the erythrocyte and is absent in some African populations. These maps are open source and made available by the Malaria Atlas Project (http://www.map.ox.ac.uk/map/) under the Creative Commons Attribution 3.0 Unported License. (*Reproduced from* [*A*] Gething PW, Patil AP, Smith DL, et al. A new world malaria map: plasmodium falciparum endemicity in 2010. Malar J 2011;10:378; and [*B*] Gething PW, Elyazar IRF, Moyes CL, et al. A long neglected world malaria map: plasmodium vivax endemicity in 2010. PLoS Negl Trop Dis 2012;6(9):e1814.)

Sterilizing immunity, complete prevention of infection, does not occur. Moreover, the duration of acquired immunity is not life-long: if individuals from endemic areas are no longer exposed to infection for as little as a year, they are at risk of disease upon repeat exposure. Many cases of malaria in the United States occur when individuals from endemic countries return home to visit friends and relatives. These individuals may not realize that their immunity has decayed, making them again susceptible to high-density infection and disease.

Hemoglobinopathies alter susceptibility to malaria infection and disease. Sickle cell trait (HbAS) is estimated to afford 90% protection from severe disease, 75% protection from hospitalization with malaria, but no protection from asymptomatic infection.[5,6] This protection contributes to the persistence of HbS in African populations given the decreased life expectancy of homozygotes. Protection is also seen with hemoglobin C and alpha-thalassemia and beta-thalassemia. However, it is important to recognize that individuals with any of these hemoglobinopathies can still get malaria and have severe manifestations.

HISTORY AND PHYSICAL

During medical evaluation of patients with fever, taking a travel history and considering malaria are critical. Malaria should be suspected in any case of documented or history of fever and residence in or travel to malaria-endemic areas. Key malaria-related questions to ask on history include the following:

- *Has the patient traveled to a malaria-endemic area? Which species are present in that region?* The geographic region determines the possibility of malaria infection and the most likely species, risk of severe disease, and treatment choice based on geographic patterns of antimalarial drug resistance. See the CDC Travelers' Health Web site (http://wwwnc.cdc.gov/travel) for details on malaria epidemiology by country.
- *When did exposure occur?* The time from the bite of an infected mosquito until presentation with clinical illness of *P faliciparum* is typically 10 to 14 days but may be as short as 7 days and as long as 30 days. Presentation with clinical illness may be delayed in those with partial immunity or who were taking incomplete or ineffective prophylaxis. *P malariae* may persist at low levels for long periods of time, up to years. Because of their dormant stages, *P vivax* and *P ovale* may present months to years after initial infections. Three to 6 weeks after the initial infectious bite is the most common period for relapse of *P vivax* infection obtained in tropical areas, and most relapses have occurred by 6 months. Relapse may occur 6 to 12 months after *P vivax* infection obtained in subtropical or temperate climates.[7]
- *Has the patient used antimalarials in the last 1 to 2 months?* Drugs recently used for treatment or prophylaxis should not be used for treatment of clinical illness. Among individuals living in or emigrating from endemic areas, it is important to know if they were treated for malaria in the last 1 to 2 months, what drug was used, and if treatment was completed. Among travelers, it is important to know if they were taking malaria prophylaxis, what drug was used, and what their adherence was. Note that taking prophylaxis, even as recommended, does not definitively exclude malaria diagnosis.

Other groups in which *Plasmodium* infection should be considered in health care include asymptomatic immigrants (refugees, international adoptees, and others) from endemic areas. See the section on "Screening and Treatment of immigrants from malaria endemic areas" in later discussion.

The physical examination and initial laboratory evaluation should be used to determine the likelihood of malaria, evaluate other conditions on the differential, and determine the disease severity if malaria is likely (see **Box 2** and the section, "Assessing severity"). General physical examination should be performed with specific attention to the following organ systems:

- Ophthalmologic: Check for conjunctival pallor indicative of anemia. If seizures, altered consciousness, or other concern for cerebral malaria, consider dilated funduscopic examination by an ophthalmologist to evaluate for retinal hemorrhages, areas of retinal opacification, papilledema, cotton wool spots, or decolorization of retinal vessels.[8]
- Pulmonary: Note tachypnea, which may be related to pulmonary complications (manifested by crepitation) or to metabolic acidosis (manifested by the characteristic acidotic breathing pattern).

- Cardiac: Note tachycardia, which could be related to fever, increased cardiac output demand due to anemia, or shock. Assess capillary refill and extremity temperature variation.
- Gastrointestinal: Palpate for splenomegaly.
- Neurologic: Calculate Glasgow Coma Score if altered mental status and monitor for deterioration. Monitor for seizures. Assess for nuchal rigidity and photophobia, which would suggest meningitis rather than cerebral malaria.

DIFFERENTIAL DIAGNOSIS

Because the symptoms of malaria are nonspecific, the differential diagnosis is broad. Specific alternative diagnoses are listed in **Box 1**.

DIAGNOSIS

Malaria has the potential to be fatal. In cases where the index of suspicion is high, treatment can be started before testing results are available or even before they are performed, so that there is no delay in therapy. If presumptive treatment is initiated, diagnostic specimens should still be obtained.

Blood smear and detection by microscopy are considered the gold standard for laboratory confirmation of malaria. Thick and thin smears should be read. The CDC provides details on preparation and interpretation.[9] Briefly, smears are stained with either Wright's or ideally Giemsa stain. The thick smear is the most sensitive measure to detect low-density infection because it allows the microscopist to review a large volume of blood and is read for detection of infection. The thin smear, which allows greater resolution of the red blood cell morphology and the parasite, is used for determining the *Plasmodium* species and quantifying the specific parasite density. The later features are important for treatment and monitoring decisions. If the initial blood smears are negative but *Plasmodium* infection remains on the differential, 2 additional smears should be obtained at 12- to 24-hour intervals. Blood smears and trends in

---

Box 1
Differential diagnoses of malaria

Sepsis due to bacteremia

Encephalitis (rickettsial or viral)

Meningitis (bacterial or viral)

Pneumonia (bacterial, viral or fungal)

Typhoid fever

Dengue fever

Chikungunya

Leptospirosis

Brucellosis

Rickettsial infections

Acute schistosomiasis (Katayama fever)

Amebic liver abscess

Acute HIV

parasite quantification are also useful in following response to treatment (see later discussion).

Antigen-detecting rapid diagnostics tests (RDTs) are increasingly available for diagnosis of malaria in both resource-limited and nonendemic settings. The tests are generally cassette- or card-based lateral flow immunochromatographic assays that appear much like a pregnancy test. Labeled antibodies detect 1 of 3 *Plasmodium* antigens that may or may not be species specific depending on the test. Up-to-date information on the tests available, their mechanisms, and performance characteristics can be found on the WHO Foundation for Innovative New Diagnostics Web site.[10]

Only one RDT is approved for use in commercial and hospital laboratories in the United States. The BinaxNOW test (Alere Inc, Waltham, MA, USA) detects one antigen that is specific for *P falciparum* and another that is found in all human *Plasmodium* species. The sensitivity of detecting *P falciparum* and non-*P falciparum* infection in US or Canadian hospitals has ranged from 72% to 100% depending on the study.[11–14] This RDT is specifically less sensitive for the detection of *P malariae* and low-density infections (<200 parasites per microliter). Sensitivity for detection of *P knowlesi* is low (29%).[15] The current recommendations are that RDTs should be used in conjunction with blood smears. RDTs may significantly reduce the time required for preliminary diagnosis and, thus, are useful tools for initial diagnosis.[14] Positive RDTs should be considered significant support of *Plasmodium* infection, but blood smears are required for confirmation, definitive species identification, and quantification. Negative RDTs should not eliminate consideration of malaria, especially if there has been recent treatment or infection is due to low-density or non-*falciparum* infections. Blood smears should be performed to exclude the diagnosis.

All cases of laboratory confirmed malaria should be reported to the state health department and to the CDC (www.cdc.gov/malaria/report.html).

ASSESSMENT OF SEVERITY

Clinical disease is classified as uncomplicated or severe malaria. Uncomplicated malaria is the presence of symptoms and/or signs of malaria and a positive parasitologic test in the absence of evidence of end organ damage. Fever, the quintessential symptom of malaria, is often greater than 40°C and associated with severe rigors and chills and profuse diaphoresis as fever resolves. Although rarely observed, fever is classically periodic with the interval between fevers determined by *Plasmodium* species causing the infection. Fever as well as other common initial symptoms, including malaise, fatigue, headache, cough, abdominal pain, anorexia, nausea, vomiting, diarrhea, myalgias, and back pain, is nonspecific, requiring a high index of suspicion of malaria in anyone with possible exposure. Signs that may be associated with uncomplicated malaria include mild jaundice due to hemolysis and splenic enlargement. Laboratory abnormalities may include mild anemia, thrombocytopenia, mild coagulopathy, increased blood urea nitrogen, and elevated creatinine not meeting criteria for acute kidney injury. Uncomplicated malaria may be caused by any of the *Plasmodium* species infecting humans.

Severe malaria is most often caused by cytoadherence of *P falciparum*–infected erythrocytes in capillary beds of a wide range of organs. The presence of one or more of the features listed in **Box 2** and a positive malaria diagnostic test in the absence of an alternative cause are defined as severe malaria. These manifestations may occur alone or in combination. Specific clinical syndromes that can occur in endemic settings as well as in nonimmune travelers include but are not limited to severe anemia and cerebral malaria. Severe anemia can lead to metabolic acidosis, renal

---

Box 2
Manifestations of severe malaria adapted from World Health Organization and US Centers for Disease Control and Prevention

- *Impaired consciousness*

- *Prostration:* Generalized weakness leading to inability to sit, stand, or walk without assistance

- *Multiple convulsions:* More than 2 episodes within 24 hours

- *Acidosis:* A base deficit of greater than 8 mEq/L or, if not available, a plasma bicarbonate level of less than 15 mmol/L or venous plasma lactate ≥5 mmol/L

- *Hypoglycemia:* Blood or plasma glucose less than 2.2 mmol/L (<40 mg/dL)

- *Severe anemia:* Hemoglobin concentration ≤5 g/dL or a hematocrit of ≤15% in children less than 12 years of age; less than 7 g/dL, and less than 20%, respectively, in those ≥12 year old

- *Renal impairment:* Evidence of acute kidney injury, decreased urine output, decreased glomerular filtration rate, increased creatinine

- *Jaundice:* Plasma or serum bilirubin greater than 50 µmol/L (3 mg/dL) with a parasite count greater than 100,000/µL

- *Pulmonary edema:* Radiologically confirmed or oxygen saturation less than 92% on room air with a respiratory rate greater than 30/min, often with chest indrawing and crepitations on auscultation

- *Significant bleeding:* Including recurrent or prolonged bleeding from the nose, gums, or venipuncture sites; hematemesis or melena

- *Shock:* Compensated shock defined as capillary refill ≥3 s or temperature gradient on leg (mid to proximal limb), but no hypotension. Decompensated shock defined as systolic blood pressure less than 70 mm Hg with evidence of impaired perfusion (cool peripheries or prolonged capillary refill)

- *Hyperparasitaemia: P falciparum* or *P knowlesi* parasitemia greater than 10% (CDC uses >5% as a cutoff)

Data from US Centers for Disease Control and Prevention. Malaria diagnosis & treatment in the United States. Available at: https://www.cdc.gov/malaria/diagnosis_treatment/index.html. Accessed November 26, 2016; and World Health Organization. Guidelines for the treatment of malaria. 3rd edition. Available at: http://www.who.int/malaria/publications/atoz/9789241549127/en/. Accessed November 26, 2016.

---

impairment, and noncardiogenic pulmonary edema. Cerebral malaria can present with seizures and/or decreased consciousness, including coma, and can lead to cerebral edema, increased intracranial pressure, herniation, and death.

Laboratory tests and potential findings to use in valuation of potential complications include the following:

- Complete blood count: anemia, thrombocytopenia, leukopenia, or leukocytosis
- Chemistry panel: acidosis, acute kidney injury, and hypoglycemia
- Urinalysis: hemoglobinuria and proteinuria
- Lumbar puncture (if altered consciousness or other indication): findings may be normal or have elevated opening pressure, mildly elevated protein, or mild pleocytosis
- Blood cultures: concomitant bacteremia
- Blood gas: metabolic acidosis with or without respiratory compensation
- Type and cross-match

TREATMENT AND MANAGEMENT
Uncomplicated Malaria

In cases of malaria infection without signs of severe disease, oral treatment should be initiated as promptly as possible (**Table 1**). Hospitalization should be considered for individuals from nonendemic regions, young children, and those with high parasite density (>4%). Choice of antimalarial drug is determined by the species of *Plasmodium* causing the infection, the drug resistance patterns in the region where infection was likely acquired, and whether the patient has taken any other antimalaria drugs in the last 1 to 2 months for treatment or prevention. If the *Plasmodium* species causing the infection is not certain, then the infection should be treated as though it were *P falciparum*. In all areas, drugs that were recently used in the last 1 to 2 months for treatment or prophylaxis should not be used for treatment. Specific dosing recommendations and new updates can be found on the CDC Web site,[16] (also listed in Key Resources).

If *P vivax* or *P ovale* is identified or suspected, primaquine should be administered to prevent relapse due to dormant liver stages. However, primaquine can cause hemolytic anemia and is contraindicated in G6PD-deficient persons. G6PD screening should be done before primaquine treatment. Alternate regimens many be considered in consultation with an infectious disease or tropical medicine expert for persons with borderline or true G6PD-deficiency.

During treatment, parasite density should be monitored daily until negative.[17]

Severe Malaria

When signs or symptoms of severe diseases are present, parenteral treatment should be initiated promptly because death can occur within hours of presentation. Artesunate or quinine/quinidine should be used for treatment. Given the level of monitoring and the frequency of clinical and laboratory assessment required to manage patients with severe malaria, admission to an intensive care unit is recommended. Initial evaluation is described above. Parasite quantification every 12 hours is recommended for the first 2 to 3 days to document response to treatment and to a decrease in parasite quantification. If there is not significant decrease in parasite density by 48 to 72 hours, consider expert consultation.

Supportive care measures, such as fluid resuscitation, cardiac and respiratory monitoring, oxygen, and supportive ventilation, should be provided as clinically indicated. In addition to antimalarial treatment, management of complications may require anticonvulsants, antibiotics, antipyretics, and blood transfusions. Exchange transfusions are no longer recommended.[18,19] Clinical assessments should be repeated every 2 to 4 hours. If there is a decline in mental status after initiation of treatment, clinicians should consider new onset of seizures, hypoglycemia, or worsening anemia. Hypoglycemia is a common complication and may mimic cerebral malaria. Laboratory evaluation, including hemoglobin/hematocrit, glucose, and lactate, should be repeated every 6 hours, and supportive care should be administered based on these results.

Quinidine and artesunate are available in the United States for treatment of severe malaria. Treatment should be initiated with intravenous quinidine if it is available. Quinidine can cause arrhythmias, so intravenous administration of the drug requires close cardiac monitoring.[20] Hypotension is common and should be treated with volume expansion. Baseline electrocardiogram should be performed, and changes in the width of the QRS and length of the QTc should be monitored hourly. The infusion should be held if the QTc prolongs by more than 50% of the baseline length, but

Table 1
General malaria pediatric treatment recommendations and additional information

Syndrome and Species	Drug Resistance in the Region Acquired	Drug Recommendations () = See Notes	Notes
Uncomplicated malaria, P falciparum or species unknown	Chloroquine resistant or resistance unknown	A. Atovoquone-proguanil B. Artemether-lumefantrine C. Quinine sulfate plus doxycycline, tetracycline, or (clindamycin) D. Mefloquine	• All areas should be considered chloroquine-resistant unless specifically noted as chloroquine-sensitive below. See CDC Yellow Book for country-specific details • A, B, C equally recommended; due to increased risk of neuropsychiatric complications, D is only recommended if A, B, C are not possible • D. Also not recommended in infections acquired in SE Asia due to resistance • In C, clindamycin is recommended when doxycycline and tetracycline are contraindicated, eg, children <8 y old and pregnant women
	Chloroquine sensitive	Chloroquine phosphate or hydroxychloroquine	• Chloroquine-sensitive areas are Central America west of the Panama canal, Haiti, Dominican Republic, and most of the Middle East • Regimens for chloroquine-resistant infections may be used as available, more convenient, or preferred
Uncomplicated malaria, P malariae or P knowlesi	All regions	Chloroquine phosphate or hydroxychloroquine	

Uncomplicated malaria, P ovale and P vivax (chloroquine sensitive)	All regions (except where P vivax chloroquine resistance is common, see below)	Chloroquine phosphate plus primaquine or hydroxychloroquine plus primaquine	• See text on use of primaquine • Low rates of chloroquine-resistant P vivax have been found in Myanmar, India, Central and South America; chloroquine should be initiated but monitored closely, if no response change to chloroquine-resistant regimen, and report to CDC
Uncomplicated malaria, P vivax (chloroquine resistant)	Chloroquine resistant	A. Quinine sulfate plus either doxycycline or tetracycline plus primaquine B. Atovoquone-proguanil plus primaquine C. Mefolquine plus primaquine	• Chloroquine-resistant P vivax is well documented in Papua New Guinea and Indonesia
Severe malaria	All regions	Quinidine gluconate plus doxycycline, tetracycline, or clindamycin Investigational new drug (contact CDC): artesunate followed by atovaquone-proguanil, doxycycline, or mefloquine	• Monitor for hypotension, hypoglycemia, and cardiac complications (widening of QRS or lengthening of the QTc interval); see text • Monitor parasite density every 12 h during the first 48–72 h; should decrease 90% in first 48 h • Once parasitemia <1%, may transition to oral regimen: quinine plus oral partner drug OR complete oral course of atovaquone-proguanil or artemether-lumefantrine • Total course for quinidine/quinine based on area of infection origin: 7 d for southeast Asia, 3 d for Africa or South America

Adapted from CDC. Guidelines for the treatment of malaria in the US Centers for Disease Control and Prevention. Malaria diagnosis & treatment in the United States. Available at: https://www.cdc.gov/malaria/diagnosis_treatment/index.html. Accessed November 26, 2016.

may be restarted when the QTc is no more than 25% longer than its original length. Additional side effects and toxicities include hypoglycemia, tinnitus, reversible hearing loss, dizziness, vision changes, nausea, and vomiting.

Artesunate is available as an investigational new drug through the CDC. Criteria for access to artesunate are confirmed cases of malaria requiring parenteral therapy because of severe malaria, parasitemia greater than 5%, or inability to tolerate oral therapy. In addition, one of the following must be true: artesunate is more readily available than quinidine; quinidine is contraindicated; or there was intolerance to or failure of quinidine.[21] A retrospective case series of participants in this experimental protocol showed that artesunate is safe and clinically beneficial.[22] Clinical trials in endemic settings and a systematic review show significantly lower rates of mortality using artesunate compared with quinine.[23–25] The CDC Malaria Hotline (contact information in "When to Refer" section) should be called for access to and use of artesunate.

After parenteral therapy for at least 24 hours, parasite density is less than 1%, and the patient can tolerate oral medications, treatment may be transitioned to an oral regimen (see **Table 1**). Complete courses of atovaquone-proguanil or lumefantrine-artemether may be used and may be preferred given they are better tolerated than oral quinine.

WHEN TO REFER

All suspected malaria cases should be seen in consultation with an infectious disease expert. Cases with any manifestations of severe disease may require management in an intensive care setting. The CDC staffs a malaria hotline and can provide additional consultation (Monday-Friday 9 AM to 5 PM EST, call either (770) 488-7788 or (855) 856-4713; after hours, weekends, and holidays call (770) 488-7100 and ask for the malaria clinician on call).

SCREENING AND TREATMENT OF IMMIGRANTS FROM MALARIA-ENDEMIC AREAS

In medical evaluations of asymptomatic immigrants (refugees, international adoptees, and others) from endemic areas, any history of malaria infection and treatment should be noted and signs of chronic infection evaluated, such as anemia and splenomegaly. If these signs of chronic infection are detected, then malaria diagnostic tests should be performed and any detected infections should be treated with oral medication, as described above.

In the absence of evidence of acute or chronic infection, the CDC provides guidelines for the treatment of these populations, which are summarized here.[26] More details may be found on the Web site listed in **Box 3**.

Box 3
Key guidelines and sources for malaria diagnosis and treatment

World Health Organization
  Diagnosis and treatment guidelines: http://www.who.int/malaria/areas/treatment/en/

US Centers for Disease Control and Prevention
  General information: https://www.cdc.gov/malaria/
  Diagnosis and treatment guidelines: https://www.cdc.gov/malaria/diagnosis_treatment/index.html
  Prophylaxis: http://wwwnc.cdc.gov/travel/yellowbook/2016/table-of-contents
  Immigrant and refugee health: http://www.cdc.gov/immigrantrefugeehealth/guidelines/domestic/malaria-guidelines-domestic.html

---

Refugees from malaria-endemic areas in sub-Saharan Africa without evidence of acute or chronic infection: Refugees should have received presumptive malaria treatment before departure for the United States. If documentation of predeparture treatment is not available, then postarrival presumptive treatment should be considered. Children weighing less than 5 kg and pregnant women may have been screened for

Table 2
Drugs for malaria prophylaxis currently available in the United States

	Pros	Cons	Regimen
Atovaquone-proguanil	• Minimal side effects • Good for short trips given short posttravel duration of treatment	• Contraindicated in pregnancy, children <5 kg, severe renal impairment • Increases effect of warfarin • More expensive than other options	Pretravel: 1–2 d During travel: Daily Posttravel: 7 d
Doxycycline	• Inexpensive • Readily available • May prevent other infections as well, eg, rickettsial infections and leptospirosis	• Photosensitivity • Risk of *Candida* vaginitis • Esophagitis and gastrointestinal side effects: Take with meal or sufficient fluids, do not take just before bed • Contraindicated in pregnancy and children <8 y old	Pretravel: 1–2 d During travel: Daily Posttravel: 4 wk
Mefloquine	• Recommended choice for pregnant women traveling to areas with chloroquine resistance	• Rare but serious neuropsychiatric side effects • Contraindicated in people with some psychiatric conditions, seizure disorders, and cardiac conduction abnormalities	Pretravel: ≥2 wk During travel: Weekly Posttravel: 4 wk
Chloroquine	• Minimal side effects • Safe in pregnancy	• Limited geographic range (Central America west of the Panama canal, Haiti, Dominican Republic, and most of the Middle East)	Pretravel: 1–2 wk During travel: Weekly Posttravel: 4 wk
Primaquine	• Most effective choice for short trips to areas where >90% of infection is caused by *P vivax*	• G6PD testing required • Contraindicated in people with G6PD-deficiency and pregnancy	Primary prophylaxis Pretravel: 1–2 d During travel: Daily Posttravel: 7 d Terminal prophylaxis following use of other regimen for primary prevention Posttravel: 14 d

infection and only treated if positive. Presumptive treatment or screening and treatment are not recommended for refugees from other areas.

International adoptees without evidence of acute or chronic infection: In contrast to refugees, guidelines for international adoptees do not recommend presumptive treatment or screening. However, a recent study of asymptomatic *Plasmodium* infection in international adoptees from Ethiopia found 14% had infection, leading the investigators to suggest that screening with polymerase chain reaction be recommended.[27]

PROPHYLAXIS

Prophylaxis against malaria is recommended for all travelers to malaria-endemic areas. Specific recommendations are updated every 2 years and can be found in the CDC Yellow Book (see link in **Box 3**). The 5 drugs currently available in the United States for malaria prophylaxis are listed in **Table 2**. Choice of drug is determined primarily by the species distribution and drug-resistance patterns in the destination and patient characteristics.

SUMMARY

- Globally, there has been a significant decrease in *Plasmodium* infection and reduction of malaria-related morbidity and mortality in the last 15 years.
- The number of cases of malaria imported to the United States continues to increase likely due to increased global travel.
- Prompt provision of effective treatment is critical to limiting the complications of malaria.
- Understanding *Plasmodium* species variation and the epidemiology and drug resistance patterns in the geographic area where infection was acquired is important for determining the most appropriate treatment regimens.
- Easy-to-use and up-to-date guidelines for the treatment and management of malaria in endemic areas and in the United States are accessible online from key reference organizations.

REFERENCES

1. Prato M, Giribaldi G, Polimeni M, et al. Phagocytosis of hemozoin enhances matrix metalloproteinase-9 activity and TNF-alpha production in human monocytes: role of matrix metalloproteinases in the pathogenesis of falciparum malaria. J Immunol 2005;175(10):6436–42.
2. World Health Organization. World malaria report 2015. 2016. Available at: http://www.who.int/malaria/publications/world-malaria-report-2015/report/en/. Accessed November 25, 2016.
3. Newby G, Bennett A, Larson E, et al. The path to eradication: a progress report on the malaria-eliminating countries. Lancet 2016;387(10029):1775–84.
4. Cullen KA, Mace KE, Arguin PM. Malaria surveillance—United States, 2013. MMWR Surveill Summ 2016;65(2):1–22.
5. Hill AV, Allsopp CE, Kwiatkowski D, et al. Common west African HLA antigens are associated with protection from severe malaria. Nature 1991;352(6336):595–600.
6. Williams TN, Mwangi TW, Wambua S, et al. Sickle cell trait and the risk of Plasmodium falciparum malaria and other childhood diseases. J Infect Dis 2005;192(1):178–86.
7. White NJ. Determinants of relapse periodicity in Plasmodium vivax malaria. Malar J 2011;10:297.

8. Lewallen S, Bronzan RN, Beare NA, et al. Using malarial retinopathy to improve the classification of children with cerebral malaria. Trans R Soc Trop Med Hyg 2008;102(11):1089–94.

9. U.S. Centers for Disease Control and Prevention. DPDx - malaria - diagnostic findings. Available at: http://www.cdc.gov/dpdx/malaria/dx.html. Accessed November 25, 2016.

10. World Health Organization. WHO-FIND malaria RDT evaluation programme. Available at: http://www.who.int/malaria/areas/diagnosis/rapid-diagnostic-tests/rdt-evaluation-programme/en/. Accessed November 25, 2016.

11. Farcas GA, Zhong KJY, Lovegrove FE, et al. Evaluation of the Binax NOW ICT test versus polymerase chain reaction and microscopy for the detection of malaria in returned travelers. Am J Trop Med Hyg 2003;69(6):589–92.

12. DiMaio MA, Pereira IT, George TI, et al. Performance of BinaxNOW for diagnosis of malaria in a U.S. hospital. J Clin Microbiol 2012;50(9):2877–80.

13. Bobenchik A, Shimizu-Cohen R, Humphries RM. Use of rapid diagnostic tests for diagnosis of malaria in the United States. J Clin Microbiol 2013;51(1):379.

14. Ota-Sullivan K, Blecker-Shelly DL. Use of the rapid BinaxNOW malaria test in a 24-hour laboratory associated with accurate detection and decreased malaria testing turnaround times in a pediatric setting where malaria is not endemic. J Clin Microbiol 2013;51(5):1567–9.

15. Foster D, Cox-Singh J, Mohamad DSA, et al. Evaluation of three rapid diagnostic tests for the detection of human infections with Plasmodium knowlesi. Malar J 2014;13:60.

16. U.S. Centers for Disease Control and Prevention. Malaria diagnosis & treatment in the United States. Available at: https://www.cdc.gov/malaria/diagnosis_treatment/index.html. Accessed November 26, 2016.

17. Griffith KS, Lewis LS, Mali S, et al. Treatment of malaria in the United States. JAMA 2007;297(20):2264.

18. U.S. Centers for Disease Control and Prevention. Malaria - exchange transfusion for treatment of severe malaria no longer recommended. Available at: http://www.cdc.gov/malaria/new_info/2013/exchange_transfusion.html. Accessed November 29, 2016.

19. Tan KR, Wiegand RE, Arguin PM. Exchange transfusion for severe malaria: evidence base and literature review. Clin Infect Dis 2013;57(7):923–8.

20. White NJ. Cardiotoxicity of antimalarial drugs. Lancet Infect Dis 2007;7(8):549–58.

21. U.S. Centers for Disease Control and Prevention. New medication for severe malaria available under an investigational new drug protocol. Available at: http://www.cdc.gov/mmWR/preview/mmwrhtml/mm5630a5.htm. Accessed November 26, 2016.

22. Twomey PS, Smith BL, McDermott C, et al. Intravenous artesunate for the treatment of severe and complicated malaria in the United States: clinical use under an investigational new drug protocol. Ann Intern Med 2015;163(7):498.

23. Dondorp AM, Fanello CI, Hendriksen ICE, et al. Artesunate versus quinine in the treatment of severe falciparum malaria in African children (AQUAMAT): an open-label, randomised trial. Lancet 2010;376(9753):1647–57.

24. Dondorp A, Nosten F, Stepniewska K, et al. South East Asian QUININE Artesunate Malaria Trial (SEAQUAMAT) group. Artesunate versus quinine for treatment of severe falciparum malaria: a randomised trial. Lancet 2005;366(9487):717–25.

25. Sinclair D, Donegan S, Isba R, et al. Artesunate versus quinine for treating severe malaria. Cochrane Database Syst Rev 2012;6:CD005967.

26. U.S. Centers for Disease Control and Prevention. Domestic malaria guidelines immigrant and refugee health. Available at: http://www.cdc.gov/immigrantrefugeehealth/guidelines/domestic/malaria-guidelines-domestic.html. Accessed November 25, 2016.

27. Adebo SM, Eckerle JK, Andrews ME, et al. Asymptomatic malaria and other infections in children adopted from Ethiopia, United States, 2006–2011. Emerg Infect Dis 2015;21(7):1227–9.

The Global State of Helminth Control and Elimination in Children

Jill E. Weatherhead, MD[a,b,*], Peter J. Hotez, MD, PhD[a,b,c,d], Rojelio Mejia, MD[a,b,*]

KEYWORDS

- Soil-transmitted helminths • Schistosomiasis • Mass drug administration
- Anthelmintics • Vaccine

KEY POINTS

- Soil-transmitted helminths and schistosomiasis are some of the most common infections found in children and adolescents worldwide and cause significant morbidity and chronic disability.
- Current strategies to reduce morbidity associated with soil-transmitted helminths and schistosomiasis include mass drug administration (MDA) and programs of water, sanitation, and hygiene (WASH).
- Although MDA and WASH are reducing the overall prevalence of helminth infections, global elimination remains elusive because of low drug efficacies and reinfection.
- Alternative strategies, including improved diagnostics, improved worm prevalence and resistance monitoring, new anthelmintics diagnostics, therapies, and vaccines, are required.

Disclosure Statement: Authors deny conflict of interest or any relationship with a commercial company that has a direct financial interest in subject matter or materials discussed in article or with a company making a competing product.

[a] Department of Pediatrics, Section of Tropical Medicine, Baylor College of Medicine, Feigin Research Building, 1102 Bates Avenue, Suite 550, Houston, TX 77030, USA; [b] National School of Tropical Medicine, Baylor College of Medicine, One Baylor Plaza, MS: BCM-113, Houston, TX 77030, USA; [c] Department of Molecular Virology and Microbiology, Baylor College of Medicine, One Baylor Plaza, MS: BCM-385, Houston, TX 77030, USA; [d] Sabin Vaccine Institute and Texas Children's Hospital (TCH), Center for Vaccine Development, Feigin Research Building, 1102 Bates Avenue, Suite 550, Houston, TX 77030, USA

* Corresponding author. Department of Pediatrics, Section of Tropical Medicine, Baylor College of Medicine, Feigin Research Building, 1102 Bates Avenue, Suite 550, Houston, TX 77030.
E-mail addresses: weatherh@bcm.edu; rmejia@bcm.edu

Pediatr Clin N Am 64 (2017) 867–877
http://dx.doi.org/10.1016/j.pcl.2017.03.005
0031-3955/17/© 2017 Elsevier Inc. All rights reserved.

pediatric.theclinics.com

INTRODUCTION

Helminth infections, including hookworm (*Necator americanus, Ancylostoma duedenale*), roundworm (*Ascaris lumbricoides*), and whipworm (*Trichuris trichiura*), collectively known as intestinal (or soil) transmitted helminths, as well as schistosomiasis, are among the most common infections found in children worldwide, infecting almost 2 billion people (**Table 1**).[1,2] Although intestinal helminth infections and schistosomiasis are not the only major parasites affecting children, their overwhelming numbers in terms of pediatric cases globally requires special attention. New estimates from the Global Burden of Disease Study 2015 indicate that together these helminth infections resulted in more than 6 million disability-adjusted life-years (DALYs), a number roughly equivalent to the DALYs caused by measles, *Haemophilus influenzae* type B meningitis, or other better-known pediatric conditions.[2] However, even these DALY estimates may represent "low-ball" figures based on revised estimates of more than 4 million DALYs from hookworm alone.[3] Thus, although intestinal helminth infections are not leading causes of death,[4] they are profoundly important causes of childhood disability and even future economic disrupters, with calculated adverse effects on future wage earning. Overwhelmingly, these worms affect children living in extreme poverty, particularly those living in rural communities or urban communities that lack adequate water, sanitation, and hygiene (WASH).[5] Contrary to previous assumptions, helminths and other neglected tropical diseases are not restricted exclusively to resource-limited countries. For some worm infections, there is a significant burden of disease found in poor communities living in countries with robust economies, including areas of the United States.[6]

The most common and most profound disabilities resulting from each of the major intestinal helminth infections and schistosomiasis are shown in **Table 2**. Children acquire their primary infection as they begin interacting with the environment during their preschool years and reach maximum worm burden for roundworm and whipworm (transmission via oral ingestion of embryonated eggs) by school age, whereas for hookworm and schistosomiasis (transmission via direct percutaneous invasion of larvae) in adolescence or young adulthood.[8,9] Overall, children infected with intestinal helminths and/or schistosomiasis often suffer from restrictions in cognitive development, impairment in memory, and reduced education attendance and performance.[5,9,10] These deficits lead to impaired school achievement.[9,11] Preschool- and school-aged children are at

Table 1
Prevalence and impact of major helminth infections, soil-transmitted helminths, and schistosomiasis, globally

	Major Human Species	Estimated Prevalence (Cases)	DALYs (Millions)	Deaths	References
Roundworm (Ascariasis)	*Ascaris lumbricoides*	761.9 million	1.075	2700	2,4,7
Whipworm (Trichuriasis)	*T trichiura*	463.7 million	0.653	None specified	2,4,7
Hookworm	*N americanus* and *Ancylostoma* sp	428.2 million	1.758	None specified	2,4,7
Blood Fluke (Schistosomiasis)	*S haematobium, S mansoni*	252.3 million	2.613	4400	2,4,7
Total		>1.9 billion	6.096	7100	—

Table 2
Transmission, symptoms, and treatment strategies for soil transmitted helminths in children

	Mode of Transmission	Major Symptoms	Treatment	References
Hookworm	Direct percutaneous invasion of larvae in contaminated soil	Growth stunting, cognitive restriction, iron deficiency anemia, and protein losses	Albendazole 400 mg once or mebendazole 100 mg bid × 3 d	8,9,20
Roundworm	Oral ingestion of eggs in contaminated soil	Growth stunting, cognitive restriction, vitamin A malabsorption, intestinal obstruction, asthma	Albendazole 400 mg once or mebendazole 100 mg bid × 3 d	8,9,20
Whipworm	Oral ingestion of eggs in contaminated soil	Growth stunting, cognitive restriction, trichuris colitis, trichuris dysentery syndrome	Albendazole 400 mg po for 3–7 d or mebendazole 100 mg bid for 3–7 d	8,9,20
Schistosomiasis	Direct percutaneous invasion of larvae in fresh water	Growth stunting, cognitive restriction, bladder cancer, liver fibrosis, hematuria, renal failure, female genital schistosomiasis	Praziquantel 20 mg/kg twice a day for 1 d	8,9,20

particular risk of poor long-term outcomes because they harbor the greatest burden of worms.[5] Children infected with roundworm are at increased risk of abdominal pain, abdominal distention, vitamin A deficiency, wheezing, and asthma, whereas children with whipworm may have colitis and other forms of inflammatory bowel disease (IBD) or Trichuris dysentery syndrome.[9] These findings go against the commonly held, but erroneous, belief that somehow worms protect children from asthma or IBD.[12] Children with hookworm experience iron-deficiency and iron-deficiency anemia, in addition to intestinal protein losses.[3] Young adults are also at risk of significant morbidity secondary to helminths. In resource-poor areas, women of reproductive age or those that are pregnant are at high risk of hookworm-induced iron-deficiency anemia.[5,13] In Africa and elsewhere, hookworm-induced anemia is also exacerbated by malaria coinfections.[14] Similarly, schistosomiasis is a major cause of chronic pediatric inflammation and anemia.[15] In addition, schistosomiasis caused by *Schistosoma haematobium* causes lesions in the female genital tract that result in a 2.9-to 4-fold increase in HIV transmission and increased risk of progress to AIDS.[13] Schistosomiasis has also been linked to female infertility and the development of noncommunicable diseases such as cancer.[16–18] Because these infections commonly have subclinical symptoms in children and young adults, the evidence of morbidity may not become apparent until adulthood, leading to limitations in adult workforce capability and wage potential, creating a cycle of poverty within the community.[1] Beyond poverty, pediatric helminth infections can exhibit a devastating social impact within communities.[19]

Previously, in the United States and other wealthy nations, helminth infections were thought to be isolated to immigrant communities, refugees, and adoptees from endemic regions. In refugees settling in North America, the prevalence of soil-transmitted helminths and schistosomiasis has been documented as high as 86%.[21] However, with the expansion of global networking and international travel and a high prevalence of worms in children living in poverty within wealthy countries, the pediatric clinician practicing within North America and Europe must be increasingly aware of the impact of worm infections in children. Two pediatric populations need to be considered. First, children and young adults with appropriate epidemiologic risk factors and geographic origins from Africa, Asia, and Latin America who present with acute symptoms, such as abdominal distention, abdominal pain, and wheezing, as well as more chronic symptoms, such as asthma, colitis, HIV, and bladder cancer, should be evaluated for helminth infections. Second, helminth infection transmission may be more common in North America and Europe than previously thought.[6] For example, toxocariasis, a zoonotic helminth infection from dogs, is widespread in the Southern United States and Eastern Europe,[22–24] whereas the intestinal helminth infections highlighted above may still occur in the Southern United States and parts of Europe,[24,25] and schistosomiasis transmission was recently documented in Corsica.[26]

DIAGNOSIS AND TREATMENT

The diagnosis of helminths has traditionally been based on serologic evaluation for schistosomiasis or visualization of eggs, in stool for intestinal helminth and intestinal schistosomiasis (*Schistosoma mansoni* or *Schistosoma japonicum*), or in urine for urogenital schistosomiasis (*S haematobium*), using microscopy. The subjective declaration of eggs and/or larvae can be a fickle and arduous task that suffers from laborious preparation, the need for skilled microscopists, with sensitivities that range from 50% to 85%.[27] Modern molecular techniques have revolutionized helminth diagnoses with greatly improved detection rates and 10-fold increases in detection of 2 or more parasitic infections (polyparasitism).[28,29] By using multiparallel quantitative real-time polymerase chain reaction with a stool bead beating DNA extraction method to reduce the cost, the assay can be used in a capacity-building setting in resource-limited countries.[28–30] Newer techniques continue to be developed allowing for more rapid, sensitive diagnostics particularly in settings of polyparasitism and low worm burden.[28]

Current therapy for children with helminth infections is based on adult dosing and adult formulations, including benzimidazoles and praziquantel. For treatment of hookworm or roundworm administration of either albendazole 400 mg orally once taken with food or mebendazole 100 mg orally twice a day for 3 days is recommended. For whipworm, albendazole 400 mg orally for 3 to 7 days or mebendazole 100 mg for 3 to 7 days is required, and for schistosomiasis, treatment consists of praziquantel 20 mg/kg orally twice a day for 1 day (see **Table 2**).[9,20]

It is evident that as the global community becomes smaller, worm infections in children may become a more common occurrence in pediatric clinics within the United States and other wealthy countries. As a result, it is imperative for the pediatric clinician to understand the historic, current, and prospective landscape of helminth disease in children around the world.

INTRODUCTION TO MASS DRUG ADMINISTRATION

The significant life-long morbidity of helminths has led to the commitment of public and private leaders to address controlling and even eliminating these pathogens globally.[5] Early goals focused primarily on WASH through improved sanitation, reducing soil and water contamination, and implementing health education within communities.[5] These strategies to improve community infrastructure incurred high cost without immediate, noticeable change, prompting a shift toward mass drug administration (MDA), also now referred to by the World Health Organization (WHO) as preventive chemotherapy.[5] MDA programs are centered on the regular, repeated administration of preventive chemotherapies, such as benzimidazoles (albendazole, mebendazole) for intestinal helminth infections, ivermectin or diethylcarbamazine citrate for filarial worms, and praziquantel for schistosomiasis.[31] It has been anticipated that repeated MDA at regular intervals will reduce worm burden to reduce morbidity, and in areas with low prevalence possibly even inhibit transmission and eventually allow for elimination of helminth infection.[5] Early precedent for a mass treatment approach was seen in the United States in the early 1900s.[32] In 1910, the Rockefeller Sanitary Commission for the Eradication of Hookworm Disease (RSC) estimated 40% of the population of Southern United States was infected with hookworm. The RSC sponsored treatment administration for more than 400,000 individuals through mobile dispensaries, implemented education campaigns, invested in public health infrastructure, and completed disease mapping among 11 southern states in efforts to reduce hookworm disease.[33] Interestingly, in school systems with the highest levels of hookworm burden, children that received therapeutic intervention were found to have greater increases in school enrollment, school attendance, and literacy by 1920. Furthermore, as children that received treatment for hookworm aged into adulthood, they had a substantial gain in income.[34] However, the success of this program was multifactorial, relying not only on MDA but also on changes in education, shifts away from agrarian activities toward urbanization, and overall economic development of the Southern United States.[34–36] Similar economic reforms led to reductions in intestinal helminth infections in Japan and South Korea beginning in the 1950s, as well as in Eastern China beginning in the 1990s.[6]

MASS DRUG ADMINISTRATION PHASE 1 (2001): REDUCTION IN MORBIDITY

Anthelmintics MDA programs gained momentum in 2001, after the release of the 2000 Millennium Development goals,[17] and with the adoption of a World Health Assembly Resolution specifically committed to intestinal helminth infections and schistosomiasis.[37] Initially, MDA programs focused on controlling worm burden within a community to reduce morbidity within an individual.[38] In order to accomplish this goal, a joint statement by WHO and UNICEF in 2004 supported the target of "high-risk" communities, including preschool- and school-aged children, adolescent girls, and women of childbearing age based on worm prevalence.[10] Because young children often harbor the greatest burden of worms, focusing on these "high-risk" communities was predicted to generate the greatest impact on morbidity while minimizing the cost for clinical diagnosis.[5,39–41] To achieve worm control, the WHO estimated that at least 75% of all school-aged children in endemic regions were in need of regular treatment or approximately 875 million children.[5,16,42] Early programs administered a single dose of benzimidazole (albendazole or mebendazole) for the treatment of soil-transmitted helminths and a single dose of praziquantel for the treatment of schistosomiasis.[38] The medications were found to be generally well tolerated and often administered by community health workers or teachers in school-based programs.[38] Furthermore, administration of regular anthelmintics treatment to high-risk groups was found to be affordable and sometimes sustainable.[10] However, it has been noted that a single-dose mebendazole or albendazole can exhibit low efficacy against whipworm or hookworm in some settings,[43,44] and in some cases, paradoxic drug failure[45] or diminished efficacy with repeated use.[46] Possibly, some of these findings explain why a Cochrane analysis of randomized clinical trials using MDA approaches failed to conclusively confirm child-health benefits in terms of nutritional benefits, hemoglobin, and school performance.[47]

MASS DRUG ADMINISTRATION PHASE 2 (2005): INTEGRATIVE CONTROL WITH THE "RAPID-IMPACT PACKAGE"

Polyparasitism in children is common due to the geographic overlap of soil-transmitted helminths and schistosomiasis globally. Because of this geographic overlap, MDA programs in high-risk communities were administering multiple therapies to control multiple infections. Furthermore, poor efficacy of monotherapy benzimidazoles, specifically for hookworm or whipworm, highlighted the need for an integrative treatment approach.[31] The "rapid-impact" package, the next step in MDA evolution and integration, was a low-cost mechanism proposed in 2005 to distribute multiple drugs to treat multiple parasites simultaneously.[48,49] Implementation of the rapid impact package included 4 drug classes: benzimidazoles (albendazole or mebendazole), ivermectin (or diethylcarbamazine citrate in some areas), praziquantel, and azithromycin, allowing for concurrent treatment of soil-transmitted helminths, filarial diseases, schistosomiasis, and trachoma, respectively.[5,49] In addition, collateral benefits for yaws, scabies, and other neglected tropical diseases were noted.[50] Another advantage of combining albendazole with ivermectin within the medication package was increased drug efficacy for whipworm secondary to cross-reactivity of medications[51] and the possibility of slowing the development of resistance to individual drug classes.[5,52] Although emergence of anthelmintics drug resistance has not yet been proven for human intestinal helminths or schistosomes, veterinary medicine has demonstrated that widespread, frequent, prolonged administration of anthelmintics chemotherapy within a population increases the risk of drug resistance.[53] With this precedent in the veterinary world, the growing evidence of decreased efficacy of mebendazole for whipworm and hookworm[46] as well as decreased efficacy of praziquantel for schistosomiasis after repeated use is of increasing concern.[54]

MASS DRUG ADMINISTRATION PHASE 3 (2012): SCALE-UP PROGRAMS FOR ELIMINATION

Despite private and public efforts, the 2010 goal to provide MDA to at least 75% of school-aged children at risk was not met.[5] By 2010, only 32.6% of children requiring coverage for soil-transmitted helminths and 14.4% of children requiring coverage for schistosomiasis received adequate therapy. Failure to meet these goals was thought to be secondary to cost-prohibitive programs and the intermittent availability of anthelmintics therapies.[52,55] In the early 2010s, the London Declaration of Stakeholders Working Group and the WHO 2020 roadmap advocated for scale-up of MDA programs to not only control infections by providing therapy to 75% of children but also add a new focus on elimination and eradication by interrupting transmission by 2020.[16,42,56,57] Emphasis was placed on collaborative and coordinated efforts by both public and private groups to provide funds for expanded coverage combined with commitments by helminth-endemic countries to focus on improvements in community infrastructure.[16,42,56,57] Programs were expected to place a larger emphasis on national funding and improvements in national health infrastructure to ensure sustainability.[42] Through such renewed commitments, new estimates by the WHO indicate that globally in 2015 more than 60% and 40% of school-aged children receive benz-imidazoles and praziquantel, respectively, on an annual basis.[58]

MASS DRUG ADMINISTRATION AS A PATHWAY TOWARD HELMINTH ELIMINATION

Despite the global commitment to global helminth control and elimination, there are significant hurdles toward achieving these goals solely through current MDA ap-proaches. To date, the Global Burden of Disease 2015 has shown only modest reduc-tions in the global prevalence of intestinal helminth infections since MDA was integrated beginning in 2005, with the greatest reductions in ascariasis (12% reduction in prevalence and 20% reduction in age standardized rates) presumably due to its high sensitivity to single-dose albendazole or mebendazole, whereas the gains have been more modest for trichuriasis and hookworm possibly due to reduced efficacies when these drugs are used in a single dose.[2] Another factor is the finding that, although ascariasis and trichuriasis intensities are highest among school-aged children, it is common to find both high-prevalence and high-intensity hookworm and schistosomi-asis infections among adults. Therefore, MDA for preschool- and school-aged chil-dren would not be expected to have an impact on elimination for either hookworm or schistosomiasis. Accordingly, there have been calls to expand MDA to treat entire communities in order to simultaneously target both adults and children.[59,60] However, it is unclear whether the concerns highlighted earlier, including paradoxically low drug efficacies or diminished efficacy with increasing use, or even drug resistance would make elimination efforts unattainable even in the setting of community-wide treat-ments. A survey of several hundred experts in neglected tropical diseases indicated a high degree of uncertainty of achieving elimination targets for intestinal helminth in-fections or schistosomiasis through MDA alone.[61]

As global MDA efforts continue to expand and reach the 75% to 100% targets adopted by the 54th World Health Assembly in 2001, a parallel program of research and development is needed to not only improve existing anthelmintics drugs to include pediatric formulations but also develop new innovative anthelmintics drug classes, particularly for whipworm and hookworm. Among those under development are tribendimidine, a cholinergic drug that also works against human liver fluke infec-tion,[62] and Cry5B, a *Bacillus thuringiensis*–derived toxin, known to activate the p38 mitogen–activated protein kinase pathway in both hookworm and ascariasis.[63,64] Overall, the pace of human anthelmintics drug development has been slow due to the orphan and neglected status of its disease target. Still another approach has been the development of anthelmintics vaccines, possibly used in combination with existing or new drugs.[65] Toward that goal, a human hookworm vaccine is in phase 1 clinical trials, as are 2 new vaccines for schistosomiasis. Vaccine development pro-grams evaluating the possibility of a multivalent anthelmintics vaccine targeting mul-tiple pathogens would additionally provide significant benefit in areas with helminthic geographic overlap.[65] Unfortunately, global efforts to advance these vac-cines through clinical development and ultimately licensure have also been slowed by the absence of prioritization by the global community relative to vaccines for pandemic disease threats such as Ebola and influenza.

SUMMARY

Helminth infections, soil-transmitted helminths and schistosomiasis, adversely affect the lives of millions of children around the world. With the increase in globalization, pe-diatricians in wealthy nations are increasingly likely to encounter these infections in their clinic. It is imperative to understand the epidemiology, transmission dynamics, and treatment options for these children in order to prevent significant long-term morbidity. The evolution of the MDA movement has progressed from control to integrative elimination programs specifically targeting young children. Scale-up approaches to include whole communities (including adults) have been proposed with the goal to ultimately achieve interruption in transmission. However, the question remains whether these programs will be efficacious and if repeated treatment within the communities will have a lasting impact on drug resistance. As a result of this uncertainty, there remains a significant need for diagnostic innovation, therapeutic development including new drugs and vaccines, as well as drug resistance monitoring to aid in the control and elimination efforts of helminth infections globally.

REFERENCES

1. Pullan RL, Smith JL, Jasrasaria R, et al. Global numbers of infection and disease burden of soil transmitted helminth infections in 2010. Parasit Vectors 2014;7:37.
2. GBD 2015 Disease and Injury Incidence and Prevalence Collaborators. Global, regional, and national incidence, prevalence, and years lived with disability for 310 diseases and injuries, 1990-2015: a systematic analysis for the Global Burden of Disease Study 2015. Lancet 2016;388(10053):1545–602.
3. Bartsch SM, Hotez PJ, Asti L, et al. The global economic and health burden of human hookworm infection. PLoS Negl Trop Dis 2016;10(9):e0004922, de Silva N, editor.
4. GBD 2015 Disease and Injury Incidence and Prevalence Collaborators. Global, regional, and national life expectancy, all-cause mortality, and cause-specific mortality for 249 causes of death, 1980–2015: a systematic analysis for the Global Burden of Disease Study 2015. Lancet 2016;388(10053):1459–544. Available at: http://linkinghub.elsevier.com/retrieve/pii/S0140673616310121.
5. Tchuem Tchuenté LA. Control of soil-transmitted helminths in sub-Saharan Africa: diagnosis, drug efficacy concerns and challenges. Acta Trop 2011;120(Suppl): S4–11.
6. Hotez P. Blue Marble Health: an innovative plan to fight diseases of the Poor amid wealth. Baltimore (MD): Johns Hopkins University Press; 2016. p. 244.
7. GBD 2015 Disease and Injury Incidence and Prevalence Collaborators. Global, regional, and national disability-adjusted life-years (DALYs) for 315 diseases and injuries and healthy life expectancy (HALE), 1990–2015: a systematic analysis for the Global Burden of Disease Study 2015. Lancet 2016;388(10053): 1603–58.
8. Hotez PJ, Bundy DAP, Beegle K, et al. Helminth infections: soil-transmitted helminth infections and schistosomiasis. New York: Oxford University Press; 2006.
9. Weatherhead JE, Hotez PJ. Worm infections in children. Pediatr Rev 2015;36(8): 341–52 [quiz: 353–4].
10. World Health Organization Expert Committee. Prevention and control of schistosomiasis and soil-transmitted helminthiasis. World Health Organ Tech Rep Ser 2002;912:1–57.
11. Miguel E, Kremer M. Worms: identifying impacts on education and health in the presence of treatment externalities. Econometrica 2004;72(1):159–217.
12. Briggs N, Weatherhead J, Sastry KJ, et al. The hygiene hypothesis and its inconvenient truths about helminth infections. PLoS Negl Trop Dis 2016;10(9): e0004944. Cooper PJ, editor.
13. Hotez P, Whitham M. Helminth infections: a new global women's health agenda. Obstet Gynecol 2014;123(1):155–60.

14. Brooker S, Akhwale W, Pullan R, et al. Epidemiology of plasmodium-helminth co-infection in Africa: populations at risk, potential impact on anemia, and prospects for combining control. Am J Trop Med Hyg 2007;77(6 Suppl):88–98.

15. King CH, Dangerfield-Cha M. The unacknowledged impact of chronic schistoso-miasis. Chronic Illn 2008;4(1):65–79.

16. World Health Organization. Investing to overcome the global impact of neglected tropical diseases. 2015. Available at: http://apps.who.int/iris/bitstream/10665/152781/1/9789241564861_eng.pdf. Accessed October 6, 2016.

17. Hotez PJ, Molyneux D, Hotez P, et al. NTDs V.2.0: "Blue Marble Health"—neglected tropical disease control and elimination in a shifting health policy landscape. PLoS Negl Trop Dis 2013;7(11):e2570. Knopp S, editor.

18. Brindley PJ, Costa da JM, Sripa B, et al. Why does infection with some helminths cause cancer? Trends Cancer 2015;1(3):174–82.

19. Liu C, Luo R, Yi H, et al. Soil-transmitted helminths in Southwestern China: a cross-sectional study of links to cognitive ability, nutrition, and school performance among children. PLoS Negl Trop Dis 2015;9(6):e0003877. Gray DJ, editor.

20. Kappagoda S, Singh U, Blackburn B. Antiparasitic therapy. Mayo Clin Proc 2011;86(6):561–83.

21. Diseases USD of H and HSNC for E and ZI. Guidelines for the U.S. Domestic Medical Examination for Newly Arrived Refugees. 2013. Available at: http://www.cdc.gov/immigrantrefugeehealth/guidelines/domestic/domestic-guidelines.html. Accessed April 12, 2017.

22. Lee RM, Moore LB, Bottazzi ME, et al. Toxocariasis in North America: a systematic review. PLoS Negl Trop Dis 2014;8(8):e3116.

23. Borecka A, Kłapeć T. Epidemiology of human toxocariasis in Poland - a review of cases 1978-2009. Ann Agric Environ Med 2015;22(1):28–31.

24. Hotez PJ, Gurwith M. Europe's neglected infections of poverty. Int J Infect Dis 2011;15(9):e611–9.

25. Starr MC, Montgomery SP. Soil-transmitted helminthiasis in the United States: a systematic review - 1940-2010. Am J Trop Med Hyg 2011;85(4):680–4.

26. Berry A, Fillaux J, Martin-Blondel G, et al. Evidence for a permanent presence of schistosomiasis in Corsica, France, 2015. Euro Surveill 2016;21(1):30100.

27. Mosli M, Gregor J, Chande N, et al. Nonutility of routine testing of stool for ova and parasites in a tertiary care Canadian centre. Can J Microbiol 2012;58(5):653–9.

28. Mejia R, Vicuña Y, Broncano N, et al. A novel, multi-parallel, real-time polymerase chain reaction approach for eight gastrointestinal parasites provides improved diagnostic capabilities to resource-limited at-risk populations. Am J Trop Med Hyg 2013;88(6):1041–7.

29. Cimino RO, Jeun R, Juarez M, et al. Identification of human intestinal parasites affecting an asymptomatic peri-urban Argentinian population using multi-parallel quantitative real-time polymerase chain reaction. Parasit Vectors 2015;8:380.

30. Pilotte N, Papaiakovou M, Grant JR, et al. Improved PCR-based detection of soil transmitted helminth infections using a next-generation sequencing approach to assay design. PLoS Negl Trop Dis 2016;10(3):e0004578. Albonico M, editor.

31. Hotez PJ, Molyneux DH, Fenwick A, et al. Control of neglected tropical diseases. N Engl J Med 2007;357(10):1018–27.

32. World Health Organization. Controlling disease due to helminth infections. In: Crompton DWT, Montresor A, Nesheim MC, et al, editors. Geneva (Switzerland): World Health Organization; 2003. Available at: http://apps.who.int/iris/bitstream/10665/42707/1/9241562390.pdf. Accessed November 21, 2016.

33. Rockefeller Foundation. 100 Years: The Rockefeller Foundation | Eradicating Hookworm Health. Available at: http://rockefeller100.org/exhibits/show/health/eradicating-hookworm. Accessed November 18, 2016.

34. Bleakley H. Disease and development: evidence from hookworm eradication in the American South. Q J Econ 2007;122(1):73–117.

35. Humphreys M. How four once common diseases were eliminated from the American South. Health Aff (Millwood) 2009;28(6):1734–44.

36. Martin MG, Humphreys ME. Social consequence of disease in the American South, 1900-world War. South Med J 2006;99(8):862–4.

37. Fifty-Fourth World Health Assembly. WHA54.19 Schistosomiasis and soil-transmitted helminth infections. 2001. Available at: http://apps.who.int/gb/archive/pdf_files/WHA54/ea54r19.pdf?ua=1. Accessed November 18, 2016.

38. Urbani C, Albonico M. Anthelminthic drug safety and drug administration in the control of soil-transmitted helminthiasis in community campaigns. Acta Trop 2003;86(2):215–21.

39. Truscott J, Turner H, Anderson R. What impact will the achievement of the current World Health Organisation targets for anthelmintic treatment coverage in children have on the intensity of soil transmitted helminth infections? Parasit Vectors 2015; 8:551.

40. Hicks JH, Kremer M, Miguel E. The case for mass treatment of intestinal helminths in endemic areas. PLoS Negl Trop Dis 2015;9(10):e0004214.

41. Anderson R, Truscott J, Hollingsworth TD. The coverage and frequency of mass drug administration required to eliminate persistent transmission of soil-transmitted helminths. Philos Trans R Soc Lond B Biol Sci 2014;369(1645): 20130435.

42. World Health Organization. Accelerating work to overcome the global impact of neglected tropical disease: a roadmap for implementation. WHO Press, World Health Organization; 2012. Available at: http://www.who.int/neglected_diseases/NTD_RoadMap_2012_Fullversion.pdf. Accessed August 10, 2016.

43. Keiser J, Utzinger J. Efficacy of current drugs against soil-transmitted helminth infections: systematic review and meta-analysis. JAMA 2008;299(16):1937–48.

44. Soukhathammavong PA, Sayasone S, Phongluxa K, et al. Low efficacy of single-dose albendazole and mebendazole against hookworm and effect on concomitant helminth infection in Lao PDR. PLoS Negl Trop Dis 2012;6(1):e1417. Prichard RK, editor.

45. De Clercq D, Sacko M, Behnke J, et al. Failure of mebendazole in treatment of human hookworm infections in the southern region of Mali. Am J Trop Med Hyg 1997;57(1):25–30.

46. Albonico M, Bickle Q, Ramsan M, et al. Efficacy of mebendazole and levamisole alone or in combination against intestinal nematode infections after repeated targeted mebendazole treatment in Zanzibar. Bull World Health Organ 2003;81(5): 343–52.

47. Taylor-Robinson DC, Maayan N, Soares-Weiser K, et al. Deworming drugs for soil-transmitted intestinal worms in children: effects on nutritional indicators, haemoglobin, and school performance. Cochrane Database Syst Rev 2015;23(7): CD000371.

48. Prichard RK, Basá Ñ Ez M-G, Boatin BA, et al. A research agenda for helminth diseases of humans: intervention for control and elimination. PLoS Negl Trop Dis 2012;6(4):e1549.

49. Molyneux DH, Hotez PJ, Fenwick A. "Rapid-impact interventions": how a policy of integrated control for Africa's neglected tropical diseases could benefit the poor. PLoS Med 2005;2(11):e336.

50. Hotez PJ, Velasquez RM, Wolf JE. Neglected tropical skin diseases: their global elimination through integrated mass drug administration? JAMA Dermatol 2014; 150(5):481–2.

51. Hotez P. Mass drug administration and integrated control for the world's high-prevalence neglected tropical diseases. Clin Pharmacol Ther 2009;85(6):659–64.

52. WHO Regional Committee. Fifty-ninth Session of the WHO Regional Committee (AFR/RC59/19). 2009. Available at: http://www.afro.who.int/en/fifty-ninth-session. html. Accessed April 12, 2017.

53. Geerts S, Gryseels B. Anthelmintic resistance in human helminths: a review. Trop Med Int Health 2001;6(11):915–21.

54. Crellen T, Walker M, Lamberton PHL, et al. Reduced efficacy of praziquantel against schistosoma mansoni is associated with multiple rounds of mass drug administration. Clin Infect Dis 2016;63(9):1151–9.

55. Chami GF, Kontoleon AA, Bulte E, et al. Profiling nonrecipients of mass drug administration for schistosomiasis and hookworm infections: a comprehensive analysis of praziquantel and albendazole coverage in community-directed treatment in Uganda. Clin Infect Dis 2016;62(2):200–7.

56. Uniting to Combat Neglected Tropical Diseases. Delivering on promises and driving progress: uniting to combat neglected tropical diseases. Available at: http://unitingtocombatntds.org/resource/promises-progress-first-report-londondeclaration-ntds. Accessed August 17, 2016.

57. London Declaration on Neglected Tropical Diseases. Uniting to combat neglected tropical diseases. 2012. Available at: http://unitingtocombatntds.org/. Accessed August 17, 2016.

58. Global programme to eliminate lymphatic filariasis: progress report, 2015. Weekly Epidemiol Rec 2016;91:441–60. Available at: http://www.who.int/wer. Accessed November 18, 2016.

59. Anderson RM, Turner HC, Farrell SH, et al. Studies of the transmission dynamics, mathematical model development and the control of schistosome parasites by mass drug administration in human communities. Adv Parasitol 2016;94:199–246.

60. Truscott JE, Turner HC, Farrell SH, et al. Soil-transmitted helminths: mathematical models of transmission, the impact of mass drug administration and transmission elimination criteria. Adv Parasitol 2016;94:133–98.

61. Keenan JD, Hotez PJ, Amza A, et al. Elimination and eradication of neglected tropical diseases with mass drug administrations: a survey of experts. PLoS Negl Trop Dis 2013;7(12):e2562.

62. Robertson AP, Puttachary S, Buxton SK, et al. Tribendimidine: mode of action and nAChR subtype selectivity in ascaris and oesophagostomum. PLoS Negl Trop Dis 2015;9(2):e0003495. Keiser J, editor.

63. Urban JF, Hu Y, Miller MM, et al. Bacillus thuringiensis-derived Cry5B has potent anthelmintic activity against ascaris suum. PLoS Negl Trop Dis 2013;7(6):e2263. Geary TG, editor.

64. Cappello M, Bungiro RD, Harrison LM, et al. A purified Bacillus thuringiensis crystal protein with therapeutic activity against the hookworm parasite Ancylostoma ceylanicum. Proc Natl Acad Sci U S A 2006;103(41):15154–9.

65. Hotez PJ, Strych U, Lustigman S, et al. Human anthelminthic vaccines: rationale and challenges. Vaccine 2016;34:3549–55.

Pediatric Human Immunodeficiency Virus Continuum of Care

A Concise Review of Evidence-Based Practice

Megan E. Gray, MD[a], Phillip Nieburg, MD, MPH[b], Rebecca Dillingham, MD, MPH[a],*

KEYWORDS

- HIV • AIDS • Children • Adolescents • Prevention • Adherence

KEY POINTS

- HIV remains a major public health crisis in children and adolescents across the world.
- There are 2 key populations of youth living with HIV, those who acquire HIV perinatally and those who acquire HIV through risk behaviors later in childhood or adolescence.
- Beyond technical and scientific advances, effective prevention of new HIV infections requires addressing a complex combination of social, economic, behavioral, structural, and logistic obstacles.
- For youth living with HIV to achieve viral suppression and optimal health outcomes, providers should be aware of and address age-specific barriers to HIV testing, linkage to care, ART adherence, and retention in care.

INTRODUCTION

Since the discovery of human immunodeficiency virus (HIV) in 1983, momentous advances in the recognition, treatment, and prevention of HIV infection have averted an estimated 9 million deaths so far in the new millennium.[1] HIV/AIDS remains, however, one of the largest international public health crises. Children and adolescents are especially vulnerable populations, and the identification and care of youth living with HIV present unique challenges.

There are 2 distinct populations of youth living with HIV. There are those who acquired HIV through perinatal transmission and require HIV care from the time of their birth and those who acquired HIV through risk behaviors in adolescence, such as

Disclosure Statement: The authors have no disclosures.
[a] Division of Infectious Diseases and International Health, University of Virginia, PO Box 801340, Charlottesville, VA 22908-1340, USA; [b] Department of Pediatrics, University of Virginia, 1215 Lee Street, Charlottesville, VA 22908, USA
* Corresponding author.
E-mail address: RD8V@hscmail.mcc.virginia.edu

unprotected sexual encounters or injection drug use. Both populations of HIV-seropositive youth require tailored approaches for their care to be successful. The cascade of care for individuals living with HIV begins with diagnosis, counseling, linkage to care, and initiation of antiretroviral therapy (ART), at which point the work of patients and providers has only just begun. Strict adherence to ART, persistence in ART, and retention in care are necessary for viral suppression and require collaboration of patients, health care staff, social workers, and physicians.[2]

As of 2016, 1.8 million children under the age of 15 are living with HIV and 87% of these children live in sub-Saharan Africa.[3] At the end of 2013, 1999 children under the age of 13 lived with HIV in the United States, and 73% of these children acquired the infection through perinatal transmission.[4] Approximately three-quarters of adolescents living with HIV worldwide represent those that were infected at birth, which is evidence of the positive impact of ART on life expectancy of perinatally infected children.[5] The rates of perinatal HIV infection in the United States are very low and the majority of adolescents living with HIV in this country acquired the virus through risk behaviors. Of the approximately 2 million adolescents living with HIV across the world, only 1% is from the United States.[6] This adolescent 1% accounts for 22% of all new HIV infections nationally.[4] Young male, transgender African American adolescents are the highest risk group.[7] Globally, however, girls and young women are at highest risk due to culture-specific gender norms, sexual abuse,[8] intergenerational sexual relationships,[7] and enhanced biologic suceptibility.[9]

Refugees and immigrants represent another special population because up to 14% are leaving countries of high HIV prevalence.[10] High rates of pregnancy were noted in 1 cohort of HIV-infected refugees in Rhode Island, highlighting the need for preventative HIV perinatal care.[11] Among approximately 7000 children adopted internationally over a 15-year period (1990–2005), 12 children were found infected with HIV.[12]

In 2016, only 50% of perinatally exposed children globally were tested within the recommended 2 months.[1] Of the children who tested positive for HIV, only 50% are receiving treatment,[1] although this varies by country and region. Compared with Europe and Central Asia, where more than 95% of children younger than 15 years old living with HIV are receiving ART, sub-Saharan Africa has 1.83 million or 73% of their children living with HIV who are untreated.[3] In the rest of Africa and the Middle East, 86% of children living with HIV are untreated. For infants born with HIV, treatment is crucial to prevent rapid progression to AIDS in the early years of life. Without ART, half of these children will die by age 2 years old.[7]

Statistics are similarly bleak for youth who acquire HIV later in life. In the United States 44% of young people living with HIV are unaware of their diagnosis.[4] Adolescents in sub-Saharan Africa are even less informed of their HIV infection status, with only 13% of adolescent girls and 9% of adolescent boys receiving testing in the most recent 12 months.[1] HIV is the number 2 cause of death of adolescents globally, and it is the number 1 cause of death of adolescents in Africa.[1] Disturbingly, since the year 2000, deaths have tripled among adolescents with AIDS, which is in stark contrast to other affected groups that have seen improved mortality rates.[6] Disparities in resources, health care, and infrastructure; stigmatizing cultural influences; and a poor understanding of HIV infection all play a role in the current state of HIV care.[13]

PREVENTING HUMAN IMMUNODEFICIENCY VIRUS/AIDS IN CHILDREN AND ADOLESCENTS

The Joint United Nations Programme on AIDS (UNAIDS) and the World Health Organization (WHO) are leading a global program with a goal to end AIDS by 2030, a goal that requires both a greater focus on ART for people already living with HIV infection and a renewed emphasis on preventing new HIV infections.[7]

Overall funding for global HIV/AIDS programs has increased over the past several years, with the US President's Emergency Plan for AIDS Relief (PEPFAR) the largest global funding source for effective prevention programs.[14] The proportion of HIV/AIDS resources available for prevention of new HIV infections, however, has fallen slightly over that period, in part because the number of people living with HIV who are receiving lifelong treatment with relatively expensive ART has been increasing rapidly. As a consequence, global progress toward the prevention goal of fewer than 500,000 new HIV infections per year is considered off-track.[7] Although progress toward the ultimate prevention goal of a successful HIV vaccine has not yet met expectations, the prevention of mother-to-child transmission of HIV (MTCT) has been both a US and a global success story.

Preventing Mother-to-Child Transmission of Human Immunodeficiency Virus in Pregnancy and in the Perinatal Period

Globally, MTCT accounts for more than 90% of new HIV infections among children. The WHO has put forward a comprehensive approach to prevention of MTCT (**Box 1**).[15] Although overall global progress has been sporadic, significant progress has been made in certain countries. For example, in 21 priority African countries, the proportion of known HIV-infected pregnant women who received ART in pregnancy increased from 36% in 2009 to 80% in 2015.[16] The numbers of HIV-infected children fell correspondingly by 48% between the years 2009 and 2014.[17] Six of these priority countries reduced MTCT by at least 90% over that period. Finally, by 2016, Cuba, Belarus, Armenia, and Thailand each reduced MTCT to the point that it is no longer considered a significant public health problem in those countries.

Without any intervention for HIV-infected pregnant women, the risk of MTCT ranges from 15% to 45%. Effective interventions, however, can reduce this transmission risk to less than 5%. Within the United States, although approximately 8500 HIV-infected women give birth annually,[4] the number of children who are HIV-infected in utero or in the perinatal period is now fewer than 100 per year. The lower rate of perinatal transmission is in part a result of high rates of antenatal HIV testing and counseling. In addition, HIV-infected pregnant women in the United States have good access to antiretroviral medicines during pregnancy and delivery.[18,19] It is recommended that pregnant women who do not have maximally suppressed HIV viral loads at the time

---

Box 1
World Health Organization comprehensive approach to mother-to-child transmission of HIV among adolescents and other women of childbearing age

1. Prevent HIV infections among adolescents and other women of childbearing age.

2. Help HIV-infected adolescents and other women avoid unintended pregnancy.

3. Prevent HIV transmission from HIV-infected adolescents and other women to their infants.

4. Provide appropriate treatment care and support to mothers living with HIV and their children.

From World Health Organization. PMTCT strategic vision 2010-2015 preventing mother-to-child transmission of HIV to reach to the UNGASS and millennium development goals. 2010. Available at: http://www.who.int/hiv/pub/mtct/strategic_vision/en/. Accessed December 10, 2016.

of labor should have a cesarean section delivery to further reduce the HIV transmission risk to their newborns.

Prevention of Mother-to-Child Transmission of Human Immunodeficiency Virus Through Breast Milk

MTCT may still occur beyond the perinatal period due to HIV transmitted via breast milk. Although the HIV transmission risk is lower if breastfeeding mothers are on ART, more than half of all MTCT HIV infections in 2013 were attributed to breast milk transmission.[17] Infant formula feeding is the optimal way to eliminate that risk. Infant formula use, however, may not be possible in all circumstances due to the cost of formula and poor access to clean water. In such cases, exclusive breastfeeding rather than mixed feeding (the latter is associated with greater HIV transmission risk) should continue until weaning. Mothers should continue ART to keep their breast milk viral load suppressed and infants should receive their own ART until they reach 6 weeks old.

Preventing Human Immunodeficiency Virus Infections Among Adolescents

In contrast to perinatal infections and infections in older adults, where HIV infection and mortality rates have been falling, the adolescent age group has seen increasing rates of both HIV infection and HIV-related mortality. Approximately two-thirds of these new HIV infections and deaths are occurring in female adolescents. Effective prevention of new HIV infections among adolescents is a complex issue because the causes of HIV transmission vary in different cultural, social, economic, and geographic settings. Appropriately, there is a broad range of prevention strategies, which include

1. Raising awareness of HIV/AIDS, its transmission mechanisms, and its behavioral components
2. Encouraging community-based and school-based sex education
3. Increasing use of male and female condoms
4. Increasing uptake of VMMCs
5. Increasing use of harm reduction interventions, such as clean injection equipment
6. Increasing uptake of pre-exposure (drug) prophylaxis (PrEP) and other ART use to lower viral load
7. Use of vaginal microbicides
8. Approaches to reduce child marriage
9. Other structural approaches to address gender inequality and gender-based violence

Although each of these individual interventions has been demonstrated as efficacious in one setting or another, the optimal combination in any one location necessarily is dictated by local circumstances.

Recently, a group of United Nations agencies along with the US PEPFAR program launched the "ALL IN! to End Adolescent AIDS" agenda. This agenda will help address and implement interventions similar to those recently begun by the DREAMS Innovation Challenge supported by the US PEPFAR program in collaboration with the Bill & Melinda Gate Foundation, several drug companies, and other nongovernmental organizations.[20] The DREAMS Innovation Challenge is focused on (1) keeping girls in school, (2) strengthening the service delivery capacity of community-based organizations, (3) linking men to services; (4) supporting the use of PrEP, (5) linking adolescents to employment opportunities, and (6) increasing the use of data to inform policy.

Voluntary Medical Male Circumcision

Medical male circumcision may be of particular interest to pediatricians as a prevention strategy. After a compellingly high (>55%) efficacy of voluntary male medical circumcision (VMMC) was demonstrated to reduce men's risk of acquiring HIV infection in several randomized controlled trials, use of that intervention was recommended by the WHO and UNAIDS.[21] By late 2015, approximately 12 million adolescent men and boys had been circumcised in 14 priority African countries. Current program efforts are focused on further integrating VMMC services within routine health systems, investigating safe alternatives to surgical circumcisions, and providing sufficient counseling to ensure that circumcision recipients understand that protection from HIV is not absolute and still requires condom use and avoiding other high-risk behaviors. Expanded use of infant male circumcision as an HIV prevention intervention is also being investigated in several African countries.

ANTIRETROVIRAL THERAPY ADHERENCE

Unlike other chronic diseases where even partial adherence to medications may be adequate treatment, poor adherence to ART risks creating resistant HIV strains that are difficult or impossible to treat and may then be transmitted. Adherence rates more than 90% have been considered necessary to achieve viral suppression.[22,23] Adherence rates among adolescents, however, range from 65% to 90%,[24] with 1 study in the United States reporting adherence rates of 65%.[25] Where ART is available and accessible there are still approximately a quarter of children and adolescents who are not taking their pills regularly. Evidence-based strategies to improve adherence in adolescents are critical for individual health and to prevent transmission.[26] Development of these strategies requires understanding of age-specific barriers to adherence.

Barriers in Antiretroviral Therapy Adherence Specific to Infants and Children

For infants and very young children, many logistical factors impede adherence despite the best intentions of caregivers. Liquid ART formulations are often bitter and poorly tolerated[27]; their cost is up to 4 times higher than tablets; and the bulk and weight of multiple months of liquid ART makes them conspicuous and difficult to transport and store.[28] Dosing of liquid formulations requires medication dispensers with markings, which may present a challenge for caregivers with poor vision or lack of education. For children over the age of 2, tablets are preferred to liquid formulations.[28] To avoid liquid formulations, some caregivers report crushing tablets or opening capsules to sprinkle them over food, which may result in inadequate dosing of ART.[27] Gastrostomy tubes have been used to provide a more reliable route of administration. Studies showed that gastrostomy tubes were associated with improved adherence in young children and decreased the time required to administer ART.[29,30] They may also be used for nutritional supplementation, which has been shown to increase weight and was associated with decreased hospital visits and mortality. The routine use of gastrostomy tubes, however, is not recommended given the cost, practical limitations, and related risks.[31]

For children old enough to swallow nonliquid formulations, other barriers remain. Taking ART on an empty stomach can be uncomfortable and lack of food is a reality for many children and adolescents. In a study in Uganda, 25% of children refused to take their medication if food was not available.[32] Children reported that lack of assistance from adult caregivers and forgetfulness were reasons for nonadherence.[32–34] Children with caregivers reporting substance abuse, lower levels of education, or poor understanding of ART also had lower adherence.[33] Although adolescents may have more weighty social and emotional challenges associated with their HIV-positive status, younger children are not unaffected. Young children also reported hopelessness, depression, and fear of taking medications in front of other children, which is of special concern in the orphan population or among children at boarding schools.[32,34] Living in a rural setting is a risk for decreased ART adherence,[24] with 1 study showing that children and adolescents who live more than 10 km from medical care are more than twice as likely to be nonadherent to ART.[33]

Disclosure of Human Immunodeficiency Virus Status to Seropositive Youth

Children may be too young to understand their HIV-positive status and knowing the appropriate time and setting for disclosure is understandably often a challenge for caregivers. The WHO recommends that children of school age should be informed of their HIV-positive status and that younger children should be told in an incremental manner in relation to their cognitive capabilities.[35] In the context of a supportive caregiver relationship, disclosure has been shown to improve medication adherence,[32,33,36,37] although full disclosure is only performed 17% to 31% of the time.[38] Complicated family and social factors can also play a major role. Orphans are more likely to be given full disclosure and studies have shown that biological parents have fear of disclosing to their children due to feelings of culpability. Caregivers' fear of stigmatization, negative emotional impacts on the affected child, or uncertainty of how to disclose HIV positive status are some of the major motivations for partial disclosure or nondisclosure.[38] Physicians should be aware of the challenges of disclosure and address this as part of a social history assessment to provide guidance and refer caregivers to available resources.

Adolescent-Specific Barriers to Adherence

Adolescence presents myriad challenges for children transitioning into adulthood, including discovery of sexuality, independence, and self-identity. HIV infection in adolescents adds an enormous burden and without adequate social support by family or caregivers adherence to ART is jeopardized. Disclosure to other family members, health care providers, and sexual partners is anxiety provoking and has been reported as a reason for nonadherence.[24] In the United States, adolescents who acquire HIV through risk behaviors reported higher rates of nonadherence than those who acquired HIV perinatally.[25] Many perinatally infected adolescents have been linked to care since an early age and are more likely to have an involved caregiver and access to health care services, such as medication delivery.[25] Regardless of the means of transmission, caregivers reported that depression, poor self-image, and peer pressure all affected adolescents' likelihood of taking their ART regimen. Anticipated or experienced stigma was reported as the main barrier to adherence in adolescents living with HIV.[24] Stigmatizing attitudes regarding HIV are prominent throughout the world and youth living with HIV often face discrimination. Several misconceptions about HIV exist that discourage voluntary testing, taking medications in public, or going to regular health care appointments. These misapprehensions include the belief that HIV is a result of divine punishment or a result of licentious sexual practices.[39]

Facilitators of Adherence

Several themes reappear in discussions of adherence for children and adolescents. Awareness of HIV-positive status and understanding the implications and importance of ART are fundamental to fostering good habits and finding a supportive community. Social support is one of the most important facilitators of adherence,[33] which can come from caregivers, other family members, health care workers, or other peers living with HIV. Newer resources include online support groups, where those living with HIV can communicate anonymously with others and offer encouragement or ask questions.[40] Strategic planning of location, timing, and method of ART consumption is helpful for many children and adolescents. Examples given by families included using alarms and log books as reminders as well as keeping ART in a consistent location that is convenient and safe.[32] Extra support from health care facilities is also helpful for many, including transportation services, telephone calls and text message reminders for appointments, and food services.[24]

ACCESS TO CARE

Many complex factors must work in concert for successful HIV care to be delivered to children and adolescents living with HIV. A breakdown in any area of care can lead to loss of follow-up and poor outcomes for youth (**Table 1**).[5,41–46] Accessible clinics, adequately trained health care providers, funding for ART and laboratory testing, and psychosocial and adherence support are all critical components for linkage to and retention in HIV care.

The cost of care is a major barrier in resource poor countries. Laboratory reagents, in particular nucleic acid amplification tests, are expensive and may not always be available. In some African countries, poor reliability of drug supply chains for ART makes perinatal prophylaxis and consistent treatment of HIV infections impossible.[43] Even if ART and laboratory testing are free and available, delivery of these services in a setting that is realistic for patients is still needed. In Burkina Faso, a study evaluating a MTCT prevention program described pregnant women being tested for HIV in 1 prenatal HIV clinic and being referred for testing and treatment in 3 separate health care facilities before returning for further prenatal counseling.[47] Shortages in health care workers and inadequate health care training can result in insufficient services. For example, HIV testing for infants may only be offered on 1 day of each month despite recommended testing at specific time intervals after birth.[47]

In the United States, the Ryan White HIV/AIDS Program reaches 52% of all people diagnosed with HIV by providing primary medical care and support services to those who are uninsured or underinsured. Part D of the Ryan White HIV/AIDS Program focuses on providing services to women, infants, children, and adolescents. In 2015, 6.7 million Part D grant dollars were allocated to health care centers across the country, making this an invaluable resource for youth living with HIV in the United States.[48]

Human Immunodeficiency Virus Therapy

The guidelines for specific ART regimens for infants, children, and young adolescents are complex and depend on age, weight, and stage in sexual maturity. The WHO and the United States guidelines now recommend that all individuals living with HIV should initiate ART at the time of diagnosis and this should be done independent of CD4 count, viral load, or presence of clinical symptoms. Decisions regarding ART regimens should take into account HIV resistance, palatability, dosing frequency and complexity, available formulations, and practical considerations, including the volume and weight of liquid formulations. As in adults, adherence counseling should be performed routinely before initiating ART.[41]

In a study evaluating ART outcomes in children in Asia and Africa, approximately 95% of health care sites were able to provide access to first-line ART at no cost to patients. Second-line ART was provided at no cost in 88% of health care sites. Free access to treatments for opportunistic infections was less consistent, ranging from 41% to 100%. Free ART has a significant impact on retention in care. Loss to follow-up was

Table 1
Evidence-based recommendations regarding management of HIV in children and adolescents

Perinatal Transmission	Transmission Through Risk Behaviors	
Prevention	• Initiation of lifelong ART for all pregnant women living with HIV • Six weeks of antepartum ART prophylaxis for exposed newborns • Avoidance of breastfeeding for mothers without HIV viral suppression if other feeding options are available	• HIV testing and counseling • Safe condom use • Pre-exposure prophylaxis • Addressing gender norms that perpetuate inequalities • VMMC

Diagnosis	• Immunologic testing should not be performed in children younger than 18 mo of age.
	• Virologic testing is recommended in exposed infants at 14–21 d, 1–2 mo, and 4–6 mo.
	• CD4 T-lymphocyte count and plasma HIV RNA should be tested at the time of diagnosis if the child is not on active ART.
	• Testing for resistance is recommended.
	• Laboratory monitoring should occur every 3 mo.
		• HIV testing is recommended:
		  1. For key populations in all settings
		  2. For all adolescents in generalized epidemics
		  3. Should be made accessible to all adolescents in low and concentrated epidemics
		• Testing should be done in concert with pretest and posttest counseling and linkage to care.
		• Youth-friendly testing centers
		• Physician and staff knowledge of consent laws, which vary by country

Linkage to care	• Home-based HIV testing and counseling result in improved linkage to care. • Special attention should be given to high risk groups: adolescent boys who have sex with men, those who are sexually exploited, injection drug users, transgender adolescents, young girls, and orphans who may face stigma or legal consequences when seeking health care.	
ART access	• ART should be available to all children and adolescents at no cost. • Dispersible tablets, scored tablets, and avoidance of liquid/syrup formulations are recommended when possible to avoid underdosing.	
ART adherence	• Caregivers should be counseled on disclosure of HIV-positive status to the affected child as knowledge of HIV-positive status improves adherence. • Community-based approaches, including specific training of health care workers, to help address treatment adherence is recommended.	

(continued on next page)

Table 1 (continued)	
Perinatal Transmission	**Transmission Through Risk Behaviors**
Retention and engagement in care	• Community-based service delivery is associated with improved retention and reduced exposure to stigma. • All counseling and supportive services should also address sexual education. • Adolescent sexuality should be treated in a nonjudgmental and positive way. • Adolescents should be counseled about the health benefits and risks of disclosure to others and supported throughout this process.

Transitions in care	• Optimization of provider communication between adolescent and adult clinics
	• Engagement in regular multidisciplinary case conferences between adult and adolescent care providers.
	• Implementation of support groups and mental health consultation services
	• Incorporation of a family planning component into clinical care
	• Preparation of youth for life-skills development:
	  ○ Proper use of primary care physicians
	  ○ Appointment management
	  ○ Symptom recognition
	  ○ Self-efficacy with medication and insurance management

Data from Refs.[5,41–46]

5 times higher in patients who were required to pay for ART than in those who were provided ART free of cost.[43]

The Inter-Agency Task Team for Prevention and Treatment of HIV Infection in Pregnant Women, Mothers and Children and the WHO have created an Optimal Formulary and Limited-use List to guide ART use in treatment of infants and children living with HIV. The Optimal Formulary includes 2 liquid nucleoside reverse transcriptase inhibitors (NRTIs) and 1 liquid protease inhibitor. In addition, several tablets are dispersible and/or scored for more diverse dosing possibilities and methods of administration.[49] The WHO also recommends using fixed-dose combinations and dispersible tablets when these formulations are available. To avoid excessive volumes and the potential underdosing of ART, it is also recommended that liquids and syrups be avoided and caution be used when transitioning to adult formulations that may require splitting of tablets.[41] For treatment-naïve children, a 3-drug regimen consisting of a non-NRTI (NNRTI) with a boosted protease inhibitor or a dual NRTI/NNRTI backbone with an integrase strand inhibitor is recommended. For infants younger than 14 days old, there is no guideline available regarding dosing of ART.[41] Much of the available data used to develop guidelines for ART selection and dosing in children and infants rely heavily on clinical trials done in adult populations. Considering the complexity of HIV therapy for children and adolescents, it is expected that general pediatric practitioners seek additional resources and assistance from infectious disease subspecialists. Certain national resources are available, such as the Clinician Consultation Center, through the University of California, San Francisco, which provides free phone consultation from experts regarding HIV/AIDS management and perinatal HIV/AIDS.[50]

Transitions in Care

Because HIV is now a manageable chronic disease in the context of ART adherence, youth living with HIV age into an adult population. Transitioning to adult health care is a challenge because many adolescents have developed strong relationships with their pediatric HIV health care providers. Fragmentation of adult health care is difficult for adolescents with comorbid psychiatric conditions, and transitions may result in some degree of loss of anonymity or involuntary disclosure that expose youth to discrimination and stigmatizing attitudes. Several models have been proposed to standardize transition of care and prevent loss of follow-up or nonadherence. All models advise early and repeated discussions with adolescents about transitioning care. Several models include a visit to an adult physician while still being seen by the pediatric or adolescent care provider.[5]

SUMMARY

Children and adolescents are significantly and distressingly affected by the HIV pandemic. HIV treatment in the context of linkage and retention in care can provide the opportunity for HIV-positive youth to grow and thrive into adulthood. HIV care is multifaceted and challenging, but coordinated efforts to prevent HIV transmission, promote adherence to ART, and retain youth in care can, with current tools, make HIV infection a manageable chronic disease and hopefully a disappearing one.

REFERENCES

1. UNICEF. Children and aids 2016 statistical update: executive summary. 2016. Available at: http://www.childrenandaids.org/sites/default/files/Stats_Exec_Summary_IAS_July_2016.pdf. Accessed December 14, 2016.

2. Gardner EM, McLees MP, Steiner JF, et al. The spectrum of engagement in HIV care and its relevance to test-and-treat strategies for prevention of HIV infection. Clin Infect Dis 2011;52(6):793–800.

3. World Health Organization. Paediatric HIV data and statistics. Paediatric HIV Data and Statistics. 2016. Available at: http://www.who.int/hiv/topics/paediatric/data/en/. Accessed December 14, 2016.

4. Centers for Disease Control and Prevention (CDC). HIV/AIDS: HIV by group. HIV Among Pregnant Women, Infants, and Children and HIV Among Youth Web site. 2016. Available at: https://www.cdc.gov/hiv/group/gender/pregnantwomen/index.html. Accessed December 14, 2016.

5. Dowshen N, D'Angelo L. Health care transition for youth living with HIV/AIDS. Pediatrics 2011;128(4):762–71.

6. UNICEF data: monitoring the situation of children and women. 2016. Available at: https://data.unicef.org/topic/hivaids/adolescents-young-people/#. Accessed November 2, 2016.

7. Joint United Nations Programme on HIV/AIDS (UNAIDS). Global AIDS update 2016. 2016. Available at: http://www.unaids.org/sites/default/files/media_asset/global-AIDS-update-2016_en.pdf. Accessed December 14, 2016.

8. Moore AM, Awusabo-Asare K, Madise N, et al. Coerced first sex among adolescent girls in sub-saharan africa: Prevalence and context. Afr J Reprod Health 2007;11(3):62–82.

9. Arnold KB, Burgener A, Birse K, et al. Increased levels of inflammatory cytokines in the female reproductive tract are associated with altered expression of

proteases, mucosal barrier proteins, and an influx of HIV-susceptible target cells. Mucosal Immunol 2016;9(1):194–205.

10. Centers for Disease Control and Prevention (CDC). Immigrant and refugee health: screening for HIV infection during the refugee domestic medical examination. 2012. Available at: https://www.cdc.gov/immigrantrefugeehealth/guidelines/domestic/screening-hiv-infection-domestic.html. Accessed December 20, 2016.

11. Blood E, Beckwith C, Bazerman L, et al. Pregnancy among HIV-infected refugees in Rhode Island. AIDS Care 2009;21(2):207–11.

12. Schwarzwald H. Illnesses among recently immigrated children. Semin Pediatr Infect Dis 2005;16(2):78–83.

13. Fox MP, Rosen S. Systematic review of retention of pediatric patients on HIV treatment in low and middle-income countries 2008-2013. AIDS 2015;29(4):493–502.

14. Joint United Nations Programme on AIDS (UNAIDS). Prevention gap report. 2016. Available at: http://www.unaids.org/en/resources/documents/2016/prevention-gap. Accessed December 10, 2016.

15. World Health Organization. PMTCT strategic vision 2010-2015 preventing mother-to-child transmission of HIV to reach to the UNGASS and millennium development goals. 2010. Available at: http://www.who.int/hiv/pub/mtct/strategic_vision/en/. Accessed December 10, 2016.

16. AVERT: Prevention of mother-to-child transmission (PMTCT) of HIV. 2016. Available at: http://www.avert.org/professionals/hiv-programming/prevention/prevention-mother-child. Accessed December 10, 2016.

17. Joint United Nations Programme on HIV/AIDS (UNAIDS). 2015 progress report on the global plan towards the elimination of new HIV infections among children and keeping their mothers alive. 2015. Available at: http://www.unaids.org/en/resources/documents/2015/JC2774_2015ProgressReport_GlobalPlan. Accessed December 10, 2016.

18. Centers for Disease Control and Prevention. HIV Surveillance Report. 2016(27). Available at: http://www.cdc.gov/hiv/library/reports/hiv-surveillance.html. Accessed December 18, 2016.

19. Nesheim S, Taylor A, Lampe MA, et al. A framework for elimination of perinatal transmission of HIV in the united states. Pediatrics 2012;130(4):738–44.

20. DREAMS innovation challenge. 2016. Available at: http://dreamschallenge.org. Accessed December 10, 2016.

21. Moses S. Male circumcision: a new approach to reducing HIV transmission. CMAJ 2009;181(8):E134–5.

22. World Health Organization. Adherence to long term therapies: Evidence for action. HIV and AIDS. 2003. Available at: http://www.who.int/chp/knowledge/publications/adherence_full_report.pdf. Accessed November 7, 2016.

23. Sethi AK, Celentano DD, Gange SJ, et al. Association between adherence to antiretroviral therapy and human immunodeficiency virus drug resistance. Clin Infect Dis 2003;37(8):1112–8.

24. Nabukeera-Barungi N, Elyanu P, Asire B, et al. Adherence to antiretroviral therapy and retention in care for adolescents living with HIV from 10 districts in Uganda. BMC Infect Dis 2015;15:520.

25. Chandwani S, Koenig LJ, Sill AM, et al. Predictors of antiretroviral medication adherence among a diverse cohort of adolescents with HIV. J Adolesc Health 2012;51(3):242–51.

26. Cohen MS, Smith MK, Muessig KE, et al. Antiretroviral treatment of HIV-1 prevents transmission of HIV-1: Where do we go from here? Lancet 2013;382(9903):1515–24.

27. Schlatter AF, Deathe AR, Vreeman RC. The need for pediatric formulations to treat children with HIV. AIDS Res Treat 2016;2016:1654938.
28. Nahirya-Ntege P, Cook A, Vhembo T, et al. Young HIV-infected children and their adult caregivers prefer tablets to syrup antiretroviral medications in africa. PLoS One 2012;7(5):e36186.
29. Shingadia D, Viani RM, Yogev R, et al. Gastrostomy tube insertion for improvement of adherence to highly active antiretroviral therapy in pediatric patients with human immunodeficiency virus. Pediatrics 2000;105(6):E80.
30. Temple ME, Koranyi KI, Nahata MC. Gastrostomy tube placement in nonadherent HIV-infected children. Ann Pharmacother 2001;35(4):414–8.
31. Miller TL, Awnetwant EL, Evans S, et al. Gastrostomy tube supplementation for HIV-infected children. Pediatrics 1995;96(4 Pt 1):696–702.
32. Fetzer BC, Mupenda B, Lusiama J, et al. Barriers to and facilitators of adherence to pediatric antiretroviral therapy in a sub-saharan setting: insights from a qualitative study. AIDS Patient Care STDS 2011;25(10):611–21.
33. Arage G, Tessema GA, Kassa H. Adherence to antiretroviral therapy and its associated factors among children at South Wollo Zone Hospitals, Northeast Ethiopia: a cross-sectional study. BMC Public Health 2014;14:365.
34. Kikuchi K, Poudel KC, Muganda J, et al. What makes orphans in kigali, rwanda, non-adherent to antiretroviral therapy? Perspectives of their caregivers. J Int AIDS Soc 2014;17:19310.
35. Krauss B, Letteney S, De Baets A, et al. Guideline on HIV disclosure counselling for children up to 12 years of age. The World Health Organization 2011;9–10. Available at: http://apps.who.int/iris/bitstream/10665/44777/1/9789241502863_eng.pdf.
36. Bikaako-Kajura W, Luyirika E, Purcell DW, et al. Disclosure of HIV status and adherence to daily drug regimens among HIV-infected children in uganda. AIDS Behav 2006;10(4 Suppl):S85–93.
37. Mellins CA, Brackis-Cott E, Dolezal C, et al. The role of psychosocial and family factors in adherence to antiretroviral treatment in human immunodeficiency virus-infected children. Pediatr Infect Dis J 2004;23(11):1035–41.
38. Atwiine B, Kiwanuka J, Musinguzi N, et al. Understanding the role of age in HIV disclosure rates and patterns for HIV-infected children in southwestern uganda. AIDS Care 2015;27(4):424–30.
39. Adejumo OA, Malee KM, Ryscavage P, et al. Contemporary issues on the epidemiology and antiretroviral adherence of HIV-infected adolescents in sub-saharan africa: a narrative review. J Int AIDS Soc 2015;18:20049.
40. Flickinger TE, DeBolt C, Waldman AL, et al. Social support in a virtual community: analysis of a clinic-affiliated online support group for persons living with HIV/AIDS. AIDS Behav 2016. [Epub ahead of print].
41. AIDSinfo. Guidelines for the use of antiretroviral agents in pediatric HIV infection. 2016. Available at: https://aidsinfo.nih.gov/guidelines/html/2/pediatric-arv-guidelines/444/regimens-recommended-for-initial-therapy-of-antiretroviral-naive-children. Accessed December 8, 2016.
42. Bobat R, Archary M, Lawler M. An update on the HIV treatment cascade in children and adolescents. Curr Opin HIV AIDS 2015;10(6):411–9.
43. Leroy V, Malateste K, Rabie H, et al. Outcomes of antiretroviral therapy in children in Asia and Africa: a comparative analysis of the IeDEA pediatric multiregional collaboration. J Acquir Immune Defic Syndr 2013;62(2):208–19.
44. Luzuriaga K, Mofenson LM. Challenges in the elimination of pediatric HIV-1 infection. N Engl J Med 2016;374(8):761–70.

45. Van Rooyen HE, Strode AE, Slack CM. HIV testing of children is not simple for health providers and researchers: legal and policy frameworks guidance in south africa. S Afr Med J 2016;106(5):37–9.

46. World Health Organization. HIV and adolescents: Guidance for HIV testing and counselling and care for adolescents living with HIV: Recommendations for a public health approach and considerations for policy-makers and managers. 2013. Available at: http://apps.who.int/iris/bitstream/10665/94334/1/9789241506168_eng.pdf. Accessed December 14, 2016.

47. Coulibaly M, Meda N, Yonaba C, et al. Missed opportunities for early access to care of HIV-infected infants in burkina faso. PLoS One 2014;9(10):e111240.

48. Health Resource and service Administration. About the Ryan white HIV/AIDS program. Part D: Services for Women, Infants, Children, and Youth Web site. 2016. Available at: https://hab.hrsa.gov/about-ryan-white-hivaids-program/part-d-services-women-infants-children-and-youth. Accessed December 14, 2016.

49. Inter-Agency Task Team (IATT) for Prevention and Treatment of HIV Infection in Pregnant Women, Mother and Children. IATT paediatric ARV formulary and limited-use list: 2016 update. August 2016:1–9. Available at: http://emtct-iatt.org/wp-content/uploads/2016/10/Updated-Ped-ARV-Formulary-List-5-Sept-2016-1.pdf.

50. Clinician Consultation Center: Clinician consultation. 2016. Available at: http://nccc.ucsf.edu/. Accessed December 20, 2016.

Tuberculosis in Children

Tania A. Thomas, MD, MPH

KEYWORDS

- Tuberculosis • Global epidemiology • Latent infection • Diagnosis • Management
- Prevention • Advocacy

KEY POINTS

- Although tuberculosis (TB) is a preventable condition, it remains a major cause of childhood morbidity and mortality worldwide.
- Young children are at especially high risk of progressing to active TB after exposure.
- Because an accurate diagnostic test for TB in children does not exist, making a confirmatory diagnosis is challenging and requires clinical acumen.
- TB treatment is lengthy, and child-friendly drug formulations are urgently needed.

INTRODUCTION

Despite achieving great public health strides to control tuberculosis (TB) within the United States, it remains an enormous public health issue worldwide. Accurate statistics on pediatric TB cases are difficult to obtain for a multitude of reasons, including under-recognition, challenges in confirming the diagnosis, and under-reporting to national TB programs. The clinical and radiographic manifestations are less specific in children compared with adults and are often confused with bacterial pneumonia. Microbiologic confirmation of disease is limited by the paucibacillary nature of TB in children. In general, TB cultures and newer rapid molecular tests are positive in the minority of children, generally less than 25% to 40% of children with TB disease.[1,2] Additionally, there are often logistic challenges in obtaining adequate specimens from young children. However, in the era of multidrug-resistant TB, in which the organism is resistant to isoniazid and rifampin (the 2 most potent first-line agents), there is an increasing need to attempt culture-confirmation on all children suspected of having TB to inform treatment decisions. Among children who are started on TB therapy, families struggle with proper dose administration due to the lack of pediatric drug formulations and there are programmatic gaps in notifying the national TB programs, leading to under-reporting by the World Health Organization (WHO). Yet, with proper

Disclosure Statement: T.A. Thomas reports no financial conflicts of interest. T.A. Thomas is supported by NIH K23 AI097197.
Division of Infectious Diseases and International Health, University of Virginia, PO Box 801340, Charlottesville, VA 22908-1340, USA
E-mail address: tat3x@virginia.edu

management, including timely treatment initiation with appropriate drug dosages, treatment outcomes are generally favorable.

EPIDEMIOLOGY

The global distribution of childhood TB mirrors that of adults (**Fig. 1**), with a heavy burden of disease in sub-Saharan Africa and Asia.[3] The United States is considered a low-incidence country with less than 4 cases per 100,000 population. Domestically, most TB cases are associated with foreign birth.[4] Between 2008 and 2010, there were 2660 children and adolescents diagnosed with TB.[5] Among them, 31% were foreign born youth. Of the remaining US-born cases, 66% had at least 1 parent who was foreign-born. These trends suggest that most domestic TB cases in children may be exposed in international settings or through foreign-born parents, thus highlighting an opportunity for increased prevention efforts.

Only recently have systematic attempts been made to quantify the disease burden of TB in children on a global scale. In response to increasing attention and demand, the WHO published pediatric-specific disease estimates for the first time in 2012, reporting approximately 500,000 cases of TB among children younger than 15 years of age.[6] However, these were based on extrapolations from adult data, which were heavily weighted on sputum-smear positivity and did not incorporate sufficient adjustments to account for underdetection and under-reporting in pediatric populations.[7] Subsequent modifications to the mathematical models have been incorporated, relying more on transmission dynamics, household demographics, and population-based age structures.[8–10] As a result, the WHO estimates for pediatric TB in the ensuing years doubled: in 2015, the children made up approximately 1 million (10%) of the 10.4 million incident cases.[3] This immense variation in estimated disease burden highlights the challenges in detecting and reporting pediatric TB cases and stresses the importance in resolving these gaps to inform resource allocation and public health efforts.

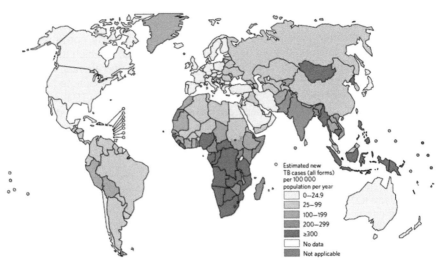

Fig. 1. Estimated TB incidence rates in 2015. (*From* WHO Global Tuberculosis Report 2016; with permission.)

Similarly, the estimated pediatric mortality burden from TB is poorly quantified. The WHO estimated 210,000 deaths from TB among children in 2015, 24% of whom were coinfected with human immunodeficiency virus (HIV).[3] In many high-burden regions, deaths from TB are often generalized as being due to pneumonia or meningitis. In a recent systematic review from the Child Health Epidemiology Reference Group (CHERG), established by the WHO and the United Nations Children's Fund (UNICEF), using vital registration and verbal autopsy data, TB was not included as a specific cause of mortality in children younger than 5 years of age.[11] However, it has long been known that TB disproportionately affects young children:

- Mortality from TB is highest among the very young (0–4 years of age) compared with any other age group.[12]
- Infants and young children carry a higher risk of disseminated disease, including TB meningitis and miliary TB, each with associated mortality.[13–15]

The global TB community is working toward "zero TB deaths in children"[16] and meeting this goal relies on coordinated efforts to improve awareness, diagnosis, reporting, and treatment outcomes.

PATHOGENESIS

M tuberculosis complex organisms, which include *M africanum*, *M bovis*, *M bovis* Bacille Calmette-Guerin (BCG), and *M canetti* (and others that do not typically affect humans), are transmitted via the respiratory route when small (1–5 μm) infected droplet nuclei are aerosolized from people with pulmonary or laryngeal TB and inhaled into the alveoli by close contacts.[17] There are many unknown details about the biological events that transpire during early stages of exposure and infection. Alveolar macrophages and dendritic cells are among the first cells to detect and ingest the mycobacteria. Along with additional innate antimicrobial mediators, they trigger a cascade of innate immunologic events to activate complement pathways, stimulate chemokine and proinflammatory cytokine production, including interferon-gamma (IFN-γ) and tumor necrosis factor-alpha (TNF-α), and augment opsonization and phagocytosis to clear or control the infection.[18] If this fails or is insufficient, the mycobacteria can invade the lung parenchyma. Adaptive immune responses are triggered when macrophages and dendritic cells present *M tuberculosis* antigens to T cells, including helper T (Th)-1 type CD4+ T-cells, CD8+ cytotoxic T cells, and gamma-delta (γδ) T cells, which further potentiate key cytokine secretion for *M tuberculosis* control.[19] Historically, B cells were not considered to be an important component in TB immunopathogenesis; however, there is growing evidence to suggest that B cells mediate protection through antigen presentation, cytokine production, and antibody production via interactions with T cells.[20,21] Ultimately, clinicians rely on measuring the T-cell–mediated immune responses as an indication of TB infection, through the IFN-γ release assays (IGRAs) and the tuberculin skin test (TST).

Effective immune responses may lead to complete clearance of the pathogen, or containment in a quiescent state. Inadequate or inappropriate immune responses lead to continued replication of the pathogen with progression to pulmonary disease and possible dissemination to extrapulmonary sites. Age and immunologic function are the biggest drivers of progressive disease. Infants and young children have the highest propensity to progress to active, disseminated disease due to the age-related deficiencies and/or downregulation of key immunologic factors (**Fig. 2**).[22,23] Importantly, the risk of TB disease follows a bimodal pattern. Although children between the ages of 5 to 10 years are at the lowest risk of progressing to disease,

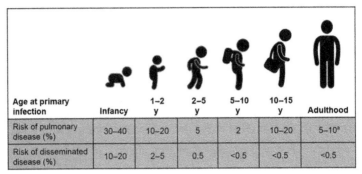

Age at primary infection	Infancy	1–2 y	2–5 y	5–10 y	10–15 y	Adulthood
Risk of pulmonary disease (%)	30–40	10–20	5	2	10–20	5–10[a]
Risk of disseminated disease (%)	10–20	2–5	0.5	<0.5	<0.5	<0.5

Fig. 2. Age-related risks of TB disease after primary infection in the prechemotherapy era.[a] Lifetime risk. (*Adapted from* Marais BJ, Gie RP, Schaaf HS, et al. The clinical epidemiology of childhood pulmonary tuberculosis: a critical review of literature from the pre-chemotherapy era. Int J Tuberc Lung Dis 2004;8(3):278–85.)

adolescents carry higher risks, including reactivation of *M tuberculosis* manifesting as active disease after years of successful containment.[5,23]

Additional factors that affect progression of disease include

- Time since exposure, with greatest risk in the first 2 years after exposure
- Mycobacterial burden of exposure
- The virulence of the mycobacterial strain.

Host and environmental risk factors associated with progression include

- Immunocompromising states such as HIV with acquired immune deficiency syndrome (AIDS), malignancy, and chronic renal disease[24,25]
- Socioeconomic conditions such as malnutrition and overcrowding[26,27]
- Environmental exposure to tobacco and indoor air pollutants.[27–29]

NATURAL HISTORY OF DISEASE

TB is often oversimplified as having 2 possible clinical states: latent TB infection (LTBI) or active disease. However, as global targets to end the TB epidemic by 2030 are neared,[30] there is a renewed appreciation for the historically described spectrum of manifestations, including pathogen clearance, dormant states of infection, subclinical disease, nonsevere disease, and severe TB disease[31,32] (**Fig. 3**). A better understanding of the spectrum of TB may improve resource allocation by focusing treatment and prevention efforts on susceptible individuals, thereby bringing TB control closer.

Immediately after exposure and primary infection from an infectious TB case, there are generally no clinical or radiologic manifestations. It may be possible for humans to clear the pathogen after close contact with infectious sources.[31] Clearance of the pathogen may be attributed to genetic resistance to infection or other innate immune responses.[33–36] If clearance occurs through T-cell independent mechanisms, IGRA and TST results should be negative. However, clearance may also occur through T-cell–mediated immunity, which would manifest with positive IGRA and TST results. This latter phenomenon may explain why some people who are diagnosed as having LTBI ultimately have a low likelihood of ever developing active TB disease.[31] However, how often this truly occurs in young children is not well documented.

As per historical description of the timetable of primary TB in children by pediatrician Arvid Wallgren,[37] it takes approximately 4 to 12 weeks after exposure for the

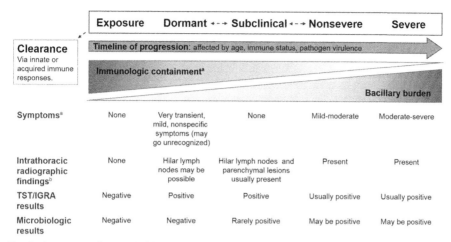

Fig. 3. Spectrum of TB in children. [a] Symptomatology may reflect the intense immunologic reaction to the bacilli, rather than the bacillary burden itself. [b] Findings may not be present if a child has extra-thoracic TB.

adaptive immune responses to reflect evidence of TB infection, as measured by the IGRA and TST. During this period, there is local extension of the infection into the lung parenchyma, termed a Ghon focus, which can manifest clinically with mild, self-limiting, and nonspecific respiratory symptoms, including hypersensitivity reactions such as fevers, erythema nodosum, or phlyctenular conjunctivitis.[23] As demonstrated in contact tracing reports, chest radiographs at this time may also demonstrate transient lymphadenopathy in the hilar and/or mediastinal regions; together with the Ghon focus this is termed a Ghon complex.[38,39] From the regional lymph nodes, the mycobacteria are capable of traversing through the lymphatics into the systemic circulation, allowing for occult hematogenous spread and seeding of distant sites that may serve as a nidus for future disease. Yet, in the absence of effective immunologic control, this stage confers great risk of developing miliary TB and TB meningitis, although the exact pathogenesis of the latter is still under debate.[40,41] In the approximate 6 months that ensue, intrathoracic lymph node enlargement and/or parenchymal disease may develop; older children may develop pleural effusions. These manifestations can be associated with respiratory and systemic symptoms. In some children, calcifications may develop approximately 1 to 2 years after primary infection; this is associated with a reduced risk of further disease progression.[37,38] However, late manifestations of TB, including reactivation of TB within the lungs or at extrapulmonary sites, do occur.[42]

CLINICAL MANIFESTATIONS OF DISEASE

M tuberculosis is capable of infecting nearly any organ (**Table 1**); however, the most common clinical manifestations of disease are found within the thoracic cavity and peripheral lymph nodes.

Common intrathoracic manifestations include mediastinal or hilar lymphadenopathy and pulmonary parenchymal lesions. Less commonly, the pleura or pericardium become involved. Isolated intrathoracic lymphadenopathy may be detected early after

Table 1 Extrathoracic manifestation of tuberculosis disease	
Organ System	**Potential Disease Manifestations**
Central nervous system	Meningitis, tuberculoma, stroke
Ocular	Uveitis, phlyctenular conjunctivitis[a]
Otic or nasopharyngeal	Chronic suppurative otitis media, mastoiditis, tonsillitis, laryngeal involvement
Cardiac	Pericardial effusion, secondary right-sided heart failure from extensive pulmonary disease and bronchiectasis
Abdominal	Peritonitis, enteritis, involvement of lymph nodes, visceral involvement (especially liver and spleen)
Genitourinary[b]	Genital involvement possible for females > males, interstitial nephritis, glomerulonephritis
Osteoarticular	Vertebral osteomyelitis, other skeletal involvement possible (especially tubular and flat bones), dactylitis, joint effusions or arthritis (less common), reactive arthritis (Poncet disease)
Lymphatic	Peripheral (cervical > axillary > inguinal region) or central adenopathy
Cutaneous	Numerous manifestations from exogenous infection (chancres, warts) or endogenous spread (lupus vulgaris, pustulonodular lesions), Erythema induratum of Bazin

[a] Hypersensitivity reaction.
[b] Uncommonly seen in young children due to long latency for reactivation in these organs.

infection and is often not associated with symptoms. However, as these inflammatory reactions progress and lymph nodes enlarge, complications can ensue:

- Small airways may become obstructed or compressed, which may manifest with cough, wheezing, or dyspnea.
- Lymph nodes may caseate or necrose, erupting into the airway, leading to bronchopneumonia and manifesting with cough, dyspnea, malaise, and fever.
- Hypersensitivity reactions may also occur, including pleural effusions, which may provoke symptoms of chest pain, fever, and reduced endurance.

The symptomatology is largely nonspecific and thus can easily be confused with bacterial or viral causes of pneumonia. The classic description of a chronic cough may apply, but it is also important to recognize that young children have a propensity to progress rapidly to disease after exposure. Indeed, TB as a cause of acute pneumonia among young, immunocompromised children is under-recognized.[43] Systematic reviews report *M tuberculosis* as a culture-confirmed pathogen in 7.5% to 12% of children younger than 5 years of age with pneumonia from TB-endemic areas.[43,44] This is a notable finding given the paucibacillary nature of pediatric TB disease.

Extrathoracic manifestations make up approximately 20% to 40% of TB cases, although concomitant overlap with pulmonary disease can occur. The most commonly involved extrathoracic sites are the peripheral lymph nodes or the central nervous system. Lymphadenitis often manifests in the cervical regions with enlarged, painless lymph nodes. Examination typically reveals a solitary rubbery node that lacks erythema or warmth. Over time, adjacent nodes may become palpable and the lesion grows matted and fixed; sinus fistulas may also form. Especially in countries with low TB incidence, other nontuberculous mycobacteria (NTM) are capable of manifesting with lymphadenitis.

Disease within the central nervous system represents the most serious complication of TB, with significant morbidity or mortality occurring in approximately 50% of cases.[45,46] Contributing to the devastating consequences of disease are the subacute onset and nonspecific systemic symptoms during the early stages, such as irritability, fever, and anorexia, and possible focal respiratory or gastrointestinal symptoms. As disease progresses, findings of meningitis become apparent, including vomiting, altered consciousness, convulsions, meningismus, cranial nerve palsies, or signs of raised intracranial pressure. Complications include hydrocephalus, cerebrovascular disease such as stroke and vasculitis, tuberculoma, and coma.[47] Early diagnosis is the key to improved outcomes. However, in the absence of reliable diagnostic tools, a high index of clinical suspicion is required, not only in TB-endemic regions but also in low-TB-burden countries with migrant populations.[48]

DISEASE IN SPECIAL POPULATIONS

Perinatal infection from *M tuberculosis* is thought to be a rare but serious event. It can occur from hematogenous spread of the bacilli from an infected mother through the placenta, which typically results in primary infection of the fetal liver, or directly into the amniotic fluid with subsequent aspiration and infection of the lungs or gastrointestinal tract.[49] TB of the reproductive organs was historically associated with infertility; however, direct extension of TB to the uterus is increasingly being described as a mechanism for congenital TB in the era of improved assistive reproductive technology.[50] Additionally, respiratory transmission may occur postnatally. Symptoms of disease are nonspecific and are indistinguishable from bacterial sepsis or congenital viral infections, and may manifest as early as 2 to 3 weeks of age. A high clinical index of suspicion is required for this relatively uncommon event.

Adolescence represents another uniquely susceptible time for TB progression (see **Fig. 2**). Disease presentation can digress from typical childhood manifestations to include aspects of adult-type TB, including cavitary pulmonary TB or extrathoracic manifestations that are associated with longer incubation periods, such as genitourinary TB.[51] Health care providers should inquire about concurrent substance abuse because this may call for additional counseling or monitoring that is not routinely conducted for younger children. Anxiety and depression may be common, exacerbated by infection control and contact investigation procedures, as well as stigma associated with the diagnosis.[52] These factors, combined with behavioral aspects, add to the vulnerabilities in this population and may lead to poor outcomes, including challenges related to adherence and follow-up.[53,54]

Across the world, HIV infection is the strongest risk factor for TB. Children experience indirect as well as direct effects of HIV. Children who are HIV-uninfected but exposed to others who are HIV-positive also bear an increased risk of TB infection and disease.[55,56] Those who are infected with HIV have impaired cell-mediated immunity to control TB infection, conferring a higher risk of progression to active TB disease after exposure; of reactivation of latent infection; and of severe disease manifestations.[57] Timely recognition of HIV and initiation of antiretroviral therapy (ART) is essential for immune restoration and improved TB control; also important are repeated screening for TB in the early months of ART, as well as provision of isoniazid preventive therapy (in all children who have been ruled out for active TB) and cotrimoxazole therapy.[58–61]

DIAGNOSIS

There are various challenges in confirming the diagnosis of TB in children, which stem from the subtle or nonspecific radiographic findings and the paucibacillary nature of disease.[16,62,63] To date, an accurate diagnostic test for pediatric TB does not exist.

Thus, it is essential for clinicians to note that TB is often a clinical diagnosis and, given the poor sensitivity of current diagnostic tools, a negative test does not rule out disease in children.

Confirmatory Tests

A confirmatory diagnosis relies on detecting the pathogen directly; alternative approaches include detecting the histopathologic or host immune response to the pathogen. Direct pathogen-based tests include TB culture, nucleic acid amplification tests (NAATs), and smear microscopy:

- Mycobacterial culture is the gold-standard test for TB, with a limit of detection (LOD) of approximately 10 to 100 colony forming units per milliliter (CFU/mL) in solid or liquid culture media.
  - The sensitivity is generally only 7% to 40% in children due to the paucibacillary nature of disease in this subpopulation.[1,64–66]
  - The time required (up to 6 weeks for positive growth) is sometimes too lengthy to be clinically useful; however, this is a necessary step to conduct phenotypic drug susceptibility testing.
  - When M tuberculosis is isolated, it is important to perform drug-sensitivity testing against first-line TB drugs as a start, and against second-line TB drugs as needed.
- Although smear microscopy and NAATs are much faster than culture, these assays are also contingent on the bacillary burden and the sensitivity is even further reduced.[67–71]
  - Smear microscopy has a LOD of approximately 10,000 CFU/mL, conferring limited utility in pediatric TB cases.
  - The newer GeneXpert MTB/RIF (Cepheid, Sunnyvale, California, USA) assay is a NAAT that detects M tuberculosis DNA and concomitant resistance to rifampicin with an LOD of 131 CFU/mL.[72] The hands-free and automated nature of this rapid cartridge-based test has contributed to its wide spread implementation throughout high-TB burden settings.[73]
  - GeneXpert only has a pooled sensitivity of approximately 66% compared with TB culture in pediatric populations.[2]
  - Repeated sampling offers incremental yield.[67,68,70]

Of course, collecting a deep respiratory specimen for TB culture from a young child brings added challenges. Most children younger than 7 years do not have the tussive force and/or the oromotor coordination to produce a good-quality expectorated sputum specimen on command. Semi-invasive techniques, such as gastric aspiration and lavage, or sputum induction with or without nasopharyngeal aspiration, may be required. With procedural training, sputum induction provides at least similar microbiologic yield compared with gastric aspiration.[64,65,74] An alternative method of obtaining respiratory specimens includes the use of the string test in which a gelatin capsule containing a nylon string is swallowed and later retrieved for TB culture. The procedure is tolerable for children who can swallow and culture yield seems comparable to sputum induction in preliminary studies.[75,76] Detecting the organism in stool may be an option where GeneXpert MTB/RIF testing is available.[77,78]

In extrapulmonary TB, site-specific specimens for TB culture are often collected, such as cerebrospinal fluid, lymph node aspirates, and other tissue specimens. However, the yield is variable. Mycobacterial blood cultures seem to be of limited yield in children compared with adults.[64,79–81] Histopathologic diagnosis is more commonly pursued in extrapulmonary TB. The overall yield is not well characterized, and depends somewhat on the experience of the proceduralist and pathologist; sensitivity and specificity may be hindered by other granulomatous processes.[82]

Screening Tests

Host immune responses can be harnessed to determine immunologic evidence of exposure to *M tuberculosis*. However, the currently available immunodiagnostics are not able to distinguish between latent infection and active disease. The TST is the oldest screening test for TB and works by measuring a delayed-type hypersensitivity reaction to various mycobacterial antigens within the purified protein derivative. It is well recognized that this test suffers from lack of sensitivity and specificity.[83] To minimize the false-negative and false-positive rates, different cutoffs are used to interpret the findings based on epidemiologic (ie, recent exposure) and individual (ie, host immune response, age) factors.

The newer IGRAs address the issue of specificity cross-reactivity by using particular antigens that are absent from *M bovis* BCG and many other NTM species; this confers a performance advantage among BCG-vaccinated children. Both of the 2 commonly used commercial assays, the T-Spot.TB (Oxford Immunotec, Abingdon, UK) and the QuantiFERON-TB Gold (Qiagen, Hilden, Germany), require a whole blood sample to measure IFN-γ secretion from CD4$^+$ T cells in response to ex vivo stimulation with RD-1 antigens; neither is preferred over the other.[84] They rely on intact cell-mediated immunity, which may hinder performance in very young children and/or children coinfected with HIV, 2 populations who would benefit most from an accurate diagnostic assay.[85] Advisory bodies have recommended caution when using IGRAs in children younger than 5 years of age due to a lack of data and favor the use of the TST.[86,87] However, increasing experience suggests potential utility in young children, particularly those between 2 to 5 years of age.[84,88]

Overall, when using these screening tests it is helpful to note that

- Each test has inherent limitations leading to false-positives or false-negatives.
- Routine screening should be avoided in favor of targeted testing among children with at least 1 risk factor for TB.
- Neither test can discriminate between latent infection and active disease.
- Among symptomatic children, a negative test (TST or IGRA) never rules out TB disease.[89]

Clearly, improved diagnostics are urgently needed for children.[63] Newer methods that have been evaluated in limited pediatric studies have focused on nonrespiratory specimens, including blood-based assays, such as the T-cell activation marker (TAM) assay, which harnesses host immune responses as a diagnostic biomarker[90]; and transcriptomic studies, which hold promise as a diagnostic and prognostic marker.[91–93] Other biomarkers that have shown promise in adult populations, such as the antibodies in lymphocyte supernatant assay (ALS) and the urinary lipoarabinomannan (LAM) assay, have not shown consistent results in pediatric populations.[94–98] Using feasibly obtained specimens, such as urine, would confer a notable advantage as a point-of-care diagnostic test, and further work in this area is warranted.

Imaging

Given the lack of accurate diagnostic assays, imaging studies serve an important role in the diagnosis of intrathoracic TB. Chest radiographs are the most commonly used method. However, the findings can be relatively nonspecific and interobserver variation may exist, even among experienced clinicians.[99,100] Suggestive findings include

- Intrathoracic lymphadenopathy, for which a lateral film may have additive yield[101]
- Complications such as airway compression
- Air-space disease, which may be indistinguishable from other causes of pneumonia
- Miliary nodules or cavitation (less common).

Computer-aided detection for pulmonary TB has shown initial promise among adults, although performance is reduced in smear-negative (ie, paucibacillary) disease[102]; this technology has not yet been validated among children. Other modalities, such as dose-reduced computed tomography (CT) scans, fluorine-18-fluorodeoxyglucose (FDG)-PET imaging, and MRI, may provide additional detail but are not routinely used in children.

MANAGEMENT

Treatment regimens for pediatric TB have been largely adapted from adults. Because of the slow growth of mycobacteria and the dormant state of many bacilli, the duration of treatment is quite lengthy. Additional considerations include

- Treatment of latent TB requires 3 to 9 months, depending on whether a monotherapy or combination therapy approach is used.
- The short-course regimen for active TB requires 6 months
- More severe forms of TB, including TB meningitis and drug-resistant TB, require 12 or more months of therapy.

Traditional treatment of LTBI typically includes 9-months of isoniazid daily with pyridoxine (for breastfeeding infants, adolescents, and others with low pyridoxine intake). The newer regimen of isoniazid and rifapentine weekly for 12 doses is safe and effective in children 2 to 17 years of age and may improve adherence rates.[103] However, it is currently only available through directly observed therapy (DOT) programs, which may not be routinely available. In attempts to improve completion rates, some experts have increasingly used the 4-month regimen of rifampin, which had typically been recommended for LTBI treatment among those exposed to isoniazid-resistant strains.[104,105]

The standard approach to drug-susceptible TB relies on combination drug therapy with isoniazid, rifampin, pyrazinamide, and ethambutol for the first 2 months, followed by 4 months of isoniazid and rifampin. DOT, typically through a public health department, is recommended to assist with delivery of medications that may be unpalatable, improve adherence, monitor for toxicity, and provide additional support. However, this brings added costs and may not be routinely available.

If drug resistance is confirmed or presumed through an epidemiologic link, treatment should be based on drug susceptibility results (using the index case's results when appropriate). A minimum of 4 active drugs should be used, including an injectable agent. Because of variable efficacy of some second-line drugs, and increased risks of toxicities, treatment decisions should be made in conjunction with a specialist.[86] Close monitoring is required to ensure culture conversion, clinical resolution, and minimize side effects and long-term sequelae.[106]

For the first time in decades, there are newer anti-TB drugs available and in the pipelines. Including children in preclinical and clinical pharmacokinetic studies and efficacy trials is imperative to meeting the goals for global TB control.[107,108] Equally urgent is the need for child-friendly first-line and second-line drugs that are palatable, easily administered, and less toxic.

PREVENTION

TB is a preventable condition that requires coordinated systematic efforts. A child with active TB represents a sentinel event, typically reflecting ongoing transmission in the community. Infection control measures conferring great strides in TB control include household contact investigation of index cases and treatment of LTBI, and these strategies are increasingly being adopted in settings with high TB burden.[30,109] In addition to these public health efforts, primary care providers have an important role in TB control by conducting annual targeted LTBI screening.[86,110]

For decades, the BCG vaccine has been widely used to protect against childhood TB. Although the vaccine is not perfect, it is estimated that 1 year of BCG vaccination prevents over 117,000 deaths per pediatric (<15 years of age) birth cohort.[111,112] However, production issues have led to sizable shortfalls in supply since 2013, which have not completely been resolved. Modeling studies have estimated that the recent shortages may contribute to nearly 20,000 excess childhood deaths from TB.[112]

The development of new and improved TB vaccines is hindered by insufficient understanding of the correlates of protection. As was realized after the modified vaccinia Ankara 85A (MVA85A) TB vaccine trial among human infants, experimental animal models have been unreliable in predicting responses in humans.[113] However, various TB vaccine strategies are under study, including modifications to replace the current BCG, novel vaccines designed to boost responses among BCG recipients, and therapeutic vaccines designed to aid those undergoing TB treatment.[114]

SUMMARY

TB remains a major threat to child health worldwide. Global migration requires that clinicians in low-incidence countries maintain awareness for TB because timely recognition is key, especially in young children. A turning point has been reached in which increased advocacy has stimulated major efforts toward recognition and control of TB in children. However, there is much to be done to meet the ambitious programmatic targets, including widespread uptake of proven prevention efforts and development of newer strategies, including effective vaccines. Dedicated research and development are need for accurate, child-friendly, and fieldable diagnostics. Pediatric-specific studies are necessary to define the best approach to childhood TB using tolerable drugs, especially for drug-resistant TB. All of this requires coordinated efforts and adequate funding. The momentum must continue to end the neglect of childhood TB.

REFERENCES

1. Starke JR. Pediatric tuberculosis: time for a new approach. Tuberculosis (Edinb) 2003;83(1–3):208–12.
2. World Health Organization. Automated real-time nucleic acid amplification technology for rapid and simultaneous detection of tuberculosis and rifampicin resistance: Xpert MTB/RIF assay for the diagnosis of pulmonary and extrapulmonary TB in adults and children. Policy update. Geneva (Switzerland): World Health Organization; 2013.
3. World Health Organization. Global tuberculosis report 2016. Geneva (Switzerland): World Health Organization; 2016.
4. CDC. Reported Tuberculosis in the United States, 2014. 2015. Available at: http://www.cdc.gov/tb/statistics/reports/2014. Accessed November 30, 2016.

5. Winston CA, Menzies HJ. Pediatric and adolescent tuberculosis in the United States, 2008-2010. Pediatrics 2012;130(6):e1425–1432.

6. World Health Organization. Global tuberculosis report 2012 (in IRIS). Geneva (Switzerland): World Health Organization; 2012.

7. Seddon JA, Jenkins HE, Liu L, et al. Counting children with tuberculosis: why numbers matter. Int J Tuberc Lung Dis 2015;19(Suppl 1):9–16.

8. Dodd PJ, Gardiner E, Coghlan R, et al. Burden of childhood tuberculosis in 22 high-burden countries: a mathematical modelling study. Lancet Glob Health 2014;2(8):e453–459.

9. Jenkins HE, Tolman AW, Yuen CM, et al. Incidence of multidrug-resistant tuberculosis disease in children: systematic review and global estimates. Lancet 2014;383(9928):1572–9.

10. World Bank. Population ages 0-14. 2015. Available at: http://data.worldbank.org/indicator/SP.POP.0014.TO.ZS. Accessed November 30, 2016.

11. Liu L, Oza S, Hogan D, et al. Global, regional, and national causes of child mortality in 2000-13, with projections to inform post-2015 priorities: an updated systematic analysis. Lancet 2015;385(9966):430–40.

12. Frost WH. The age selection of mortality from tuberculosis in successive decades. 1939. Am J Epidemiol 1995;141(1):4–9 [discussion: 3].

13. Karande S, Gupta V, Kulkarni M, et al. Prognostic clinical variables in childhood tuberculous meningitis: an experience from Mumbai, India. Neurol India 2005; 53(2):191–5 [discussion: 195–6].

14. van Toorn R, Springer P, Laubscher JA, et al. Value of different staging systems for predicting neurological outcome in childhood tuberculous meningitis. Int J Tuberc Lung Dis 2012;16(5):628–32.

15. Sharma SK, Mohan A, Sharma A, et al. Miliary tuberculosis: new insights into an old disease. Lancet Infect Dis 2005;5(7):415–30.

16. World Health Organization. Roadmap for childhood tuberculosis: towards zero deaths. Geneva (Switzerland): World Health Organization; 2013.

17. Fennelly KP, Martyny JW, Fulton KE, et al. Cough-generated aerosols of *Mycobacterium tuberculosis*: a new method to study infectiousness. Am J Respir Crit Care Med 2004;169(5):604–9.

18. Basu Roy R, Whittaker E, Kampmann B. Current understanding of the immune response to tuberculosis in children. Curr Opin Infect Dis 2012;25(3):250–7.

19. Lewinsohn DA, Gennaro ML, Scholvinck L, et al. Tuberculosis immunology in children: diagnostic and therapeutic challenges and opportunities. Int J Tuberc Lung Dis 2004;8(5):658–74.

20. Chan J, Mehta S, Bharrhan S, et al. The role of B cells and humoral immunity in *Mycobacterium tuberculosis* infection. Semin Immunol 2014;26(6):588–600.

21. Rao M, Valentini D, Poiret T, et al. B in TB: B cells as mediators of clinically relevant immune responses in tuberculosis. Clin Infect Dis 2015;61(Suppl 3): S225–34.

22. Vanden Driessche K, Persson A, Marais BJ, et al. Immune vulnerability of infants to tuberculosis. Clin Dev Immunol 2013;2013:781320.

23. Marais BJ, Gie RP, Schaaf HS, et al. The clinical epidemiology of childhood pulmonary tuberculosis: a critical review of literature from the pre-chemotherapy era. Int J Tuberc Lung Dis 2004;8(3):278–85.

24. Ekim M, Tumer N, Bakkaloglu S. Tuberculosis in children undergoing continuous ambulatory peritoneal dialysis. Pediatr Nephrol 1999;13(7):577–9.

25. Munteanu M, Cucer F, Halitchi C, et al. The TB infection in children with chronic renal diseases [abstract only]. Rev Med Chir Soc Med Nat Iasi 2006;110(2): 309–13.

26. Jaganath D, Mupere E. Childhood tuberculosis and malnutrition. J Infect Dis 2012;206(12):1809–15.

27. Chisti MJ, Ahmed T, Shahid AS, et al. Sociodemographic, epidemiological, and clinical risk factors for childhood pulmonary tuberculosis in severely malnourished children presenting with pneumonia: observation in an Urban Hospital in Bangladesh. Glob Pediatr Health 2015;2. 2333794x15594183.

28. Patra S, Sharma S, Behera D. Passive smoking, indoor air pollution and childhood tuberculosis: a case control study. Indian J Tuberc 2012;59(3):151–5.

29. Jafta N, Jeena PM, Barregard L, et al. Childhood tuberculosis and exposure to indoor air pollution: a systematic review and meta-analysis. Int J Tuberc Lung Dis 2015;19(5):596–602.

30. World Health Organization. The end TB strategy. Geneva (Switzerland): World Health Organization; 2015.

31. Dheda K, Schwander SK, Zhu B, et al. The immunology of tuberculosis: from bench to bedside. Respirology 2010;15(3):433–50.

32. Barry CE 3rd, Boshoff HI, Dartois V, et al. The spectrum of latent tuberculosis: rethinking the biology and intervention strategies. Nat Rev Microbiol 2009; 7(12):845–55.

33. Cobat A, Gallant CJ, Simkin L, et al. Two loci control tuberculin skin test reactivity in an area hyperendemic for tuberculosis. J Exp Med 2009;206(12):2583–91.

34. Thye T, Owusu-Dabo E, Vannberg FO, et al. Common variants at 11p13 are associated with susceptibility to tuberculosis. Nat Genet 2012;44(3):257–9.

35. Cobat A, Poirier C, Hoal E, et al. Tuberculin skin test negativity is under tight genetic control of chromosomal region 11p14-15 in settings with different tuberculosis endemicities. J Infect Dis 2015;211(2):317–21.

36. Fox GJ, Orlova M, Schurr E. Tuberculosis in newborns: the lessons of the "Lubeck Disaster" (1929-1933). PLoS Pathog 2016;12(1):e1005271.

37. Wallgren A. The time-table of tuberculosis. Tubercle 1948;29(11):245–51.

38. Davies PD. The natural history of tuberculosis in children. A study of child contacts in the Brompton Hospital Child contact clinic from 1930 to 1952. Tubercle 1961;42(Suppl):1–40.

39. Marais BJ, Gie RP, Schaaf HS, et al. A proposed radiological classification of childhood intra-thoracic tuberculosis. Pediatr Radiol 2004;34(11):886–94.

40. Donald PR, Schaaf HS, Schoeman JF. Tuberculous meningitis and miliary tuberculosis: the Rich focus revisited. J Infect 2005;50(3):193–5.

41. Janse van Rensburg P, Andronikou S, van Toorn R, et al. Magnetic resonance imaging of miliary tuberculosis of the central nervous system in children with tuberculous meningitis. Pediatr Radiol 2008;38(12):1306–13.

42. Perez-Velez CM, Marais BJ. Tuberculosis in children. N Engl J Med 2012;367(4): 348–61.

43. Chisti MJ, Ahmed T, Pietroni MA, et al. Pulmonary tuberculosis in severely-malnourished or HIV-infected children with pneumonia: a review. J Health Popul Nutr 2013;31(3):308–13.

44. Oliwa JN, Karumbi JM, Marais BJ, et al. Tuberculosis as a cause or comorbidity of childhood pneumonia in tuberculosis-endemic areas: a systematic review. Lancet Respir Med 2015;3(3):235–43.

45. Chiang SS, Khan FA, Milstein MB, et al. Treatment outcomes of childhood tuberculous meningitis: a systematic review and meta-analysis. Lancet Infect Dis 2014;14(10):947–57.

46. Bang ND, Caws M, Truc TT, et al. Clinical presentations, diagnosis, mortality and prognostic markers of tuberculous meningitis in Vietnamese children: a prospective descriptive study. BMC Infect Dis 2016;16(1):573.

47. van Toorn R, Solomons R. Update on the diagnosis and management of tuberculous meningitis in children. Semin Pediatr Neurol 2014;21(1):12–8.

48. van Well GT, Paes BF, Terwee CB, et al. Twenty years of pediatric tuberculous meningitis: a retrospective cohort study in the western cape of South Africa. Pediatrics 2009;123(1):e1–8.

49. Peng W, Yang J, Liu E. Analysis of 170 cases of congenital TB reported in the literature between 1946 and 2009. Pediatr Pulmonol 2011;46(12):1215–24.

50. Flibotte JJ, Lee GE, Buser GL, et al. Infertility, in vitro fertilization and congenital tuberculosis. J Perinatol 2013;33(7):565–8.

51. Cruz AT, Hwang KM, Birnbaum GD, et al. Adolescents with tuberculosis: a review of 145 cases. Pediatr Infect Dis J 2013;32(9):937–41.

52. Franck C, Seddon JA, Hesseling AC, et al. Assessing the impact of multidrug-resistant tuberculosis in children: an exploratory qualitative study. BMC Infect Dis 2014;14:426.

53. Blok N, van den Boom M, Erkens C, et al. Variation in policy and practice of adolescent tuberculosis management in the WHO European Region. Eur Respir J 2016;48:943–6.

54. Enane LA, Lowenthal ED, Arscott-Mills T, et al. Loss to follow-up among adolescents with tuberculosis in Gaborone, Botswana. Int J Tuberc Lung Dis 2016; 20(10):1320–5.

55. Marquez C, Chamie G, Achan J, et al. Tuberculosis infection in early childhood and the association with HIV-exposure in HIV-uninfected children in rural Uganda. Pediatr Infect Dis J 2016;35(5):524–9.

56. Cotton MF, Slogrove A, Rabie H. Infections in HIV-exposed uninfected children with focus on sub-Saharan Africa. Pediatr Infect Dis J 2014;33(10):1085–6.

57. Verhagen LM, Warris A, van Soolingen D, et al. Human immunodeficiency virus and tuberculosis coinfection in children: challenges in diagnosis and treatment. Pediatr Infect Dis J 2010;29(10):e63–70.

58. Anigilaje EA, Aderibigbe SA, Adeoti AO, et al. Tuberculosis, before and after antiretroviral therapy among HIV-infected children in Nigeria: what are the risk factors? PLoS One 2016;11(5):e0156177.

59. Zar HJ, Cotton MF, Strauss S, et al. Effect of isoniazid prophylaxis on mortality and incidence of tuberculosis in children with HIV: randomised controlled trial. BMJ 2007;334(7585):136.

60. Bwakura-Dangarembizi M, Kendall L, Bakeera-Kitaka S, et al. A randomized trial of prolonged co-trimoxazole in HIV-infected children in Africa. N Engl J Med 2014;370(1):41–53.

61. Crook AM, Turkova A, Musiime V, et al. Tuberculosis incidence is high in HIV-infected African children but is reduced by co-trimoxazole and time on antiretroviral therapy. BMC Med 2016;14:50.

62. Cuevas LE, Petrucci R, Swaminathan S. Tuberculosis diagnostics for children in high-burden countries: what is available and what is needed. Paediatr Int Child Health 2012;32(Suppl 2):S30–7.

63. Nicol MP, Gnanashanmugam D, Browning R, et al. A blueprint to address research gaps in the development of biomarkers for pediatric tuberculosis. Clin Infect Dis 2015;61(Suppl 3):S164–72.

64. Thomas TA, Heysell SK, Moodley P, et al. Intensified specimen collection to improve tuberculosis diagnosis in children from Rural South Africa, an observational study. BMC Infect Dis 2014;14:11.

65. Zar H, Hanslo D, Apolles P, et al. Induced sputum versus gastric lavage for microbiological confirmation of pulmonary tuberculosis in infants and young children: a prospective study. Lancet 2005;365(9454):130–4.

66. Nicol MP, Zar HJ. New specimens and laboratory diagnostics for childhood pulmonary TB: progress and prospects. Paediatr Respir Rev 2011;12(1):16–21.

67. Nicol MP, Workman L, Isaacs W, et al. Accuracy of the Xpert MTB/RIF test for the diagnosis of pulmonary tuberculosis in children admitted to hospital in Cape Town, South Africa: a descriptive study. Lancet Infect Dis 2011;11(11):819–24.

68. Zar HJ, Workman L, Isaacs W, et al. Rapid molecular diagnosis of pulmonary tuberculosis in children using nasopharyngeal specimens. Clin Infect Dis 2012;55(8):1088–95.

69. Rachow A, Clowes P, Saathoff E, et al. Increased and expedited case detection by Xpert MTB/RIF assay in childhood tuberculosis: a prospective cohort study. Clin Infect Dis 2012;54(10):1388–96.

70. Zar HJ, Workman L, Isaacs W, et al. Rapid diagnosis of pulmonary tuberculosis in African children in a primary care setting by use of Xpert MTB/RIF on respiratory specimens: a prospective study. Lancet Glob Health 2013;1(2):e97–104.

71. Detjen AK, DiNardo AR, Leyden J, et al. Xpert MTB/RIF assay for the diagnosis of pulmonary tuberculosis in children: a systematic review and meta-analysis. Lancet Respir Med 2015;3(6):451–61.

72. Helb D, Jones M, Story E, et al. Rapid detection of *Mycobacterium tuberculosis* and rifampin resistance by use of on-demand, near-patient technology. J Clin Microbiol 2010;48(1):229–37.

73. Lawn SD, Nicol MP. Xpert(R) MTB/RIF assay: development, evaluation and implementation of a new rapid molecular diagnostic for tuberculosis and rifampicin resistance. Future Microbiol 2011;6(9):1067–82.

74. Hatherill M, Hawkridge T, Zar HJ, et al. Induced sputum or gastric lavage for community-based diagnosis of childhood pulmonary tuberculosis? Arch Dis Child 2009;94(3):195–201.

75. Chow F, Espiritu N, Gilman RH, et al. La cuerda dulce–a tolerability and acceptability study of a novel approach to specimen collection for diagnosis of paediatric pulmonary tuberculosis. BMC Infect Dis 2006;6:67.

76. Nansumba M, Kumbakumba E, Orikiriza P, et al. Detection yield and tolerability of string test for diagnosis of childhood intrathoracic tuberculosis. Pediatr Infect Dis J 2016;35(2):146–51.

77. Marcy O, Ung V, Goyet S, et al. Performance of Xpert MTB/RIF and alternative specimen collection methods for the diagnosis of tuberculosis in HIV-infected children. Clin Infect Dis 2016;62(9):1161–8.

78. Banada PP, Naidoo U, Deshpande S, et al. A novel sample processing method for rapid detection of tuberculosis in the stool of pediatric patients using the Xpert MTB/RIF assay. PLoS One 2016;11(3):e0151980.

79. Pavlinac PB, Lokken EM, Walson JL, et al. *Mycobacterium tuberculosis* bacteremia in adults and children: a systematic review and meta-analysis. Int J Tuberc Lung Dis 2016;20(7):895–902.

80. Heysell SK, Thomas TA, Gandhi NR, et al. Blood cultures for the diagnosis of multidrug-resistant and extensively drug-resistant tuberculosis among HIV-infected patients from rural South Africa: a cross-sectional study. BMC Infect Dis 2010;10:344.

81. Gray KD, Cunningham CK, Clifton DC, et al. Prevalence of mycobacteremia among HIV-infected infants and children in northern Tanzania. Pediatr Infect Dis J 2013;32(7):754–6.

82. Fukunaga H, Murakami T, Gondo T, et al. Sensitivity of acid-fast staining for *Mycobacterium tuberculosis* in formalin-fixed tissue. Am J Respir Crit Care Med 2002;166(7):994–7.

83. Dunn JJ, Starke JR, Revell PA. Laboratory diagnosis of *Mycobacterium tuberculosis* infection and disease in children. J Clin Microbiol 2016;54(6):1434–41.

84. Starke JR, Byington CL, Maldonado YA, et al. Interferon-γ release assays for diagnosis of tuberculosis infection and disease in children. Pediatrics 2014; 134(6):e1763–73.

85. Mandalakas AM, Detjen AK, Hesseling AC, et al. Interferon-gamma release assays and childhood tuberculosis: systematic review and meta-analysis. Int J Tuberc Lung Dis 2011;15(8):1018–32.

86. American Academy of Pediatrics. Tuberculosis. In: Kimberlin D, Brady M, Jackson M, et al, editors. Pediatrics. 30th edition. Elk Grove Village (IL): American Academy of Pediatrics; 2015. p. 805–31.

87. Lewinsohn DM, Leonard MK, LoBue PA, et al. Official American Thoracic Society/Infectious Diseases Society of America/Centers for Disease Control and Prevention Clinical Practice Guidelines: Diagnosis of Tuberculosis in Adults and Children. Clin Infect Dis 2017;64(2):111–5.

88. Grinsdale JA, Islam S, Tran OC, et al. Interferon-gamma release assays and pediatric public health tuberculosis screening: the San Francisco program experience 2005 to 2008. J Pediatr Infect Dis Soc 2016;5(2):122–30.

89. Starke JR. Interferon-gamma release assays for the diagnosis of tuberculosis infection in children. J Pediatr 2012;161(4):581–2.

90. Portevin D, Moukambi F, Clowes P, et al. Assessment of the novel T-cell activation marker-tuberculosis assay for diagnosis of active tuberculosis in children: a prospective proof-of-concept study. Lancet Infect Dis 2014;14(10):931–8.

91. Anderson ST, Kaforou M, Brent AJ, et al. Diagnosis of childhood tuberculosis and host RNA expression in Africa. N Engl J Med 2014;370(18):1712–23.

92. Zak DE, Penn-Nicholson A, Scriba TJ, et al. A blood RNA signature for tuberculosis disease risk: a prospective cohort study. Lancet 2016;387(10035): 2312–22.

93. Zhou M, Yu G, Yang X, et al. Circulating microRNAs as biomarkers for the early diagnosis of childhood tuberculosis infection. Mol Med Rep 2016;13:4620–6.

94. Rekha RS, Kamal SM, Andersen P, et al. Validation of the ALS assay in adult patients with culture confirmed pulmonary tuberculosis. PLoS One 2011;6(1): e16425.

95. Thomas T, Brighenti S, Andersson J, et al. A new potential biomarker for childhood tuberculosis. Thorax 2011;66(8):727–9.

96. Chisti MJ, Salam MA, Raqib R, et al. Validity of antibodies in lymphocyte supernatant in diagnosing tuberculosis in severely malnourished children presenting with pneumonia. PLoS One 2015;10(5):e0126863.

97. Blok N, Visser DH, Solomons R, et al. Lipoarabinomannan enzyme-linked immunosorbent assay for early diagnosis of childhood tuberculous meningitis. Int J Tuberc Lung Dis 2014;18(2):205–10.

98. Nicol MP, Allen V, Workman L, et al. Urine lipoarabinomannan testing for diagnosis of pulmonary tuberculosis in children: a prospective study. Lancet Glob Health 2014;2(5):e278–84.

99. Du Toit G, Swingler G, Iloni K. Observer variation in detecting lymphadenopathy on chest radiography. Int J Tuberc Lung Dis 2002;6(9):814–7.

100. Swingler GH, du Toit G, Andronikou S, et al. Diagnostic accuracy of chest radiography in detecting mediastinal lymphadenopathy in suspected pulmonary tuberculosis. Arch Dis Child 2005;90(11):1153–6.

101. Smuts NA, Beyers N, Gie RP, et al. Value of the lateral chest radiograph in tuberculosis in children. Pediatr Radiol 1994;24(7):478–80.

102. Breuninger M, van Ginneken B, Philipsen RH, et al. Diagnostic accuracy of computer-aided detection of pulmonary tuberculosis in chest radiographs: a validation study from sub-Saharan Africa. PLoS One 2014;9(9):e106381.

103. Villarino ME, Scott NA, Weis SE, et al. Treatment for preventing tuberculosis in children and adolescents: a randomized clinical trial of a 3-month, 12-dose regimen of a combination of rifapentine and isoniazid. JAMA Pediatr 2015; 169(3):247–55.

104. Cruz AT, Starke JR. Safety and completion of a 4-month course of rifampicin for latent tuberculous infection in children. Int J Tuberc Lung Dis 2014;18(9): 1057–61.

105. Cruz AT, Martinez BJ. Childhood tuberculosis in the United States: shifting the focus to prevention. Int J Tuberc Lung Dis 2015;19(Suppl 1):50–3.

106. Seddon JA, Furin JJ, Gale M, et al. Caring for children with drug-resistant tuberculosis: practice-based recommendations. Am J Respir Crit Care Med 2012; 186(10):953–64.

107. Nachman S, Ahmed A, Amanullah F, et al. Towards early inclusion of children in tuberculosis drugs trials: a consensus statement. Lancet Infect Dis 2015;15(6): 711–20.

108. Srivastava S, Deshpande D, Pasipanodya JG, et al. A combination regimen design program based on pharmacodynamic target setting for childhood tuberculosis: design rules for the playground. Clin Infect Dis 2016;63(Suppl 3):S75–9.

109. Morrison J, Pai M, Hopewell PC. Tuberculosis and latent tuberculosis infection in close contacts of people with pulmonary tuberculosis in low-income and middle-income countries: a systematic review and meta-analysis. Lancet Infect Dis 2008;8(6):359–68.

110. van der Heijden YF, Heerman WJ, McFadden S, et al. Missed opportunities for tuberculosis screening in primary care. J Pediatr 2015;166(5):1240–5.e1.

111. Mangtani P, Abubakar I, Ariti C, et al. Protection by BCG vaccine against tuberculosis: a systematic review of randomized controlled trials. Clin Infect Dis 2014; 58(4):470–80.

112. Harris RC, Dodd PJ, White RG. The potential impact of BCG vaccine supply shortages on global paediatric tuberculosis mortality. BMC Med 2016;14(1):138.

113. Tameris MD, Hatherill M, Landry BS, et al. Safety and efficacy of MVA85A, a new tuberculosis vaccine, in infants previously vaccinated with BCG: a randomised, placebo-controlled phase 2b trial. Lancet 2013;381(9871):1021–8.

114. Principi N, Esposito S. The present and future of tuberculosis vaccinations. Tuberculosis (Edinb) 2015;95(1):6–13.

Influenza: A Global Perspective

Elizabeth T. Rotrosen, BA, Kathleen M. Neuzil, MD, MPH*

KEYWORDS

- Influenza • Influenza vaccines • Children • Vaccine policy • Antiviral medications

KEY POINTS

- The influenza virus circulates annually and causes global epidemics and occasional pandemics because of its ability to mutate via antigenic drift and shift, respectively.
- Children have high attack rates of influenza.
- Children younger than 5 years are at increased risk for severe or complicated influenza infections.
- Vaccination is the most effective means of protection against influenza.

INTRODUCTION

Influenza, a common, highly contagious, acute, febrile respiratory disease, is caused by influenza virus, which circulates globally. Influenza virus causes annual outbreaks, with or without seasonality, which are likely related to climate and other factors that influence transmission. The influenza virus undergoes frequent antigenic mutations, known as antigenic drift, that contribute to variability from year to year and present challenges for annual vaccine design and production. In addition, influenza poses a unique potential to cause pandemics when a novel virus emerges through genetic reassortment, or antigenic shift, resulting in a virus with surface glycoproteins against which there is little preexisting immunity in the population.

Influenza virus affects people of all ages and causes mild to severe illness and even death in some cases. According to the World Health Organization (WHO), annual epidemics of influenza result in an estimated 3 to 5 million cases of severe illness and between 250,000 and 500,000 deaths worldwide,[1] although the cocirculation of other pathogens and lack of diagnostic testing in many settings makes it difficult to accurately estimate the burden of influenza. As influenza is a vaccine-preventable illness, it is important from a global health standpoint to differentiate illnesses attributable to the influenza virus from influenza-like illnesses caused by other pathogens.

Those at increased risk for the most severe illness, or influenza-related complications, include the elderly, children younger than 5 years, and individuals of all ages,

The authors have no conflicts of interest or financial ties to disclose.
Center for Vaccine Development, University of Maryland, School of Medicine, 685 West Baltimore Street, Room 480, Baltimore, MD 21201, USA
* Corresponding author.
E-mail address: kneuzil@som.umaryland.edu

who are immunocompromised or have chronic underlying health conditions that predispose them to more severe disease, as well as pregnant women. Although health care workers are not at higher risk than the general population for influenza-related complications, they are a group that is often prioritized for vaccination to maintain the workforce and to prevent them from transmitting influenza to vulnerable patients.

Although treatment of influenza infection is available in certain settings, prevention is the better option. The best way to prevent influenza infection is by vaccination. Vaccination against influenza can prevent the primary influenza syndrome as well as complications, such as acute otitis media (AOM) or pneumonia.[2,3]

This article focuses on pediatric influenza and gives an overview of the influenza virus as well as the epidemiology of the disease. It includes information on influenza in children in low-resource settings, where available, and a discussion of influenza vaccines, treatments, and policy recommendations.

INFLUENZA IN CHILDREN: CLINICAL CHARACTERISTICS AND DISEASE BURDEN

In otherwise healthy children, influenza is typically a mild to moderate disease and, in most children, resolves without complications.[4] The most common signs and symptoms of influenza in children are sudden onset of fever, cough, and rhinorrhea. Influenza is most severe in younger children.[5–7] Symptoms, such as sore throat, headache, myalgia, and fatigue, are reported less commonly in children than adults.[8] This difference may be due in part to the inability of young children to describe these complaints. Because the signs and symptoms of influenza are not unique to this disease and the presentation of certain signs and symptoms varies among individuals, it can be difficult to diagnose influenza by clinical presentation alone; thus, a firm diagnosis generally requires laboratory confirmation.

Clinical attack rates and morbidity from influenza infection vary considerably from year to year and across geographies. When compared with adults, influenza attack rates are consistently higher in children and may reach 30% or more during selected seasons.[7,9] Data from the United States show the importance of laboratory testing in fully understanding the burden of influenza illness. Among young children, few influenza infections are recognized by clinical signs and symptoms alone; in one population-based US study of children younger than 5 years, only 17% of outpatient and 28% of inpatient cases of laboratory-confirmed influenza (LCI) received a clinical diagnosis of influenza from their health care provider before laboratory results were known.[4]

Although influenza-related hospitalization and death, discussed later, do occur, outpatient visits are far more common for all age groups. With increasing age, more children with influenza can be managed as outpatients, whereas with younger children, influenza tends to be more severe and more often requires hospitalization. In one population-based study in the United States, annual influenza-attributable outpatient visit rates were approximately 10-, 100-, and 250-fold greater than the rates of hospitalization for children younger than 5 months, 6 to 23 months, and 24 to 59 months, respectively.[4] Antibiotic use also increases as a result of influenza infections. A retrospective cohort study of children younger than 15 years over 19 influenza seasons in the United States estimated that for every 100 children, an average of 6 to 15 outpatient visits and 3 to 9 courses of antibiotics were attributable to influenza every year.[10]

LCI-related hospitalization rates are high among young children, ranging from 0.58 to 2.4 hospitalizations per 1000 children younger than 5 years per year in the United States.[4,11,12] Children younger than 6 months consistently have high rates of hospitalization, and about 80% to 85% of pediatric influenza-attributable hospitalizations are accounted for by children younger than 24 months.[4,10–14] Hospitalizations due to LCI are likely underestimated for several reasons, including lack of diagnostic testing, insensitive diagnostic methods, and influenza virus being in the causal pathway to the hospitalization but no longer present at time of testing (eg, influenza virus leading to bacterial pneumonia or asthma exacerbation).[13,15]

Influenza infections can be complicated by other secondary infections, which add considerably to the burden of influenza. Clinically, AOM is the most frequent influenza-associated syndrome. Another significant, though less common, complication of influenza is pneumonia. Although pneumococcal and *Haemophilus influenzae* type B (Hib) infections were commonly identified pathogens preceding or concomitant to influenza infection in children, such secondary infections are less frequent now that pneumococcal and Hib vaccines are routinely administered to children.[5–7,16] Hospitalized children with influenza-associated bacterial pneumonia are more likely to have a severe and complicated clinical course than those hospitalized for influenza without associated pneumonia. Influenza-associated pneumonia can be particularly dangerous in children with underlying conditions and can be fatal.[17,18] In a mortality study in children hospitalized with LCI in the United States from 2004 to 2007, *Staphylococcus aureus* was the most common bacterial infection identified in children with influenza.[19]

Although death due to influenza is rare in an individual child, the annual outbreaks and high attack rates of the disease lead to demonstrable mortality at the population level. Influenza-related pediatric deaths became reportable to the US Centers for Disease Control and Prevention in 2004. From 2004 to 2016, between 37 (in the 2011–2012 influenza season) and 288 (in the 2009–2010 influenza season) annual deaths due to LCI were reported in children younger than 18 years in the United States.[20,21] These deaths are undoubtedly an underestimate given that health care workers do not routinely test for influenza, that the tests are imperfectly sensitive, and that influenza virus may initiate the sequence of events leading to death but may no longer be detectable at the time of testing. Studies in the United States have shown that among children who died of influenza, the illness progressed rapidly to death, often within 72 hours of clinical onset, further emphasizing the importance of prevention. Although children with underlying medical conditions are at increased risk for death from influenza, a substantial proportion of influenza-attributable pediatric mortality occurs in otherwise healthy children, many of whom die before they are admitted to the hospital.[19,22]

Although global surveillance for influenza is extensive, limited data are available that specifically address influenza burden in children in low-resource settings. Outside of research studies conducted in these areas, few clinical diagnoses of influenza are confirmed in the laboratory. Nevertheless, the available data show an important and disproportionately high burden of influenza among young children in low-resource settings compared with children of a similar age in more developed areas. As in temperate settings, influenza attack rates vary from year to year in tropical settings. Recent studies in young children in Bangladesh and Senegal during the 2013 season reported laboratory-confirmed clinical influenza attack rates of 24.5% and 18.0%, respectively, for all circulating strains of influenza.[23,24] Although these rates are high, comparable attack rates in young children in the United States in other nonpandemic years have been reported.[25–28] Even if attack rates of influenza are similar in young children in low- and high-resource settings, morbidity and mortality of influenza are likely to be higher in low-resource settings, given population characteristics (eg, malnutrition), reduced or delayed access to health care, and less extensive use of pneumococcal and Hib vaccines.

A worldwide meta-analysis of data collected between 1995 and 2010 reported that the number of new episodes of influenza-associated severe acute lower respiratory infections (ALRIs) in children younger than 5 years was 15-fold greater in developing countries than in developed countries.[29] That same meta-analysis estimated between

28,000 and 111,500 deaths occurred in children younger than 5 years from influenza-related ALRIs in 2008. It was estimated that up to 99% of these deaths occurred in low-income countries.[29] A study in Bangladesh between 2008 and 2010 found that children younger than 5 years are hospitalized for influenza-associated illness at substantially higher rates than adults. The study estimated that 113,000 of 19,331,302 (0.6%) children younger than 5 years are hospitalized annually for influenza, compared with 16,000 of 132,920,875 (0.01%) persons at least 5 years of age. The study also reported that rates of hospitalization for influenza among young children in Bangladesh are disproportionately high when compared with influenza hospitalization rates among children of the same age in the United States.[30]

Influenza infection in children has consequences beyond the direct medical outcomes outlined earlier. Children shed influenza virus longer and in larger amounts than adults and, thus, play a major role in the transmission of influenza in families and society.[7,9,31–37] Influenza places a high medical and societal burden on children, their families, and communities. This burden is evident in school absenteeism, parents' missed days from work, and wages lost as a result.[4,11,16] In one study in Finland, school and day-care absenteeism is highest among children younger than 3 years, and parental days missed from work are higher as well.[16] A US-based study showed a similar trend, with parents of influenza-infected children missing an average of 1 day of work for every 3 days of school missed by a child attributable to influenza.[38] These numbers are likely an underestimate of the burden of influenza, as they reflect only those children who sought medical care for their illness and do not account for illnesses that occurred on non-school days.

VACCINES

Vaccination is the leading approach for the prevention of influenza, and many influenza vaccines are available on the global market. These vaccines fall into 2 broad categories: parenterally administered nonreplicating vaccines and intranasally (IN) administered live-attenuated vaccines. Current vaccines are all designed with the same goal of inducing immunity to the hemagglutinin (HA) and/or neuraminidase (NA) surface glycoproteins of the influenza virus. As the HA and NA of the virus undergo frequent antigenic drift, the seasonal influenza vaccine is reformulated as often as twice annually to match the strains projected to circulate in the following influenza season. The WHO recommends influenza strains that should be included in the seasonal influenza vaccines (for both the Northern and Southern hemispheres' vaccine compositions) based on global epidemiologic and virologic surveillance, which has been undertaken by the Global Influenza Surveillance and Response System (GISRS) for more than 50 years. The GISRS tracks the evolution of influenza viruses as well as the emergence of influenza strains with the potential to cause pandemics.[39]

Currently marketed influenza vaccines for nonpandemic use are trivalent or quadrivalent. Trivalent vaccines contain 3 total strains: 2 influenza A strains (one H1N1 and one H3N2) as well as 1 influenza B lineage strain; quadrivalent influenza vaccines contain an additional B lineage influenza strain. It has proven difficult to predict which B lineage will circulate in a given year, and in some years both B lineages circulate concurrently.[40,41] Thus, quadrivalent influenza vaccines were developed to include both influenza B lineages (Victoria and Yamagata) that currently circulate in humans. Quadrivalent vaccines were first licensed in the United States for use in the 2013 to 2014 influenza season.

There are 2 categories of seasonal influenza vaccine currently available on the global market. Intramuscularly (IM) or intradermally (ID) injected, nonreplicating influenza virus vaccines, which can be further classified based on production substrate (egg based or cell culture based); types of preparation (whole virus, split-virion, subunit, or fully recombinant vaccines); dose (0.25-mL pediatric, 0.5-mL adult), and by presence or absence of adjuvant (MF59). The other category of approved influenza vaccine is the live-attenuated influenza vaccine (LAIV), which is administered IN. Because of the time required for influenza vaccine manufacturing, testing, packaging, and distribution, seasonal vaccines are generally available only by late summer or early fall.

This section focuses on seasonal influenza vaccines (as opposed to pandemic vaccines), licensed primarily in the United States for children, defined here as individuals younger than 18 years. Influenza vaccines are not currently licensed anywhere in the world for infants younger than 6 months. For children 6 to 23 months old, the only available vaccines are inactivated influenza vaccines (IIVs). Nonadjuvated inactivated vaccines are the only approved option for children younger than 2 years, except in Canada where an MF59-adjuvanted trivalent IIV was approved for children 6 to 23 months of age in 2015.[42,43] For children older than 2 years, an LAIV is also approved in many countries. For a summary of seasonal influenza vaccines licensed for children in the United States see **Table 1**.

INACTIVATED INFLUENZA VACCINES
Safety

Clinical trials and postlicensure surveillance have shown IIVs to be highly safe. The most common adverse events associated with IIVs in all age groups are injection site reactions. In children, injection site reactions as well as fever are the most common safety concerns of IIVs and tend to be mild and short-lived.[44–51] In 2010, a trivalent IIV produced by an Australian pharmaceuticals company was strongly correlated with increased rates of febrile seizures in children in Australia.[52] Subsequent enhanced surveillance for febrile seizures in the United States and elsewhere showed a slight increase in the rates of febrile seizures among children who had received IIVs. The febrile seizure risk among children in the United States was noted to be elevated in some years and not others and more so when IIV was coadministered with 13-valent pneumococcal conjugate vaccines or diphtheria, tetanus, and pertussis vaccines. In all cases the risk for febrile seizures in the United States was determined to be substantially lower than observed in 2010 in Australia.[45,52–54]

Although for most children IIVs are very safe, they may pose a safety risk to individuals with severe egg allergies. Residual egg protein may remain in most influenza

Table 1
Categories of pediatric vaccines licensed for prevention of seasonal influenza

	Live Attenuated	Nonreplicating Vaccines			
		Standard Inactivated	Recombinant	Intradermal Inactivated	Adjuvanted Inactivated
Route	IN	IM	IM	ID	IM
Frequency	Annual	Annual	Annual	Annual	Annual
Approved ages[a]	2–49 y	≥6 mo	≥18 y	18–64 y	6–23 mo, ≥65 y
HA (mcg/strain)	15	15	45	9	15
Substrate for production	Eggs	Eggs, cell culture	Cell culture	Eggs	Eggs, cell culture

[a] Approved ages may differ by manufacturer and country.

Adapted from Neuzil KM, Ortiz JR. Influenza vaccines and vaccination strategies. In: Bloom BR, Lambert PH, editors. The Vaccine Book. Cambridge (MA): Academic Press. p. 429; with permission.

vaccines as the virus for the vaccine is grown in embryonated hens' eggs. Eggs are not used in the production of cell culture-based vaccines; however, these vaccines may still contain trace amounts of egg proteins. There is currently one cell culture-based vaccine on the market for children at least 4 years of age. The recombinant trivalent vaccine is the only entirely egg-free vaccine, but it is not licensed for use in individuals younger than 18 years.[45,55] Nonetheless, individuals with egg allergy should receive influenza vaccines (including egg-based vaccines) unless they have had a severe reaction to a prior influenza immunization. For individuals with severe egg allergy, egg-based vaccines should be administered by a physician trained to recognize and manage allergic responses. For more detailed instructions, see **Fig. 1**.

Immunogenicity

Nonreplicating vaccines elicit an immune response primarily against the HA component of the influenza virus. HA is one of the glycoproteins on the surface of the influenza virus and functions in the attachment of the virus to the host cells. Neutralizing antibodies specific to HA are the predominant means by which IIVs confer immunity

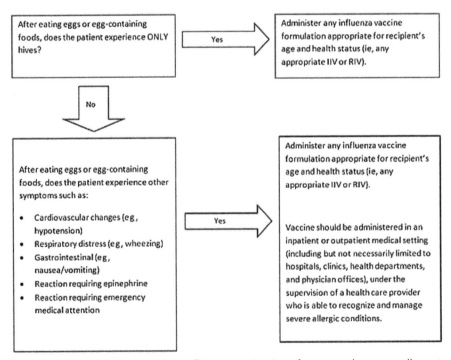

Fig. 1. Recommendations regarding influenza vaccination of persons who report allergy to eggs: Advisory Committee on Immunization Practices, United States, 2016 to 17 Influenza season. (*Data from* CDC. Flu vaccine and people with egg allergies. Available at: https://www.cdc.gov/flu/protect/vaccine/egg-allergies.htm. Accessed April 17, 2017.)

against influenza, although antibodies to the NA and other antibodies also play a role that is not as well understood.[46,47]

The immunogenicity of IIVs in children varies by influenza strain, the formulation of the vaccine, and the underlying condition and prior exposure of the recipient to similar viruses or vaccines. Depending on the degree to which the vaccine strains match the circulating strains, seasonal influenza vaccines will confer more or less protection, as antibody against influenza is for the most part strain specific. Therefore, antibody against one type or subtype of influenza may provide modest to no protection against other types or subtypes of influenza.[47]

Older children tend to have a strong antibody response, and just one dose of IIV is enough to confer protective immunity. Children younger than 9 years may have reduced antibody responses and should receive 2 doses of IIV at least 4 weeks apart the first time they are vaccinated against influenza. Once children have been primed with 2 doses of IIV, they are recommended to receive a single dose of vaccine in subsequent years. A young child may also be primed with 2 single doses of influenza vaccine across 2 influenza seasons.[47,56] For more information on vaccine priming and appropriate dosing for children, refer to **Fig. 2**.[57]

Efficacy and Effectiveness

IIVs have demonstrated efficacy and effectiveness across broad age groups and among different populations over many influenza seasons. Vaccine efficacy generally refers to the performance of a vaccine in protecting against a previously defined clinical or

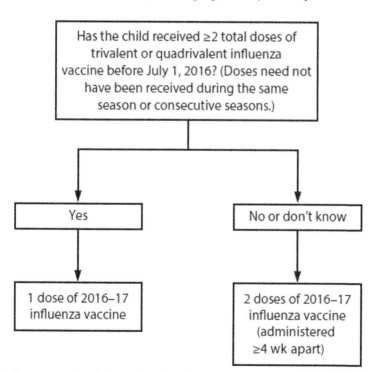

Fig. 2. Influenza vaccine dosing algorithm for children aged 6 months through 8 years: Advisory Committee on Immunization Practices, United States, 2016 to 17 influenza season. (*Data from* Grohskopf LA, Sokolow LZ, Broder KR, et al. Prevention and control of seasonal influenza with vaccines. MMWR Recomm Rep 2016;65(5):1–54.)

laboratory outcome during clinical trials. Vaccine effectiveness describes a vaccine's performance against the same outcomes in nonrandomized settings, as observed after licensure. Estimates of vaccine efficacy and effectiveness may vary between studies depending on the vaccine match, population (age and comorbid conditions), and study outcome. It is, therefore, difficult to systematically compare point estimates of vaccine efficacy across trials, unless the studies define the outcome in the same way and administer the same vaccine in the same study season. Efficacy and effectiveness tend to be greater when the vaccine virus strains more closely match the circulating virus strains.[57]

A meta-analysis of randomized controlled trials of influenza vaccine efficacy over 12 influenza seasons showed IIV had a pooled efficacy of 59% (95% confidence interval [CI], 51%–67%) among those aged 18 to 65 years.[58] Although no trials in children 2 to 17 years of age met inclusion criteria for this particular meta-analysis at the time of publication, many clinical trials have been conducted on the efficacy of seasonal influenza vaccine in children (**Table 2**). Among children aged 1 to 16 years in a multiyear study in Nashville, Tennessee, efficacy against culture-confirmed clinical influenza was 91.4% and 77.3%, respectively, during H1N1 and H3N2 years. There were too few laboratory-confirmed episodes to evaluate by narrower age strata.[59] In a randomized controlled trial in healthy children aged 6 to 23 months, vaccine efficacy was 66% (95% CI, 34%–82%) against culture-confirmed clinical illness in the first year but could not be assessed in the second year because of low influenza attack rates.[27] A clinical trial in Europe in 2007 to 2008 and 2008 to 2009 randomized healthy influenza vaccine-naïve children aged 6 months to less than 72 months to receive IIV, MF59 adjuvanted IIV, or a noninfluenza control vaccine. Vaccine efficacy was 43% and 86%, respectively, for IIV and adjuvanted IIV versus the noninfluenza control vaccine against all LCI illness across both influenza seasons.[51] In a multinational study among children 3 to 8 years of age, vaccine efficacy of a quadrivalent IIV was 55.9% against polymerase chain reaction–confirmed clinical illness of any severity.[60]

Although most studies of influenza vaccines focus on LCI illness of any severity, it is also important to look at the efficacy of influenza vaccine against more severe disease. In the multinational study of quadrivalent vaccine mentioned earlier, vaccine efficacy among children 3 to 8 years of age was 73.1% against all strains for moderate to severe LCI.[60] As severe outcomes of influenza are rare in children, they may be difficult and costly to identify in prospective studies. A case-control study design examined the effectiveness of influenza vaccine in preventing admissions to the pediatric intensive care unit (PICU). In this study, influenza vaccination reduced children's risk of life-threatening influenza and/or influenza-related admission to the PICU by 74% during influenza seasons from 2010 to 2012. In this study, there was no effectiveness demonstrated among children receiving influenza vaccine for the first time who did not receive the recommended 2 doses.[61] In a case-cohort analysis of children aged 6 months through 17 years during the 2010–2014 influenza seasons, overall influenza vaccine efficacy against death was 65% (95% CI, 54%–74%).[62]

Adjuvanted Vaccines

An adjuvant is a substance that can be formulated as a component of a vaccine to improve the immune response to the vaccine antigens. Most seasonal influenza vaccines are unadjuvanted; the only adjuvanted seasonal influenza vaccine approved for use in many countries, including the United States, uses MF59, an oil-in-water emulsion of squalene. Adjuvanted influenza vaccines are primarily licensed for individuals 65 years and older, as the adjuvant helps their weakened immune systems mount a stronger antibody response. In 2015, Canada became the first country to approve the MF59-adjuvanted influenza vaccine for use in children 6 to 23 months of age.

Table 2

Individually randomized controlled trials of influenza vaccines in children, 1985 to 2013 influenza seasons

Trials with non-influenza vaccine control group

Study Years	Study Location	Age Group	Influenza Vaccine	Vaccine Strains	Number of Doses of Vaccine	Control Vaccine	Clinical Outcome Measure	Laboratory Outcome Measure	N	Circulating Strain	Vaccine Efficacy (95% CI)	Attack Rate of Control Group (%)
1985–1990[59]	United States (Nashville, Tennessee)	1–16 y	Study y 1: bivalent inactivated vaccine[a] Study y 2–5: trivalent inactivated vaccine[a] All y: bivalent cold adapted[a]	Study y 1: A/Dunedin/6/83, A/Chile/1/83, A/Korea/1/82, A/Philippines/2/82 Study y 2: A/Texas/1/85, A/Chile/1/83, A/Bethesda/1/85, A/Mississippi/1/85 Study y 3: A/Kawasaki/9/86, A/Taiwan/1/86, A/Bethesda/1/85, A/Leningrad/360/86 Study y 4: A/Kawasaki/9/86, A/Taiwan/1/86, A/Los Angeles/2/87, A/Sichuan/2/87 Study y 5: A/Kawasaki/9/86, A/Taiwan/1/86, A/Los Angeles/2/87, A/Shanghai/11/87	1 dose of vaccine either IN or injected IM	Double control intranasal: placebo IM injection: placebo (y 1), monovalent influenza B vaccine (y 2–5)	Influenza-like illness or other upper respiratory illness	Culture	791	H1N1 y H3N2 y	Cold-adapted: 95.5 (66.7–99.4) IIV: 91.4 (63.8–98.0) Cold-adapted: 67.7 (1.1–89.5) IIV: 77.3 (20.3–93.5)	7.1 4.3

(continued on next page)

Table 2 (continued)

Study Years	Study Location	Age Group	Influenza Vaccine	Vaccine Strains	Number of Doses of Vaccine	Control Vaccine	Clinical Outcome Measure	Laboratory Outcome Measure	N	Circulating Strain	Vaccine Efficacy (95% CI)	Attack Rate of Control Group (%)
1996–1997[26]	United States	15–71 mo	LAIV (Aviron, Mountain View, California)	A/Texas/36/91-like (H1N1), A/Wuhan/359/95-like (H3N2), B/Harbin/7/94-like	1 or 2 IN doses; 2 doses given 60 d apart	Placebo	Symptomatic fever, runny nose or nasal congestion, sore throat, cough, headache, muscle aches, chills, vomiting, otitis media	Culture	*One-dose regimen* LAIV: 189 Control: 99; *2-dose regimen* LAIV: 849 Control: 410	*One-dose regimen* All strains, H3N2, B; *2-dose regimen* All strains, H3N2, B	89 (65–96), 87 (47–97), 91 (46–99); 94 (88–97), 96 (90–99), 91 (78–96)	14.1, 8.1, 6.1, 18.0, 12.0, 7.6
1996–1998[25]	United States	26–85 mo	LAIV (Aviron, Mountain View, California)	A/Shenzhen/227/95-like (H1N1), A/Wuhan/359/95 (H3N2), B/Harbin/7/94-like	1 IN dose	Placebo	Lower respiratory tract disease and/or otitis media with or without fever	Culture	*Study y 1* LAIV: 1070 Control: 532; *Study y 2* LAIV: 917 Control: 441	*Study y 1* All strains, H3N2, B; *Study y 2* All strains, H3N2 (matched), H3N2 (unmatched), B	93 (87–96), 95 (88–97), 91 (79–96); 87 (78–93), 100 (54–100), 86 (75–92), 100 (79–100)	17.7, 11.8, 6.9, 12.7, 0.9, 11.6, 0.2
1999–2001[27]	United States (Pittsburgh)	6–24 mo	IIV (Fluzone, Aventis Pasteur, Swiftwater, Pennsylvania)	Study y 1: A/Beijing/262/95 (H1N1), A/Sydney/15/97 (H3N2), B/Yamanashi/166/98 Study y 2: A/New Caledonia/20/99 (H1N1), A/Panama/2007/99 (H3N2), B/Yamanashi/166/98	2 IM injections, 4 wk apart	Placebo	Upper respiratory tract infection accompanied by fever (≥38°C) and/or AOM	Culture	*Study y 1* IIV: 273 Control: 138; *Study y 2* IIV: 252 Control: 123	*Against influenza* All strains; *Against AOM* All strains	Study y 1: 66 (34–82), Study y 2: −7 (−247–67); Study y 1: −0.28, Study y 2: −19.5	15.9, 3.3, 35.8, 59.5

2000–2002[82]	Belgium, Finland, Israel, Spain, United Kingdom	6 to <36 mo	LAIV (Wyeth Vaccines Research, Marietta, Pennsylvania)	Study y 1: A/New Caledonia/20/99 (H1N1), A/Sydney/05/97 (H3N2), B/Yamanashi/166/98 Study y 2: A/New Caledonia/20/99 (H1N1), A/Panama/2007/99 (H3N2), B/Victoria/504/2000	Study y 1: 2 IN doses, 35 ±7 d apart Study y 2: 1 IN dose	Placebo	Influenza-like illness, pneumonia, AOM	Study y 1: serology Study y 2: PCR	Study y 1: LAIV: 951 Control: 665 Study y 2 LAIV: 640 Control: 450	Study y 1 All strains	85.9 (76.3–92.0)	13.4
										All vaccine-matched strains	85.4 (74.3–92.2)	10.8
										H1N1	91.8 (80.8–97.1)	7.7
										H3N2	ND	0.2
										B	72.6 (38.6–88.9)	3.5
										Study y 2 All strains	85.8 (78.6–90.9)	30.9
										All vaccine-matched strains	88.7 (82.0–93.2)	29.1
										H1N1	90.0 (56.3–98.9)	3.1
										H3N2	90.3 (82.9–94.9)	22.4
										B	81.7 (53.7–93.9)	5.1

(continued on next page)

Table 2
(continued)

Study Years	Study Location	Age Group	Influenza Vaccine	Vaccine Strains	Number of Doses of Vaccine	Control Vaccine	Clinical Outcome Measure	Laboratory Outcome Measure	N	Circulating Strain	Vaccine Efficacy (95% CI)	Attack Rate of Control Group (%)
2000–2003[83]	China, Hong Kong, India, Malaysia, the Philippines, Singapore, Taiwan, Thailand	12 to <36 mo	LAIV (Wyeth Vaccines Research, Marietta, Pennsylvania)	*Study y 1:* A/New Caledonia/20/99 (H1N1), A/Sydney/05/97 (H3N2), B/Yamanashi/166/98 *Study y 2:* A/New Caledonia/20/99 (H1N1), A/Panama/2007/99 (H3N2), B/Yamanashi/166/98	*Study y 1:* 2 IN doses, 28 d apart *Study y 2:* 1 dose in study y 2	Placebo	Influenza-like illness as described in Belshe et al,[26] 1998	Culture	*Study y 1* LAIV: 1653 *Control:* 1111 *Study y 2* *Primed LAIV:* 881 *Unprimed LAIV:* 503 *Primed control:* 759 *Unprimed control:* 494	*Study y 1* All strains	70.1 (60.9–77.3)	16.4
										All vaccine-matched strains	72.9 (62.8–80.5)	12.5
										H1N1	80.9 (69.4–88.5)	7.3
										H3N2 (unmatched)	90.0 (71.4–97.5)	2.4
										B (matched)	44.3 (6.2–67.2)	3.2
										Study y 2 All strains	64.2 (44.2–77.3)	11.9
										All vaccine-matched strains	84.3 (70.1–92.4)	9.9
										H1N1	—	N/R
										H3N2	86.3 (71.4–94.1)	N/R
										B (unmatched)	—	N/R

									Study y 1[b] LL vs PP		N/R
2001–2002[84]	South Africa, Brazil, Argentina	6 to <36 mo	LAIV (Wyeth Vaccines, Marietta, Pennsylvania)	Study y 1: A/New Caledonia/20/99-like (H1N1), A/Panama/2007/99-like (H3N2), B/Yamanashi/166/98-like, B/Victoria/504/00-like; Study y 2: A/New Caledonia/20/99-like (H1N1), A/Panama/2007/99-like (H3N2), B/Victoria/504/00-like	Study y 1: 1 or 2 intranasal doses; Study y 2: 1 dose — Placebo	Lower respiratory tract disease and/or otitis media with or without fever	Culture	Study y 1 LL: 944 PP: 474; Study y 2 LL/L: 339 PP/P: 342	All strains	72.0 (61.9–79.8)	N/R
									All vaccine-matched strains	73.5 (63.6–81.0)	N/R
									H1N1	NC	N/R
									H3N2	72.7 (60.7–81.5)	N/R
									B (matched)	81.4 (64.2–91.2)	N/R
									Study y 2 LL/L vs PP/P		
									All strains	46.6 (14.9–67.2)	N/R
									All vaccine-matched strains	73.6 (33.3–91.2)	N/R
									H1N1	94.0 (62.0–99.9)	N/R
									H3N2	49.4 (−253.0–95.4)	N/R
									B (matched)	−102.4 (−2137.1–71.0)	N/R

(continued on next page)

Table 2 (*continued*)

Study Years	Study Location	Age Group	Influenza Vaccine	Vaccine Strains	Number of Doses of Vaccine	Control Vaccine	Clinical Outcome Measure	Laboratory Outcome Measure	N	Circulating Strain	Vaccine Efficacy (95% CI)	Attack Rate of Control Group (%)
2007–2008[51]	Germany and Finland	6 to <72 mo	*Study y 1:* ATIV (Fluad, Novartis Vaccines), subunit TIV (Aggripal S1, Novartis Vaccines) *Study y 2:* ATIV and split TIV (Influsplit SSW, GlaxoSmithKline Biologicals)	*Study y 1:* A/Solomon Islands/3/2006 (H1N1), A/Wisconsin/67/2005 (H3N2), B/Malaysia/2506/2004 *Study y 2:* A/Brisbane/59/2007 (H1N1), A/Brisbane/10/2007 (H3N2), B/Florida/4/2006	2 doses, 28 d apart	Meningococcal C conjugate vaccine (Menjugate); 6 to <12 mo; tick-borne encephalitis vaccine (Encepur children); 12 to <72 mo	Influenza-like illness	rRT-PCR	ATIV: 1937 TIV: 1772 Control: 993	All strains ATIV	86 (74–93)c	4.7
										All strains TIV	43 (15–61)	4.7
										Vaccine-matched strains ATIV	89 (78–95)	4.1
										Vaccine-matched strains TIV	45 (16–64)	4.1
2009[85]	South Africa	6–60 mo; HIV-infected	TIV (VAXIGRIP, Sanofi-Aventis, Lyon, France)	A/Brisbane/59/2007(H1N1), A/Uruguay/716/2007(H3N2), B/Florida/4/2006	2 IM doses, 1 mo apart	Placebo	Influenza-like illness	Culture and RT-PCR	TIV: 203 Control: 200	All strains	24.7 (−64.7–66.4)	8.5

Year[ref]	Location	Age	Vaccine	Strains	Dose	Comparator	Outcome	Assay	N	Category		VE % (CI)	
2010–2011[60]	Multinational study, 15 sites in Bangladesh, Dominican Republic, Honduras, Lebanon, Panama, the Philippines, Thailand, and Turkey	3–8 y	QIV (GlaxoSmithKline Vaccines)	A/California/7/2009 (H1N1), A/Victoria/210/2009 (H3N2), B/Brisbane/60/2008 (Victoria lineage), B/Florida/4/2006 (Yamagata lineage)	1 or 2 IM injections depending on priming	Hepatitis A vaccine (Havrix, GSK Vaccines)	Influenza-like illness	rRT-PCR	QIV: 2379 Control: 2398	*Any severity*	All strains	55.9 (39.1–67.3)	4.67
											All vaccine-matched strains	45.1 (9.3–66.8)	2.34
											H1N1	55.6 (21.3–74.9)	1.58
											H3N2	57.6 (28.5–74.9)	1.96
											B/Yamagata (matched)	100 (— to 100)	0.08
											B/Victoria (matched)	47.2 (12.4–68.2)	1.79
										Moderate-severe	All strains	73.1 (47.1–86.3)	2.17
											H1N1	76.5 (30.3–92.1)	0.71
											H3N2	82.4 (49.1–93.9)	0.96
											B/Yamagata (matched)	100.0 (— to 100.0)	0.04
											B/Victoria (matched)	42.1 (47.1–77.2)	0.5
2013[23]	Bangladesh	24–59 mo	LAIV (Nasovac-S, SIIL, Pune, India; lot 167E2002)	A/California/7/2009 (H1N1)-like, A/Victoria/361/2001 (H3N2)-like, B/Wisconsin/1/2010 (Yamagata lineage)-like	1 IN dose	Placebo	Symptomatic fever ($\geq 38.0°C$), upper respiratory illness, AOM, meningitis, or sepsis	rRT-PCR	LAIV: 1174 Control: 587		All strains	41.0 (28.0–51.6)	24.5
											All vaccine-matched strains	57.6 (43.6–68.0)	15.8
											H1N1	50.0 (9.2–72.5)	3.6
											H3N2	60.4 (44.8–71.6)	12.3
											B (matched)	0.0 (−1001–90.9)	0.2
											B (unmatched)	6.5 (−43.0–38.8)	5.3

(continued on next page)

Table 2 (continued)

Study Years	Study Location	Age Group	Influenza Vaccine	Vaccine Strains	Number of Doses of Vaccine	Control Vaccine	Clinical Outcome Measure	Laboratory Outcome Measure	N	Circulating Strain	Vaccine Efficacy (95% CI)	Attack Rate of Control Group (%)
2013[24]	Senegal	2 to <5 y	LAIV (Nasovac- STM, SIIL, Pune, India; lot 167E2002)	A/California/7/2009 (H1N1)-like, A/Victoria/361/2001 (H3N2)-like, B/Wisconsin/1/2010 (Yamagata lineage)-like	1 IN dose	Placebo	Fever (>37.5°C), cough, sore throat	rRT-PCR	LAIV: 1174 Control: 587	All strains	0.0 (−26.4–20.9)	18.0
										All vaccine-matched strains	−6.1 (−50.0–25.0)	8.0
										H1N1	−9.7 (−62.6–26.1)	6.2
										H3N2	—	0.0
										B (matched)	9.5 (−88.9–56.6)	1.7
										B (unmatched)	7.3 (−26.3, 31.9)	10.6
Comparative trials of influenza vaccines; no noninfluenza vaccine control group												
2002[69]	145 sites in Belgium, Finland, Germany, Greece, Israel, Italy, the Netherlands, Norway, Poland, Portugal, Spain, Switzerland, the United Kingdom	6-17 y	LAIV (Wyeth Vaccines Research, Marietta, Pennsylvania) TIV split virion (Aventis Pasteur, Lyon, France)	LAIV: A/New Caledonia/20/99 (H1N1), A/Panama/2007/99 (H3N2), B/Hong Kong/330/01 TIV: Caledonia/20/99—IVR-116, A/Panama/2007/99—RESVIR-17, B/Shanghai/7/97	1 dose IN or IM injection	None	Influenza-like illness, pneumonia, AOM	rRT-PCR	LAIV: 1111 TIV: 1109	All strains	31.9 (1.1–53.5)[d]	6.6[e]
										All vaccine-matched strains	34.7 (3.9–56.0)	6.4
										H1N1	100 (−8.4–100.0)	0.5
										H3N2	0.6 (−141.8–59.2)	1.1
										B	36.3 (0.1–59.8)	4.8

Year	Location	Age	Vaccine (Manufacturer)	Strains	Doses, Control	Case Definition	Diagnosis	Sample Size	Outcome	Efficacy % (95% CI)	Attack Rate
2002[71]	Belgium, Czech Republic, Finland, Germany, Italy, Poland, Spain, Switzerland, the United Kingdom	6–71 mo	LAIV (Wyeth Pharmaceuticals, Marietta, Pennsylvania) TIV split virion (Aventis Pasteur, Lyon, France)	LAIV: A/New Caledonia/20/99 (H1N1), A/Panama/2007/99 (H3N2), B/Hong Kong/330/01 TIV: A/Panama/2007/99 (H3N2), A/New Caledonia/20/99 (H1N1), B/Shangdong/7/97	LAIV: 2 IN doses, 35 ±7 d apart TIV: 1 IM injection, None	At least 1: fever (≥38.0°C rectal or 37.5°C axillary), shortness of breath, pulmonary congestion, pneumonia, AOM, or wheezing 2 or more: rhinorrhea, pharyngitis, cough, muscle aches, chills, headache, irritability, decreased activity, or vomiting	Serology and PCR	LAIV: 1050 TIV: 1035	All strains	52.4 (24.6–70.5)[d]	5.8[e]
									All vaccine-matched strains	52.7 (21.6–72.2)	4.8
									H1N1	100.0 (42.3–100.0)	0.8
									H3N2	−97.1 (−540.2–31.5)	0.6
									B	68.0 (37.3–84.8)	3.6
2004[70]	249 sites in the United States, 12 countries in Europe and the Middle East, and 3 countries in Asia	6–59 mo	LAIV (FluMist, MedImmune) TIV (United States and Asia: Fluogen, Aventis Pasteur; Europe and Middle East: Fluzone, Aventis Pasteur)	A/New Caledonia/20/99 (H1N1), A/Wyoming/3/2003 (H3N2)-like, B/Jilin/20/2003	1 or 2 IN (LAIV) or IM injection (TIV) doses (28–42 d apart if 2 doses), Placebo	Protocol-defined influenza symptoms	Culture	LAIV: 4179 TIV: 4173	All strains	54.9 (45.4–62.9)[d]	8.6[e]
									All vaccine-matched strains	44.5 (22.4–60.6)	2.4
									H1N1 (matched)	89.2 (67.7–97.4)	0.7
									H3N2 (matched)	—	0
									H3N2 (unmatched)	79.2 (70.6–85.7)	4.5
									B	27.3 (−4.8–49.9)	1.7

Abbreviations: ATIV, adjuvanted trivalent inactivated influenza vaccine; HIV, human immunodeficiency virus; L, one dose of live attenuated influenza vaccine; LL, two doses of live attenuated influenza vaccine; NC, not calculated; N/R, not reported; P, one dose of placebo; PCR, polymerase chain reaction; PP, two doses of placebo; QIV, quadrivalent inactivated influenza vaccine; rRT, real time Reverse Transcription; RT, Reverse Transcription; TIV, trivalent inactivated influenza vaccine; Y, years.

[a] Manufacturer not listed.

[b] Data for study years 1 and 2 for other treatment groups are available in the full publication.

[c] Study results are mainly from study year 1.

[d] Relative efficacy of LAIV compared with TIV.

[e] Attack rate is of TIV group, as there was no placebo control group in this study.

Courtesy of Kathleen Neuzil, MD, MPH, Baltimore, MD.

Recent studies on the safety, immunogenicity, and efficacy of the MF59-adjuvanted IIV in young children has shown them to be highly immunogenic and efficacious. There is evidence that the adjuvanted IIV may elicit greater reactogenicity, although adverse events associated with MF59-adjuvanted IIV vaccination were mild and transient and rates were relatively low in the clinical trial setting. One study conducted in Argentina, Australia, Chile, the Philippines, and South Africa between 2011 and 2012 showed that the adjuvanted trivalent inactivated vaccine induced significantly higher antibody titers after 2 doses than did the unadjuvanted vaccine. This superior antibody response persisted through 6 months after vaccination against both homologous and heterologous influenza strains.[63] As mentioned earlier, a study in Germany and Finland in 2007 to 2008 and 2008 to 2009 reported efficacy data for the adjuvanted trivalent inactivated vaccine. In this study, the adjuvanted trivalent IIV had absolute and relative efficacies, respectively, of 86% and 75% against all circulating influenza strains and 89% and 80%, respectively, against vaccine-matched strains when compared with unadjuvanted trivalent IIV.[51] The same study showed local and systemic reactions to vaccination to be similar in younger children vaccinated with adjuvanted trivalent IIV and trivalent IIV, although in older children the rates of systemic, but not local, reactions were higher after vaccination with adjuvanted trivalent IIV. Serious adverse events were evenly divided between the treatment groups.[51] A large trial of adjuvanted quadrivalent IIV is ongoing (NCT01964989).

LIVE-ATTENUATED INFLUENZA VACCINES

Worldwide, there are 2 types of LAIVs: one developed in the former Union of Soviet Socialist Republics and the other in the United States. The Leningrad-based LAIVs have been approved in Russia for children 3 years of age and older for many decades. More recently, a Leningrad-based LAIV has been manufactured and licensed in India for children aged 2 years and older. In the United States, an LAIV based on the Ann Arbor strain and approved under the trade name FluMist was first licensed for use in persons 5 to 49 years of age in 2003; in 2007, the age range was expanded to include children beginning at 2 years of age. LAIV is administered IN as a spray. LAIVs induce a rapid immune response in the mucosal linings of the upper respiratory tract that depend on viral replication and, initially, on activation of local immune responses. The LAIVs are based on attenuated influenza A and B vaccine viruses, called master donor viruses (MDV-A and MDV-B), which are temperature sensitive and have been rendered cold adapted, such that the virus replicates efficiently only at lower temperatures, such as in the mucosal linings of the nasopharynx, but not in the lower respiratory tract, where temperatures are relatively higher. Similar to IIVs, LAIVs are either trivalent (H1N1, H3N2, B) or quadrivalent (H1N1, H3N2, 2 B strains) according to the most recent strain recommendations. This article focuses predominantly on the US LAIV.

Safety

LAIV administration has been associated most commonly with mild upper respiratory tract reactions, such as runny nose, nasal congestion, and fever in children younger than 8 years. In clinical studies, an increased risk for wheezing illness was observed in LAIV/Ann Arbor backbone recipients aged less than 24 months (3.8% LAIV vs 2.1% IIV). An increase in hospitalizations was also observed in children aged less than 12 months after vaccination with LAIV/Ann Arbor. For these reasons, LAIV/Ann Arbor is approved for use beginning at 24 months of age. Postlicensure surveillance data from North America and Europe have not demonstrated an increased frequency of wheezing illness after administration of LAIV/Ann Arbor among healthy children older than 2 years.[44,46]

Immunogenicity

Several studies have assessed various mucosal and systemic immune responses following vaccination with LAIV.[64] Studies have also demonstrated the greater breadth of antibodies produced in response to LAIV as compared with IIV.[65] In general, when compared with IIV, LAIV induces better mucosal antibody responses and IIV induces stronger serum antibody responses.[47,66]

Overall, LAIV immunogenicity data do not correlate well with vaccine efficacy.[65–68] As there is no generally accepted correlate of immunity for LAIV, manufacturers and regulatory agencies must rely primarily on efficacy or effectiveness data for vaccine development and policy decisions.

Efficacy and Effectiveness

The efficacy of LAIV has been studied extensively. A pivotal study during the 1996 to 1997 influenza season in children 15 to 71 months of age examined the absolute efficacy of one versus 2 doses of LAIV. The one-dose regimen was 89% effective at preventing LCI illness from all influenza strains. When 2 doses of LAIV were administered 60 days apart, LAIV was 94% effective against all influenza strains.[26] Several trials comparing the efficacy of LAIV and trivalent IIV have also been conducted in children. These studies have shown LAIV to be 31.9% to 54.9% more effective against all influenza virus strains than IIV.[69–71] These head-to-head comparative trials, demonstrating superiority of LAIV to trivalent IIV in young children, led to preferential recommendations for LAIV over IIV in many countries, including the United States.

For children in low-resource countries, LAIVs are promising options given the efficacy demonstrated in comparative trials with IIV and the ease of administration. In 2013, 2 prospective placebo-controlled clinical trials were conducted on the efficacy of a single dose of the Russian-backbone LAIV in young children in Bangladesh and Senegal. In Bangladesh, LAIV was 57.6% effective against vaccine-matched influenza strains, which had an attack rate of 15.8% in the placebo group. In Senegal during the same influenza season, LAIV had zero efficacy against vaccine-matched influenza strains, despite being sufficiently powered (an attack rate of 18.0% in the placebo group) to show such an effect.[23,24] The differences in the results from these two studies are poorly understood; however, inconsistent results for the Ann Arbor backbone LAIV have also occurred in recent years, as detailed later.

ANNUAL MONITORING OF VACCINE EFFECTIVENESS AND LIVE-ATTENUATED INFLUENZA VACCINE

The increasing number of influenza vaccines, and the inherent unpredictability of influenza strain circulation, necessitates a nimble system to monitor and evaluate the impact of individual vaccines and policy decisions. A growing number of surveillance systems in the United States, Canada, Australia, and Europe monitor influenza vaccine effectiveness annually and have the ability to produce early, in-season estimates of vaccine performance.[27,72,73] The US Influenza Vaccine Effectiveness Network has shown reduced effectiveness to LAIVs during 3 influenza seasons (2013 to 2014, 2014 to 2015, and 2015 to 2016) and better performance of IIVs compared with LAIVs in children. These data contradict the head-to-head randomized trials mentioned earlier, which favored LAIVs, and data from other countries where LAIVs continue to show effectiveness.[57]

The reasons for the overall poorer performance of LAIV compared with IIV in recent influenza seasons are not well understood and should be the subject of future studies. Possible explanations of the low efficacy include (1) the suboptimal performance of the specific (H1N1) HA vaccine component included in the vaccine; (2) potential interference among viruses in the quadrivalent vaccine (ie, the additional influenza B vaccine component may affect viral replication of the A(H1N1)pdm09 virus); and (3) evaluation in a more highly vaccinated population in recent years, as compared with populations of earlier studies, in which it is likely that a higher proportion of children were vaccine naïve.[74] In light of the low effectiveness against influenza A(H1N1)pdm09 in the United States during the 2013 to 2014 and 2015 to 2016 influenza seasons, the United States and Canada have altered their vaccine recommendations for children beginning in the 2016 to 2017 season.[57,75]

INFLUENZA VACCINE POLICY

In 2012, the WHO updated its recommendations on the use of influenza vaccine.[76] For countries considering the initiation or expansion of programs for seasonal influenza vaccination, the WHO recommends that pregnant women should have the highest priority for vaccine receipt. This recommendation was based on the risk of severe disease, evidence on the safety of the vaccine during pregnancy, the potential for benefit to women and infants, and the operational feasibility. Additional groups to be considered, in no particular order of priority, are children aged 6 through 59 months, the elderly, individuals with specific medical conditions, and health care workers. It is recommended that health care workers receive influenza vaccine in many countries both to limit transmission to vulnerable patients as well as to maintain the health care workforce during influenza outbreaks.

As no vaccines are approved for children younger than 6 months of age, protection of these vulnerable infants can only be achieved through vaccination of the mother during pregnancy and vaccination of close contacts to limit transmission.[76] Randomized controlled clinical trials in Bangladesh, South Africa, and Mali have demonstrated that vaccination of pregnant women can reduce the incidence of LCI in infants.[77–79]

In temperate countries with seasonal outbreaks, influenza vaccine is given annually, before the influenza season. Influenza vaccine programs are more challenging in tropical and subtropical countries. Given the varying influenza circulation patterns in the tropics, it is not yet clear if a Southern or Northern Hemisphere vaccine administered in annual campaigns would provide year-round protection against the diverse strains that may be seen in such countries. Further, the optimal formulation or timing of immunization is still uncertain in many countries with limited historical influenza surveillance.[46]

In the United States, routine annual influenza vaccination is recommended for all persons aged 6 months and older. Children receiving influenza vaccine for the first time require 2 doses of influenza vaccine. Special effort should be made to vaccinate children at high risk for complications of influenza, American Indian and Alaskan native children, all household and close contacts of children younger than 6 months of age, pregnant and breastfeeding women, all health care personnel, and childcare providers and staff.[54,57] Although vaccines are recommended primarily to reduce influenza and its complications in the recipient, it is acknowledged that administering vaccines to children may also reduce transmission and the incidence of influenza at the household and community level.

The Advisory Committee on Immunization Practices (ACIP) and the American Academy of Pediatrics (AAP) update their influenza vaccine recommendations annually.[54,57] In light of the low effectiveness against influenza A(H1N1)pdm09 in the

United States during the 2013 to 2014 and 2015 to 2016 influenza seasons, the ACIP and AAP recommended that LAIV not be used in the 2016 to 2017 influenza season.[57] Studies are ongoing to determine whether the interim recommendation in the United States that LAIV should not be used will continue for subsequent influenza seasons. In Canada, the use of LAIV was not preferentially recommended for the 2016 to 2017 influenza season, as it had been in the past.[75]

ANTIVIRAL MEDICATIONS

Antiviral medications with activity against influenza viruses are an important adjunct to influenza vaccine in the control of influenza. These medications can be used to treat or to prevent influenza. Three influenza antiviral medications approved by the US Food and Drug Administration are recommended for use in the United States during the 2016 to 2017 influenza season: oral oseltamivir, inhaled zanamivir, and intravenous peramivir. These drugs are chemically related antiviral medications known as NA inhibitors that have activity against both influenza A and B viruses. Amantadine and rimantadine, from the adamantane class of antivirals, are licensed in the United States for the treatment of influenza A viruses. However, the adamantanes are not currently recommended because they have no intrinsic activity against influenza B viruses and there are high levels of resistance among circulating influenza A viruses.[80] Antiviral resistance is monitored carefully, and information is updated on a frequent basis throughout the season.[81]

Antiviral medications are underused for children with influenza in the United States. Trials of antiviral medications in children have shown that early treatment can shorten the duration of illness and reduce complications, including AOM, and the duration of hospitalization. The AAP and the ACIP update antiviral recommendations on an annual basis, providing specific dosage information for treatment and prophylactic use.[54,80] When indicated, antiviral treatment should be started as soon as possible after illness onset. Decisions about starting antiviral treatment should not wait for laboratory confirmation of influenza.

The AAP recommends that health care providers offer treatment as soon as possible for any child (1) hospitalized with presumed influenza; (2) hospitalized for severe, complicated, or progressive illness attributable to influenza; or (3) with presumed illness of any severity if the child is at high risk of complications. Treatment should be considered as soon as possible for any healthy child with presumed influenza or healthy children with presumed influenza who live at home with a sibling or household contact that is younger than 6 months or has a medical condition that predisposes to complications.[54]

SUMMARY

Influenza is a common respiratory illness in children and accounts for substantial morbidity and mortality on an annual basis. Influenza vaccines, the mainstay of influenza prevention and control efforts, are safe and effective. The absolute effectiveness of vaccines varies by year and is influenced by circulating virus, vaccine type, and host characteristics. The reason for recent reduced performance of LAIVs in children in the United States and elsewhere is poorly understood, and active research is ongoing. Vaccination programs are less common in tropical and subtropical countries, where unique logistical and feasibility challenges exist related to vaccine availability and more prolonged periods of virus circulation. Antiviral medications for prevention and treatment of influenza in children are an important adjunct to vaccines.

REFERENCES

1. World Health Organization. Influenza (Seasonal) fact sheet. 2014. Available at: http://www.who.int/mediacentre/factsheets/fs211/en/. Accessed September 10, 2016.
2. Grijalva CG, Zhu Y, Williams DJ, et al. Association between hospitalization with community-acquired laboratory-confirmed influenza pneumonia and prior receipt of influenza vaccination. JAMA 2015;314(14):1488–97.
3. Manzoli L, Schioppa F, Boccia A, et al. The efficacy of influenza vaccine for healthy children: a meta-analysis evaluating potential sources of variation in efficacy estimates including study quality. Pediatr Infect Dis J 2007;26(2):97–106.
4. Poehling KA, Edwards KM, Weinberg GA, et al. The underrecognized burden of influenza in young children. N Engl J Med 2006;355(1):31–40.
5. Silvennoinen H, Peltola V, Lehtinen P, et al. Clinical presentation of influenza in unselected children treated as outpatients. Pediatr Infect Dis J 2009;28(5):372–5.
6. Peltola V, Ziegler T, Ruuskanen O. Influenza A and B virus infections in children. Clin Infect Dis 2003;36(3):299–305.
7. Neuzil KM, Zhu Y, Griffin MR, et al. Burden of interpandemic influenza in children younger than 5 years: a 25-year prospective study. J Infect Dis 2002;185(2): 147–52.
8. Centre for Disease Control and Prevention. Flu symptoms and complications. 2016 Available at: http://www.cdc.gov/flu/about/disease/complications.htm. Accessed December 7, 2016.
9. Glezen WP, Couch RB. Interpandemic influenza in the Houston area, 1974-76. N Engl J Med 1978;298(11):587–92.
10. Neuzil KM, Mellen BG, Wright PF, et al. The effect of influenza on hospitalizations, outpatient visits, and courses of antibiotics in children. N Engl J Med 2000;342(4): 225–31.
11. Poehling KA, Edwards KM, Griffin MR, et al. The burden of influenza in young children, 2004-2009. Pediatrics 2013;131(2):207–16.
12. Grijalva CG, Craig AS, Dupont WD, et al. Estimating influenza hospitalizations among children. Emerg Infect Dis 2006;12(1):103–9.
13. Dawood FS, Fiore A, Kamimoto L, et al. Burden of seasonal influenza hospitalization in children, United States, 2003 to 2008. J Pediatr 2010;157(5):808–14.
14. Chaves SS, Perez A, Farley MM, et al. The burden of influenza hospitalizations in infants from 2003 to 2012, United States. Pediatr Infect Dis J 2014;33(9):912–9.
15. Gessner BD, Brooks WA, Neuzil KM, et al. Vaccines as a tool to estimate the burden of severe influenza in children of low-resourced areas (November 30-December 1, 2012, Les Pensieres, Veyrier-du-Lac, France). Vaccine 2013; 31(32):3222–8.
16. Heikkinen T, Silvennoinen H, Peltola V, et al. Burden of influenza in children in the community. J Infect Dis 2004;190(8):1369–73.
17. Dawood FS, Chaves SS, Pérez A, et al. Complications and associated bacterial coinfections among children hospitalized with seasonal or pandemic influenza, United States, 2003-2010. J Infect Dis 2014;209(5):686–94.
18. Dawood FS, Fiore A, Kamimoto L, et al. Influenza-associated pneumonia in children hospitalized with laboratory-confirmed influenza, 2003-2008. Pediatr Infect Dis J 2010;29(7):585–90.
19. Finelli L, Fiore A, Dhara R, et al. Influenza-associated pediatric mortality in the United States: increase of Staphylococcus aureus coinfection. Pediatrics 2008; 122(4):805–11.

20. Centre for Disease Control and Prevention. Influenza-associated pediatric mortality. FluView. 2016. Available at: https://gis.cdc.gov/GRASP/Fluview/PedFluDeath.html. Accessed December 16, 2016.

21. Bhat N, Wright JG, Broder KR, et al. Influenza-associated deaths among children in the United States, 2003-2004. N Engl J Med 2005;353(24):2559–67.

22. Wong KK, Jain S, Blanton L, et al. Influenza-associated pediatric deaths in the United States, 2004-2012. Pediatrics 2013;132(5):796–804.

23. Brooks WA, Zaman K, Lewis KD, et al. Efficacy of a Russian-backbone live attenuated influenza vaccine among young children in Bangladesh: a randomised, double-blind, placebo-controlled trial. Lancet Glob Health 2016;4(12):e946–54.

24. Victor JC, Lewis KD, Diallo A, et al. Efficacy of a Russian-backbone live attenuated influenza vaccine among children in Senegal: a randomised, double-blind, placebo-controlled trial. Lancet Glob Health 2016;4(12):e955–65.

25. Belshe RB, Gruber WC, Mendelman PM, et al. Efficacy of vaccination with live attenuated, cold-adapted, trivalent, intranasal influenza virus vaccine against a variant (A/Sydney) not contained in the vaccine. J Pediatr 2000;136(2):168–75.

26. Belshe RB, Mendelman PM, Treanor J, et al. The efficacy of live attenuated, cold-adapted, trivalent, intranasal influenza virus vaccine in children. N Engl J Med 1998;338(20):1405–12.

27. Hoberman A, Greenberg DP, Paradise JL, et al. Effectiveness of inactivated influenza vaccine in preventing acute otitis media in young children: a randomized controlled trial. JAMA 2003;290(12):1608–16.

28. Clover RD, Crawford S, Glezen WP, et al. Comparison of heterotypic protection against influenza A/Taiwan/86 (H1N1) by attenuated and inactivated vaccines to A/Chile/83-like viruses. J Infect Dis 1991;163(2):300–4.

29. Nair H, Brooks WA, Katz M, et al. Global burden of respiratory infections due to seasonal influenza in young children: a systematic review and meta-analysis. Lancet 2011;378(9807):1917–30.

30. Azziz-Baumgartner E, Alamgir AS, Rahman M, et al. Incidence of influenza-like illness and severe acute respiratory infection during three influenza seasons in Bangladesh, 2008-2010. Bull World Health Organ 2012;90(1):12–9.

31. Fox JP, Cooney MK, Hall CE, et al. Influenza virus infections in Seattle families, 1975-1979. II. Pattern of infection in invaded households and relation of age and prior antibody to occurrence of infection and related illness. Am J Epidemiol 1982;116(2):228–42.

32. Longini IM Jr, Koopman JS, Monto AS, et al. Estimating household and community transmission parameters for influenza. Am J Epidemiol 1982;115(5):736–51.

33. Wright P. Influenza in the family. N Engl J Med 2000;343(18):1331–2.

34. Hall CB, Douglas RG Jr. Nosocomial influenza infection as a cause of intercurrent fevers in infants. Pediatrics 1975;55(5):673–7.

35. Klimov AI, Rocha E, Hayden FG, et al. Prolonged shedding of amantadine-resistant influenzae A viruses by immunodeficient patients: detection by polymerase chain reaction-restriction analysis. J Infect Dis 1995;172(5):1352–5.

36. Frank AL, Taber LH, Wells CR, et al. Patterns of shedding of myxoviruses and paramyxoviruses in children. J Infect Dis 1981;144(5):433–41.

37. Memoli MJ, Athota R, Reed S, et al. The natural history of influenza infection in the severely immunocompromised vs nonimmunocompromised hosts. Clin Infect Dis 2014;58(2):214–24.

38. Neuzil KM, Hohlbein C, Zhu Y. Illness among schoolchildren during influenza season: effect on school absenteeism, parental absenteeism from work, and secondary illness in families. Arch Pediatr Adolesc Med 2002;156(10):986–91.

39. World Health Organization. Global Influenza Surveillance and Response System (GISRS). 2017. Available at: http://www.who.int/influenza/gisrs_laboratory/en/. Accessed January 3, 2017.

40. Brooks WA, Goswami D, Rahman M, et al. Influenza is a major contributor to childhood pneumonia in a tropical developing country. Pediatr Infect Dis J 2010;29(3):216–21.

41. Tisa V, Barberis I, Faccio V, et al. Quadrivalent influenza vaccine: a new opportunity to reduce the influenza burden. J Prev Med Hyg 2016;57(1):E28–33.

42. Gemmill I. Summary of the National Advisory Committee on Immunization (NACI) statement on seasonal influenza vaccine 2015-2016, in Canada Communicable Disease Report. 2015. p. 227–32. Available at: http://www.phac-aspc.gc.ca/publicat/ccdr-rmtc/15vol41/dr-rm41-10/ar-02-eng.php. Accessed April 18, 2017.

43. Gemmill I, Zhao L, Cochrane L. Summary of the National Advisory Committee on Immunization (NACI) statement on seasonal influenza vaccine for 2016-2017, in Canada Communicable Disease Report. 2016. p. 187–91. Available at: http://www.phac-aspc.gc.ca/publicat/ccdr-rmtc/16vol42/dr-rm42-9/ar-06-eng.php. Accessed April 17, 2017.

44. Fiore AE, Uyeki TM, Broder K, et al. Prevention and control of influenza with vaccines: recommendations of the Advisory Committee on Immunization Practices (ACIP), 2010. MMWR Recomm Rep 2010;59(RR-8):1–62.

45. Grohskopf LA, Sokolow LZ, Broder KR, et al. Prevention and control of influenza with vaccines: recommendations of the advisory committee on immunization practices, United States, 2015-16 influenza season. MMWR Morb Mortal Wkly Rep 2015;64(30):818–25.

46. Neuzil KM, Ortiz JR. Influenza vaccines and vaccination strategies. In: Bloom BR, Lambert PH, editors. The vaccine book. Cambridge (MA): USA Academic Press. p. 423–44.

47. Keitel WA, Neuzil KM, Traenor J. Immunogenicity and efficacy of inactivated/live virus seasonal and pandemic vaccines. In: Webster RG, et al, editors. Textbook of influenza. West Sussex (United Kingdom): Wiley Blackwell; 2013.

48. France EK, Glanz JM, Xu S, et al. Safety of the trivalent inactivated influenza vaccine among children: a population-based study. Arch Pediatr Adolesc Med 2004; 158(11):1031–6.

49. Hambidge SJ, Glanz JM, France EK, et al. Safety of trivalent inactivated influenza vaccine in children 6 to 23 months old. JAMA 2006;296(16):1990–7.

50. Glanz JM, Newcomer SR, Hambidge SJ, et al. Safety of trivalent inactivated influenza vaccine in children aged 24 to 59 months in the vaccine safety datalink. Arch Pediatr Adolesc Med 2011;165(8):749–55.

51. Vesikari T, Knuf M, Wutzler P, et al. Oil-in-water emulsion adjuvant with influenza vaccine in young children. N Engl J Med 2011;365(15):1406–16.

52. Global advisory committee on vaccine safety, 11-12 December 2013. Wkly Epidemiol Rec 2014;89(7):53–60.

53. Tse A, Tseng HF, Greene SK, et al. Signal identification and evaluation for risk of febrile seizures in children following trivalent inactivated influenza vaccine in the Vaccine Safety Datalink Project, 2010-2011. Vaccine 2012;30(11):2024–31.

54. Committee on Infectious Diseases. Recommendations for prevention and control of influenza in children, 2016-2017. Pediatrics 2016;138(4).

55. Centers for Disease Control and Prevention. Prevention and control of influenza with vaccines: recommendations of the Advisory Committee on Immunization Practices (ACIP)–United States, 2012-13 influenza season. MMWR Morb Mortal Wkly Rep 2012;61(32):613–8.

56. Englund JA, Walter EB, Fairchok MP, et al. A comparison of 2 influenza vaccine schedules in 6- to 23-month-old children. Pediatrics 2005;115(4):1039–47.
57. Grohskopf LA, Sokolow LZ, Broder KR, et al. Prevention and control of seasonal influenza with vaccines. MMWR Recomm Rep 2016;65(5):1–54.
58. Osterholm MT, Kelley NS, Sommer A, et al. Efficacy and effectiveness of influenza vaccines: a systematic review and meta-analysis. Lancet Infect Dis 2012;12(1): 36–44.
59. Neuzil KM, Dupont WD, Wright PF, et al. Efficacy of inactivated and cold-adapted vaccines against influenza A infection, 1985 to 1990: the pediatric experience. Pediatr Infect Dis J 2001;20(8):733–40.
60. Jain VK, Rivera L, Zaman K, et al. Vaccine for prevention of mild and moderate-to-severe influenza in children. N Engl J Med 2013;369(26):2481–91.
61. Ferdinands JM, Olsho LE, Agan AA, et al. Effectiveness of influenza vaccine against life-threatening RT-PCR-confirmed influenza illness in US children, 2010-2012. J Infect Dis 2014;210(5):674–83.
62. Flannery B, Reynolds SB, Blanton L, et al. Influenza Vaccine Effectiveness Against Pediatric Deaths: 2010-2014. Pediatrics 2017;139(5).
63. Nolan T, Bravo L, Ceballos A, et al. Enhanced and persistent antibody response against homologous and heterologous strains elicited by a MF59-adjuvanted influenza vaccine in infants and young children. Vaccine 2014; 32(46):6146–56.
64. Johnson PR, Feldman S, Thompson JM, et al. Immunity to influenza A virus infection in young children: a comparison of natural infection, live cold-adapted vaccine, and inactivated vaccine. J Infect Dis 1986;154(1):121–7.
65. Hoft DF, Babusis E, Worku S, et al. Live and inactivated influenza vaccines induce similar humoral responses, but only live vaccines induce diverse T-cell responses in young children. J Infect Dis 2011;204(6):845–53.
66. Wright PF, Hoen AG, Ilyushina NA, et al. Correlates of immunity to influenza as determined by challenge of children with live, attenuated influenza vaccine. Open Forum Infect Dis 2016;3(2):ofw108.
67. Belshe RB, Gruber WC, Mendelman PM, et al. Correlates of immune protection induced by live, attenuated, cold-adapted, trivalent, intranasal influenza virus vaccine. J Infect Dis 2000;181(3):1133–7.
68. Forrest BD, Pride MW, Dunning AJ, et al. Correlation of cellular immune responses with protection against culture-confirmed influenza virus in young children. Clin Vaccine Immunol 2008;15(7):1042–53.
69. Fleming DM, Crovari P, Wahn U, et al. Comparison of the efficacy and safety of live attenuated cold-adapted influenza vaccine, trivalent, with trivalent inactivated influenza virus vaccine in children and adolescents with asthma. Pediatr Infect Dis J 2006;25(10):860–9.
70. Belshe RB, Edwards KM, Vesikari T, et al. Live attenuated versus inactivated influenza vaccine in infants and young children. N Engl J Med 2007;356(7): 685–96.
71. Ashkenazi S, Vertruyen A, Arístegui J, et al. Superior relative efficacy of live attenuated influenza vaccine compared with inactivated influenza vaccine in young children with recurrent respiratory tract infections. Pediatr Infect Dis J 2006; 25(10):870–9.
72. Flannery B, Clippard J, Zimmerman RK, et al. Early estimates of seasonal influenza vaccine effectiveness - United States, January 2015. MMWR Morb Mortal Wkly Rep 2015;64(1):10–5.

73. Skowronski DM, Janjua NZ, De Serres G, et al. A sentinel platform to evaluate influenza vaccine effectiveness and new variant circulation, Canada 2010-2011 season. Clin Infect Dis 2012;55(3):332–42.

74. Flannery B. LAIV vs IIV effectiveness: summary of evidence since 2009. Centers for Disease Control and Prevention (CDC); 2016. Available at: https://www.cdc.gov/vaccines/acip/meetings/downloads/slides-2016-06/influenza-07-flannery.pdf. Accessed April 17, 2017.

75. National Advisor Committee on Immunization (NACI). Addendum - LAIV Use in children and adolescents. Canadian immunization guide chapter on influenza and statement on seasonal influenza vaccine for 2016-2017. 2016. Available at: http://www.phac-aspc.gc.ca/naci-ccni/flu-2016-grippe-addendum-children-enfants-eng.php. Accessed April 17, 2017.

76. WHO. Vaccines against influenza. WHO position paper. Wkly Epidemiol Rec 2012;87(47):461–76.

77. Zaman K, Roy E, Arifeen SE, et al. Effectiveness of maternal influenza immunization in mothers and infants. N Engl J Med 2008;359(15):1555–64.

78. Madhi SA, Cutland CL, Kuwanda L, et al. Influenza vaccination of pregnant women and protection of their infants. N Engl J Med 2014;371(10):918–31.

79. Tapia MD, Sow SO, Tamboura B, et al. Maternal immunisation with trivalent inactivated influenza vaccine for prevention of influenza in infants in Mali: a prospective, active-controlled, observer-blind, randomised phase 4 trial. Lancet Infect Dis 2016;16(9):1026–35.

80. CDC. Influenza antiviral medications: summary for clinicians. 2016. Available at: https://www.cdc.gov/flu/professionals/antivirals/summary-clinicians.htm. Accessed January 17, 2017.

81. CDC. Antiviral drug resistance among influenza viruses. 2016. Available at: https://www.cdc.gov/flu/professionals/antivirals/antiviral-drug-resistance.htm. Accessed January 17, 2017.

82. Vesikari T, Fleming DM, Aristegui JF, et al. Safety, efficacy, and effectiveness of cold-adapted influenza vaccine-trivalent against community-acquired, culture-confirmed influenza in young children attending day care. Pediatrics 2006;118(6):2298–312.

83. Tam JS, Capeding MR, Lum LC, et al. Efficacy and safety of a live attenuated, cold-adapted influenza vaccine, trivalent against culture-confirmed influenza in young children in Asia. Pediatr Infect Dis J 2007;26(7):619–28.

84. Bracco Neto H, Farhat CK, Tregnaghi MW, et al. Efficacy and safety of 1 and 2 doses of live attenuated influenza vaccine in vaccine-naive children. Pediatr Infect Dis J 2009;28(5):365–71.

85. Madhi SA, Dittmer S, Kuwanda L, et al. Efficacy and immunogenicity of influenza vaccine in HIV-infected children: a randomized, double-blind, placebo controlled trial. AIDS 2013;27(3):369–79.

Zika Virus Infection

Debbie-Ann T. Shirley, MBBS, MPH*, James P. Nataro, MD, PhD, MBA

KEYWORDS

- Zika • Microcephaly • Congenital • Mosquito • Travel • Sexual transmission

KEY POINTS

- Zika virus is a flavivirus related to dengue, yellow fever, and West Nile viruses, that is spread by *Aedes* mosquitoes, and has rapidly spread worldwide along the distribution of its vector.
- Zika virus was initially thought to cause asymptomatic or only mild, self-limiting symptoms, but more severe cases and the sequela of Guillain-Barré syndrome have now been recognized.
- In utero exposure has been observed to result in a congenital syndrome marked by microcephaly and a range of other brain anomalies.
- Affected infants require accurate diagnosis, close monitoring, and access to multidisciplinary care throughout childhood.
- Although vaccine development is an active area of research, there is currently no vaccine or treatment for Zika virus infection. Current preventive strategies rely on decreasing infected bites and use of barrier protection during pregnancy.

INTRODUCTION

The recent, explosive, pandemic spread of Zika virus (ZIKV) has resulted in a rapid and accelerated outpouring of collaborative research regarding this once understudied infection. ZIKV was first identified incidentally in 1947 by way of tree canopy surveillance among nonhuman primates in the Zika forest of Uganda.[1] The virus was isolated from the *Aedes* mosquito shortly after, hinting at what was later confirmed to be the principal vector of transmission. Although serologic surveillance studies from West Africa and Southeast Asia suggested that infection occurred in humans, early epidemiologic and challenge studies pointed toward only mild and self-limiting febrile illness.[2–5] The initial lack of specificity of symptoms may have allowed ongoing eastward geographic spread to be unrecognized, and little else was reported until the first large outbreak of ZIKV occurred on the island of Yap, Micronesia, in 2007, affecting

Disclosures: D.-A.T. Shirley reports that no competing interests exist.
Department of Pediatrics, University of Virginia School of Medicine, Box 800386, Charlottesville, VA 22908-0386, USA
* Corresponding author.
E-mail address: ds3ru@virginia.edu

Pediatr Clin N Am 64 (2017) 937–951
http://dx.doi.org/10.1016/j.pcl.2017.03.012
0031-3955/17/© 2017 Elsevier Inc. All rights reserved.

pediatric.theclinics.com

the vast majority of the island's population. Spread continued across the Pacific islands, with similar large outbreaks reported in French Polynesia in 2013, and the Chilean Easter Island in 2014.[6,7] ZIKV was next detected in Brazil in May 2015, with more than 1.5 million cases reported by early 2016. Six months after arrival in Brazil, a sharp increase in the prevalence of infants born with microcephaly was observed, finally bringing the alarming public health implications of this infection into focus.[8] The World Health Organization (WHO) declared a public health emergency of international concern as infection continued to spread to the rest of South and Central America and the Caribbean.[9]

Mosquito-borne transmission of ZIKV has been reported in 48 countries and territories in the Americas to date since 2015.[10] Given the location of the *Aedes* mosquito species globally, it is predicted that there will be continued spread and outbreaks in new countries.[11] Although the mechanism of entry into the Western hemisphere can be only speculated, this pandemic reminds us of the interconnectedness of our global community.[12,13] ZIKV is one of several mosquito-borne infections to have emerged as a pandemic threat over the past few decades, following behind the dengue, West Nile, and chikungunya viruses. Not only has this epidemic exemplified the ability of human international travel to accelerate the emergence and spread of potentially devastating infectious diseases,[14] it also has illustrated our ability to swiftly disseminate data and make coordinated research efforts to improve our understanding of infectious agents. New insights are continually gleaned, but despite these labors, many questions remain unanswered, including a complete description of the clinical spectrum associated with ZIKV infection. Improved rapid diagnostics and the development of effective counter-strategies for containment and prevention of infection are urgently needed to improve the impact of ZIKV infection on children globally.

ZIKA VIRUS IN THE UNITED STATES

Local transmission in the United States began in the territory of Puerto Rico,[15] with more than 34,000 locally acquired cases now reported. Local transmission was reported for the first time in the continental United States in July 2016 in Miami, Florida.[16] In November 2016, Texas became the second state to report local transmission. At this time, there have been close to 5,000 travel-associated cases, involving every state other than Alaska, and 224 locally acquired mosquito-borne cases in the continental United States; approximately one-third of all reported cases in the United States have been in pregnant women.[17] Preliminary estimates suggest that microcephaly and other brain anomalies have occurred in 6% of infants and fetuses born to women in the United States who had laboratory-confirmed evidence of ZIKV infection during pregnancy, increasing up to 15% in those women with first-trimester infection.[18]

EPIDEMIOLOGY

ZIKV is an arbovirus, within the family Flaviviridae, sharing the flavivirus genus with the yellow fever, dengue, and West Nile virues.[1] It is a single-stranded RNA virus with Asian and African lineages.[19–21] Transmission is primarily via the bite of an infected *Aedes aegypti* mosquito, which is widely distributed throughout the tropics, but also can be transmitted by other *Aedes* species, such as *Aedes albopictus,* which has a broader distribution within North America.[11] The *Aedes* mosquito has a short flight range and is well-adapted to live and breed near people and their homes, laying eggs in the stagnant water of puddles and containers. Although the bite of an infected mosquito is the principal route of infection, case studies have suggested transmission by exposure to body fluids; the virus can be detected in blood, semen, vaginal secretions, urine, cerebrospinal fluid, and saliva after resolution of symptoms (**Box 1**).

The incubation period of ZIKV disease varies from 3 to 14 days after exposure. Viremia is detected up to 10 days before symptoms develop, clearing as quickly as 2 days after symptom onset, although prolonged shedding also is known, with ZIKV RNA being detected in whole blood up to 81 days after illness. Prolonged viral detection of up to 15 weeks after illness has been reported in pregnant patients, and at least 67 days after birth in an infant.[22–26] It is presumed that congenital infection occurs via transplacental transmission, and the persistence of ZIKV RNA in the serum of pregnant patients may reflect ongoing fetal infection.[26]

Close surveillance has revealed that ZIKV is also sexually transmitted, with transmission from both infected male and infected female individuals reported, even when partners are asymptomatic.[27–30] Prolonged shedding of up to 6 months has been documented in semen, where ZIKV RNA may be up to 100,000 times that of plasma levels.[31,32] In at least 1 case, acquisition has occurred without a known risk factor, other than close contact.[33]

As ZIKV can be transmitted by blood products,[25,34,35] the US Food and Drug Administration has provided recommendations regarding universal screening of donated blood and other products.[36] The United Network for Organ Sharing also has provided guidance on issues of ZIKV infection related to organ transplantion.[37]

ZIKA VIRUS AND MICROCEPHALY

Even the earliest work on ZIKV in mice suggested a distinct neurotropism of the virus,[1] but the association in humans was not made until 2015, when a 20-fold increase in the prevalence of microcephaly was noticed among newborns in Brazil.[8,38,39] Health authorities from French Polynesia then retrospectively noted that the prevalence of central nervous system malformations in fetuses and newborns had increased to 50-fold above baseline during their own ZIKV 2013 outbreak.[8,40] Numerous similar reports have since surfaced, and based on review of the body of accumulating evidence showing associations with in utero infection, the US Centers for Disease Control and Prevention (CDC) concluded ZIKV to be a cause of congenital microcephaly and other severe brain defects in April 2016.[38–48] To date, 31 countries or territories have reported microcephaly and other central nervous system malformations potentially associated with ZIKV infection.[49]

Identification of Infection in Affected Fetuses

The ZIKV genome was completely recovered from the brain of a severely affected fetus with microcephaly, agyria, hydrocephalus, and multifocal calcifications following maternal acquisition of infection during first-trimester travel to Brazil, resulting in termination of pregnancy at 32 weeks' gestation.[46] Several other well-documented cases

---

Box 1
Modes of transmission of Zika virus

- Mosquito-borne
- Sexual contact
- Vertical
- Blood transfusion

have detected evidence of ZIKV infection by immunohistochemical staining, polymerase chain reaction (PCR), and culture within the brains of fetuses and infants with microcephaly.[24,50,51] ZIKV has been identified in the amniotic fluid and placenta of fetuses who have died, indicating an ability to infect the fetus by crossing the placental barrier.[52–54] Levels of ZIKV RNA were found to be up to 1200-fold higher in fetal/neonatal brain tissue than placental tissue, indicating active viral replication occurs in the brain.[55]

Biologic Plausibility

Murine models support vertical transmission via placental infection and injury, followed by fetal brain infection leading to the development of microcephaly.[56–59] In vitro studies of placental infection with ZIKV demonstrate spread of infection from the basal to parietal decidua, then to chorionic villi and amniochorionic membranes.[60] Placental-specific macrophages (Hofbauer cells) may help to disseminate infection to the central nervous system.[55,61] In neurospheres and brain organoids, ZIKV impairs growth of neural progenitor cells, and is associated with cell-cycle dysregulation and programmed cell death responses.[62,63] In addition to direct cytotoxicity, the possibility of immune-mediated effects, such as disruption of neurovascular development or induction of autoimmune responses against gangliosides, has been raised.[64,65] The exact mechanisms of teratogenicity and the role of contributing cofactors remain to be elucidated, but several parallels can be drawn to established congenital infections, such as cytomegalovirus and rubella, further fortifying the biologic plausibility of congenital ZIKV infection.[66]

Timing of Infection

Infections early in pregnancy have been most commonly associated with microcephaly in the infant.[40,42,67,68] Epidemiologic mapping from Brazil suggests that microcephaly best correlates with ZIKV incidence during week 17 of pregnancy (week 14 for severe microcephaly), but central nervous system anomalies have been reported in all trimesters.[13,68–70] Microcephaly cases reported in Colombia in 2016 peaked approximately 24 weeks after the peak of the ZIKV disease, further supporting that the greatest risk of microcephaly correlates with infection during the first and early second trimesters.[71] A case-control study among pregnant women from Rio de Janeiro, Brazil, found that 29% of women developing ZIKV infection at any time during pregnancy had abnormalities detectable by prenatal ultrasound; there were no abnormalities noted in the uninfected controls.[69] A larger case-control study from the same area has recently shown similar findings, with 42% of infants born to mothers infected during pregnancy having abnormal clinical or neuroimaging, although adverse outcomes occurred even in infants exposed as late as 39 weeks' gestation, indicating that effects may still occur during the latter part of pregnancy.[72] Interestingly, microcephaly has not been reported with intrapartum transmission to date.[73]

CONGENITAL ZIKA SYNDROME

Although the full range of congenital manifestations remains to be determined, a typical pattern of clinical features and imaging findings of affected infants has clearly emerged, leading to the term congenital Zika syndrome (**Box 2**).[74] Some cases have closely resembled the fetal brain disruption sequence characterized by severe microcephaly, overlapping cranial sutures, prominent occipital bone, and redundant scalp skin, hypothesized to result from decrease in intracranial pressure secondary to fetal brain volume loss.[43,75] Brain anomalies may occur without the presence of congenital

---

Box 2
Typical features of congenital Zika syndrome

- Microcephaly[a]
- Craniofacial disproportion and cutis gyrata
- Hypertonicity and hyperreflexia
- Seizures
- Irritability
- Abnormal neuroradiology findings[b]
- Dysphagia and other feeding difficulties
- Ocular abnormalities[c]
- Sensorineural hearing loss
- Arthrogryposis

[a] There is no standard definition for microcephaly. The Centers for Disease Control and Prevention define congenital microcephaly for live-born births as head circumference less than the third percentile for age and sex.[105]
[b] Reported abnormal neuroradiology findings include calcifications (mostly subcortical), ventriculomegaly, cortical thinning, abnormal gyral patterns, such as lissencephaly, hypoplasia/agenesis of the corpus callosum, decreased myelination, cerebellar hypoplasia, enlargement of the cisterna magna, and increased extra-axial fluid.[106,107]
[c] Reported ocular abnormalities include focal pigment mottling of the retina and chorioretinal atropy, optic nerve abnormalities, coloboma, lens subluxation, hemorrhagic retinopathy, abnormal vasculature of the retina, maculopathy, microphthalmia, cataracts.[41,44,53,108,109]

---

microcephaly.[76] Affected fetuses may have decreasing head circumferences documented in utero by ultrasound, but microcephaly also may develop after birth, indicating the need for ongoing evaluation in all potentially affected infants until more is known.[43,45,77]

A number of ocular anomalies have been described, predominantly of the posterior eye (see **Box 2**). First-trimester infection and smaller head circumference correlate with abnormal eye findings.[78] Ocular involvement may be bilateral in up to 70% of infants with eye disease.[79] Sensory neural hearing loss was reported in up to 6% of affected infants with microcephaly.[80] Arthrogryposis, a disorder of multiple congenital joint contractures, is likely a consequence of diminished fetal movements arising from underlying neurologic involvement. Review of 34 published reports identified 5 features that differentiate congenital Zika syndrome from other congenital infections, including severe microcephaly with partially collapsed skull, thin cerebral cortices with subcortical calcifications, macular scarring and focal pigmentary retinal mottling, congenial contractures, and marked early hypertonia.[74] Differential causes of microcephaly include other congenital infections, such as cytomegalovirus, human immunodeficiency virus, varicella-zoster, and rubella infection.[74] Rare genetic conditions, such as Aicardi-Goutières syndrome, also may share overlapping manifestations with the congenital Zika syndrome.[74]

OTHER CLINICAL MANIFESTATIONS OF ZIKA DISEASE

Outside of congenital infection, ZIKV infection in humans is mostly asymptomatic. Mild, self-limiting symptoms occur in approximately 20% of those infected. These symptoms, which overlap with the other common mosquito-borne infections of dengue virus and chikungunya virus, include pruritic maculopapular rash, fever, myalgias, arthralgias, headache, retroorbital pain, nonpurulent conjunctivitis, sore throat, petechiae, emesis, and diarrhea.[81–83] Severe infection is rare, with only occasional fatalities reported.[33,82,84,85] A strong association with ZIKV and Guillain-Barré syndrome exists. Prevalence can be 2 to 10 times or even higher above baseline in affected areas, which has allowed bilateral flaccid paralysis to serve as a sentinel marker of ZIKV during these recent outbreaks.[82,86–88] Other neurologic complications, such as acute myelitis, meningoencephalitis, and even hearing loss also have been documented.[89–91]

In children who acquire ZIKV infection postnatally, symptoms are the same as those reported in the general population.[83,92] The effects of ZIKV infection in the immunocompromised host are not yet well described. Bacterial superinfection and allograft dysfunction were noted among the complications seen in a small group of solid organ transplant recipients from Brazil.[93]

DIAGNOSIS

Diagnostic tests to confirm suspected exposure include the molecular detection of ZIKV RNA by reverse transcriptase PCR and serology. Zika virus–specific immunoglobulin (Ig)M and neutralizing antibodies typically develop toward the end of the first week of illness, but may take up to 2 weeks. IgM levels generally continue to be detectable for 12 weeks after symptom onset.[94] The specific approach to testing

---

Box 3
Laboratory tests used for the diagnosis of Zika virus infection

Test	Specimens[a]	Use	Comment
Molecular diagnostics			
RT-PCR	Serum Urine CSF	Recent infection	• PCR may be only briefly positive, hence negative results cannot always exclude recent infection
Serology			
IgM	Serum CSF	Recent infection	• Other flaviviruses can serologically cross-react, hence positive, equivocal, or inconclusive results should be confirmed by PRNT
PRNT	Serum	Confirms specificity of IgM	• 4-fold higher titer by PRNT may not always be able to discriminate between anti-Zika virus antibodies and cross-reacting antibodies in people who have been previously infected with or vaccinated against a related flavivirus • Measures mostly IgG, hence cannot distinguish between maternal and infant antibodies; repeat PRNT may be needed ≥18 mo of age, when maternal antibodies are expected to have waned

Abbreviations: RT-PCR, reverse-transcription polymerase chain reaction; Ig, immunoglobulin; PRNT plaque reduction neutralization test.
[a] Testing for other tissues and body fluids may also be available.

Adapted from Rabe IB, Staples JE, Villanueva J, et al. Interim guidance for interpretation of Zika virus antibody test results. MMWR Morb Mortal Wkly Rep 2016;65(21):543–6. Available at: https://www.cdc.gov/mmwr/volumes/65/wr/mm6521e1.htm.

will vary depending on available resources, but testing should be considered in patients who present with typical clinical manifestations of ZIKV disease in the setting of an associated epidemiologic risk factor (such as residence in, or travel to, an area where mosquito-borne transmission of ZIKV has been reported or unprotected sexual contact with a person who has). The CDC recommends that pregnant women in the United States be assessed for possible ZIKV exposure at each prenatal care visit, and tested if there has been possible exposure. Similarly, the CDC recommends laboratory testing of infants born to mothers with known or possible ZIKV infection or infants found to have abnormal clinical or neuroimaging findings that could be compatible with congenital Zika syndrome in the setting of a maternal epidemiologic link.[73] Samples should be collected directly from the infant, ideally within in the first 2 days of life, to help distinguish between congenital, peripartum, and postnatal timing of infection.[73] Maternal testing should be considered simultaneously, if not previously carried out. Like recommendations for the general population, postnatal testing of children should be performed if a child presents with compatible symptoms of acute infection, but testing of asymptomatic children is not needed if there is no concern for congenital infection. There are several general caveats to interpretation (**Box 3**), pointing to the urgent need for more precise and scalable diagnostic tests. In the meantime, laboratory diagnosis of congenital infection must be interpreted in the context of suspected timing of infection during pregnancy, serology results, and compatible clinical findings. Specific guidance on testing pregnant women and infants born to mothers with possible ZIKV infection during pregnancy should be checked periodically for revisions to these guidelines as updates become available.[73,95]

MANAGEMENT

There is no specific antiviral treatment for ZIKV infection. General management for acute symptomatic infections is supportive with rest, hydration, and analgesics/antipyretics. Use of aspirin should be avoided in children, given the association with Reye syndrome, and nonsteroidal anti-inflammatory medications should be avoided in symptomatic postnatal infection until dengue can been excluded, to decrease the risk of hemorrhagic complications.[96] For those with neurologic symptoms, management also is supportive, including intensive care as needed. For pregnant women with positive or inconclusive ZIKV laboratory testing, serial monitoring with

---

Box 4
Recommendations for travel to areas with ongoing Zika virus transmission

- Check travel advisories for updated guidance and travel notices

- Prevent mosquito bites:
  - Wear long-sleeved shirts and pants
  - Use of insect repellants registered by the Environmental Protection Agency
  - Stay in screened or air-conditioned lodgings
  - Use bed nets
  - Use permethrin-treated clothing and gear

- Counsel on standard measures to prevent sexual transmission, including condom use, as appropriate
  - Men: for 6 months from symptom onset or last potential exposure
  - Women: for 2 months from symptom onset or last potential exposure

Adapted from CDC Zika Travel Information Web site. Available at: https://wwwnc.cdc.gov/travel/page/zika-information.

ultrasonography is recommended.[95] Once born, the management of infants born to mothers with confirmed or possible ZIKV infection during pregnancy includes precise measurement of the occipitofrontal head circumference, comprehensive physical examination noting abnormal neurologic and dysmorphic findings, infant laboratory testing as discussed previously, and postnatal head ultrasonography and audiology screen.[73] Close follow-up will be required throughout early childhood, with the incorporation of detailed developmental and growth, neurologic, visual, and audiologic assessments. A multidisciplinary approach is needed to manage infants and children with congenital Zika syndrome, and input from several subspecialty areas may be required.[73] In addition, affected children and families must be provided with ongoing psychosocial support. The CDC has established a pregnancy registry to collect information about ZIKV infection during pregnancy and congenital ZIKV infection as well as the Zika Care Connect program aimed at helping families to access recommended healthcare services.[73] The American Academy of Pediatrics has created ZIKV support videos for both families and pediatricians caring for families to also assist with meeting psychosocial needs (https://www.aap.org/en-us/advocacy-and-policy/aap-health-initiatives/Zika/Pages/Zika-Videos.aspx).

Although ZIKV has been detected in breast milk, no cases of ZIKV infection associated with breastfeeding have been reported to date, leading health authorities to recommend that women with ZIKV infection during pregnancy be supported to breastfeed their infants.[73,97] One report suggests that ZIKV can be inactivated in human breast milk after prolonged storage and with pasteurization.[98] Public health recommendations will continue to be informed as our understanding of ZIKV advances and so guidelines should be periodically checked for updates on management. The long-term outcomes of congenital ZIKV infection have yet to be determined, especially for those with undetectable or milder symptoms at birth, although severe neurologic impairment is inevitably anticipated for those affected by microcephaly and other major brain anomalies.

PREVENTION

Primary infection is believed to convey immunity to subsequent infection, and hence expedited efforts to develop a vaccine are under way. Three different vaccine platforms, using an inactivated virus vaccine, a plasmid DNA vaccine, and adoptive transfer were all shown to provide protection against ZIKV challenge in rhesus monkeys.[99] Phase 1 and 2 trials of a vaccine containing Zika purified inactivated virus and a DNA vaccine are under way, while monovalent live-attenuated, pentavalent (ZIKV and dengue virus) live-atenuated and mRNA vaccine trials are scheduled to begin in 2017.[100] Development of a safe and effective ZIKV vaccine could protect pregnant women and prevent future outbreaks, similar to the successful elimination of endemic transmission of rubella and the congenital rubella syndrome in the Americas, after widespread implementation of rubella vaccination programs.[101]

Current public health prevention strategies rely on surveillance, vector control, and prevention of mosquito bites. Providers caring for children who may be traveling with families to areas with active ongoing ZIKV transmission are encouraged to check public health advisories for travel notices (see **Box 4**). Avoidance of nonessential travel to areas with ongoing risk of mosquito transmission for women who are pregnant or plan on becoming pregnant has been advised, with both preconception and postconception guidance available to decrease the risk of sexual transmission during pregnancy.[28,95,102] Health authorities also have made recommendations to delay pregnancy for women living in some areas of active mosquito-borne transmission, although such recommendations bear their own challenges for widespread adherence.[103]

SUMMARY

Our understanding of ZIKV and the congenital syndrome resulting from infection with this virus is rapidly evolving, as ongoing research efforts continually inform our knowledge. Given the location of the mosquito vectors of ZIKV, it is likely that vector-borne transmission will remain ongoing in the Americas for years to come. With more than 41 million US residents traveling abroad to Mexico, South America, Central America, and the Caribbean per year, travel-related cases will continue to be seen in the United States.[104] The potential for local transmission exists within the United States wherever the *Aedes* vector can be found. Hence, it is important for pediatric providers to be able to provide anticipatory guidance to families regarding the risk factors and clinical manifestations of ZIKV. Microcephaly is the most dramatic feature of congenital infection, but it is anticipated that more subtle effects may be discovered during early childhood. Pediatric providers should be prepared to identify infants at risk, and to provide appropriate diagnostic evaluation and multidisciplinary care along with psychosocial support to affected infants and families, while we optimistically await development of a safe and effective preventive vaccine. As discussed elsewhere in this issue, ZIKV will increase the population of children with special needs, a growing population that cannot be neglected in resource-poor settings.

REFERENCES

1. Dick GW, Kitchen SF, Haddow AJ. Zika virus. I. isolations and serological specificity. Trans R Soc Trop Med Hyg 1952;46(5):509–20.
2. Dick GW. Zika virus. II. pathogenicity and physical properties. Trans R Soc Trop Med Hyg 1952;46(5):521–34.
3. Bearcroft WG. Zika virus infection experimentally induced in a human volunteer. Trans R Soc Trop Med Hyg 1956;50(5):442–8.
4. Macnamara FN. Zika virus: a report on three cases of human infection during an epidemic of jaundice in Nigeria. Trans R Soc Trop Med Hyg 1954;48(2):139–45.
5. Olson JG, Ksiazek TG, Suhandiman, et al. Zika virus, a cause of fever in central Java, Indonesia. Trans R Soc Trop Med Hyg 1981;75(3):389–93.
6. Alera MT, Hermann L, Tac-An IA, et al. Zika virus infection, Philippines, 2012. Emerg Infect Dis 2015;21(4):722–4.
7. Tognarelli J, Ulloa S, Villagra E, et al. A report on the outbreak of zika virus on Easter Island, South Pacific, 2014. Arch Virol 2016;161(3):665–8.
8. Pan American Health Organization, World Health Organization. Neurological syndrome, congenital malformations, and zika virus infection. Implications for public health in the Americas. 2015. Available at: http://www2.paho.org/hq/index.php?option=com_docman&task=doc_view&Itemid=270&gid=32405&lang=en.
9. World Health Organization (WHO). WHO statement on the first meeting of the international health regulations (2005) (IHR 2005) emergency committee on zika virus and observed increase in neurological disorders and neonatal malformations. 2016. Available at: http://www.who.int/mediacentre/news/statements/2016/1st-emergency-committee-zika/en/.
10. Pan American Health Organization/World Health Organization. Zika epidemiological update, 17 November. Washington, DC: PAHO/WHO; 2016.

11. Bogoch II, Brady OJ, Kraemer MU, et al. Potential for zika virus introduction and transmission in resource-limited countries in Africa and the Asia-Pacific region: a modelling study. Lancet Infect Dis 2016;16(11):1237–45.

12. Lednicky J, Beau De Rochars VM, El Badry M, et al. Zika virus outbreak in Haiti in 2014: molecular and clinical data. PLoS Negl Trop Dis 2016;10(4):e0004687.

13. Faria NR, Azevedo Rdo S, Kraemer MU, et al. Zika virus in the Americas: early epidemiological and genetic findings. Science 2016;352(6283):345–9.

14. Fauci AS, Morens DM. Zika virus in the Americas–yet another arbovirus threat. N Engl J Med 2016;374(7):601–4.

15. U.S. Department of Health & Human Services. HHS declares a public health emergency in Puerto Rico in response to zika outbreak. 2016. Available at: http://www.hhs.gov/about/news/2016/08/12/hhs-declares-public-health-emergency-in-puerto-rico-in-response-to-zika-outbreak.html. Accessed November 18, 2016.

16. Centers for Disease Control and Prevention (CDC). Florida investigation links four recent zika cases to local mosquito-borne virus transmission. 2016. Available at: https://www.cdc.gov/media/releases/2016/p0729-florida-zika-cases.html. Accessed November, 18, 2016.

17. CDC. Case counts in the US. Arbonet, January 1, 2015-April 26, 2017. Available at: https://Www.cdc.gov/zika/geo/united-states.html. Accessed May 2, 2017.

18. Reynolds MR, Jones AM, Petersen EE, et al. Vital Signs: Update on Zika Virus–Associated Birth Defects and Evaluation of All U.S. Infants with Congenital Zika Virus Exposure – U.S. Zika Pregnancy Registry, 2016. MMWR Morb Mortal Wkly Rep 2017;66:366–73.

19. Kuno G, Chang GJ. Full-length sequencing and genomic characterization of bagaza, kedougou, and zika viruses. Arch Virol 2007;152(4):687–96.

20. Haddow AD, Schuh AJ, Yasuda CY, et al. Genetic characterization of zika virus strains: geographic expansion of the Asian lineage. PLoS Negl Trop Dis 2012; 6(2):e1477.

21. Faye O, Freire CC, Iamarino A, et al. Molecular evolution of zika virus during its emergence in the 20(th) century. PLoS Negl Trop Dis 2014;8(1):e2636.

22. Oliveira DB, Almeida FJ, Durigon EL, et al. Prolonged shedding of zika virus associated with congenital infection. N Engl J Med 2016;375(12):1202–4.

23. Murray KO, Gorchakov R, Carlson AR, et al. Prolonged detection of zika virus in vaginal secretions and whole blood. Emerg Infect Dis 2017;23(1). http://dx.doi.org/10.3201/eid2301.161394.

24. Driggers RW, Ho CY, Korhonen EM, et al. Zika virus infection with prolonged maternal viremia and fetal brain abnormalities. N Engl J Med 2016;374(22): 2142–51.

25. Musso D, Nhan T, Robin E, et al. Potential for zika virus transmission through blood transfusion demonstrated during an outbreak in French Polynesia, November 2013 to February 2014. Euro Surveill 2014;19(14):20761.

26. Suy A, Sulleiro E, Rodo C, et al. Prolonged zika virus viremia during pregnancy. N Engl J Med 2016;375(26):2611–3.

27. Brooks RB, Carlos MP, Myers RA, et al. Likely sexual transmission of zika virus from a man with no symptoms of infection—Maryland, 2016. MMWR Morb Mortal Wkly Rep 2016;65(34):915–6.

28. Petersen EE, Meaney-Delman D, Neblett-Fanfair R, et al. Update: Interim guidance for preconception counseling and prevention of sexual transmission of zika virus for persons with possible zika virus exposure—United States, September 2016. MMWR Morb Mortal Wkly Rep 2016;65(39):1077–81.

29. Davidson A, Slavinski S, Komoto K, et al. Suspected female-to-male sexual transmission of zika virus—New York City, 2016. MMWR Morb Mortal Wkly Rep 2016;65(28):716–7.

30. Deckard DT, Chung WM, Brooks JT, et al. Male-to-male sexual transmission of zika virus–Texas, January 2016. MMWR Morb Mortal Wkly Rep 2016;65(14): 372–4.

31. Mansuy JM, Dutertre M, Mengelle C, et al. Zika virus: high infectious viral load in semen, a new sexually transmitted pathogen? Lancet Infect Dis 2016;16(4):405.

32. Nicastri E, Castilletti C, Liuzzi G, et al. Persistent detection of zika virus RNA in semen for six months after symptom onset in a traveller returning from Haiti to Italy, February 2016. Euro Surveill 2016;21(32). http://dx.doi.org/10.2807/1560-7917.ES.2016.21.32.30314.

33. Brent C, Dunn A, Savage H, et al. Preliminary findings from an investigation of zika virus infection in a patient with no known risk factors—Utah, 2016. MMWR Morb Mortal Wkly Rep 2016;65(36):981–2.

34. Kuehnert MJ, Basavaraju SV, Moseley RR, et al. Screening of blood donations for zika virus infection—Puerto Rico, April 3-June 11, 2016. MMWR Morb Mortal Wkly Rep 2016;65(24):627–8.

35. Motta IJ, Spencer BR, Cordeiro da Silva SG, et al. Evidence for transmission of zika virus by platelet transfusion. N Engl J Med 2016;375(11):1101–3.

36. FDA news release. FDA advises testing for zika virus in all donated blood and blood components in the US. 2016. Available at: http://www.fda.gov/NewsEvents/Newsroom/PressAnnouncements/ucm518218.htm. Accessed November 18, 2016.

37. UNOS. Guidance for organ donation and transplantation professional regarding the zika virus. 2016. Available at: https://www.transplantpro.org/news/opos/guidance-for-organ-donation-and-transplantation-professionals-regarding-the-zika-virus/. Accessed November 18, 2016.

38. Pan American Health Organization, World Health Organization. Epidemiological alert. Increase of microcephaly in the northeast of Brazil. 2015. Available at: Http://Www.paho.org/hq/index.php?option=com_docman&task=doc_view&Itemid=270&gid=32396&lang=en. Accessed November 11, 2016

39. Soares de Araujo JS, Regis CT, Gomes RG, et al. Microcephaly in north-east Brazil: a retrospective study on neonates born between 2012 and 2015. Bull World Health Organ 2016;94(11):835–40.

40. Cauchemez S, Besnard M, Bompard P, et al. Association between zika virus and microcephaly in French Polynesia, 2013-15: A retrospective study. Lancet 2016; 387(10033):2125–32.

41. Oliveira Melo AS, Malinger G, Ximenes R, et al. Zika virus intrauterine infection causes fetal brain abnormality and microcephaly: tip of the iceberg? Ultrasound Obstet Gynecol 2016;47(1):6–7.

42. Schuler-Faccini L, Ribeiro EM, Feitosa IM, et al. Possible association between zika virus infection and microcephaly—Brazil, 2015. MMWR Morb Mortal Wkly Rep 2016;65(3):59–62.

43. Moura da Silva AA, Ganz JS, Sousa PD, et al. Early growth and neurologic outcomes of infants with probable congenital zika virus syndrome. Emerg Infect Dis 2016;22(11):1953–6.

44. van der Linden V, Filho EL, Lins OG, et al. Congenital zika syndrome with arthrogryposis: retrospective case series study. BMJ 2016;354:i3899.

45. Van der linden V, Pessoa A, Dobyns W, et al. Description of 13 infants born during october 2015–January 2016 with congenital zika virus infection without

microcephaly at birth—Brazil. MMWR Morb Mortal Wkly Rep 2016;65(47): 1343–8.

46. Mlakar J, Korva M, Tul N, et al. Zika virus associated with microcephaly. N Engl J Med 2016;374(10):951–8.

47. Melo AS, Aguiar RS, Amorim MM, et al. Congenital zika virus infection: beyond neonatal microcephaly. JAMA Neurol 2016;73(12):1407–16.

48. The Centers for Disease Control and Prevention(CDC). CDC concludes zika causes microcephaly and other birth defects. 2016. Available at: https://www.cdc.gov/media/releases/2016/s0413-zika-microcephaly.html.

49. WHO. World Health Organization zika situation report. 2017. Available at: http://www.who.int/emergencies/zika-virus/situation-report/10-march-2017/en/. Accessed May 2, 2017.

50. Martines RB, Bhatnagar J, Keating MK, et al. Notes from the field: Evidence of zika virus infection in brain and placental tissues from two congenitally infected newborns and two fetal losses–Brazil, 2015. MMWR Morb Mortal Wkly Rep 2016;65(6):159–60.

51. Meaney-Delman D, Hills SL, Williams C, et al. Zika virus infection among U.S. pregnant travelers—August 2015-February 2016. MMWR Morb Mortal Wkly Rep 2016;65(8):211–4.

52. Noronha L, Zanluca C, Azevedo ML, et al. Zika virus damages the human placental barrier and presents marked fetal neurotropism. Mem Inst Oswaldo Cruz 2016;111(5):287–93.

53. Calvet G, Aguiar RS, Melo AS, et al. Detection and sequencing of zika virus from amniotic fluid of fetuses with microcephaly in Brazil: a case study. Lancet Infect Dis 2016;16(6):653–60.

54. van der Eijk AA, van Genderen PJ, Verdijk RM, et al. Miscarriage associated with zika virus infection. N Engl J Med 2016;375(10):1002–4.

55. Bhatnagar J, Rabeneck DB, Martines RB, et al. Zika virus RNA replication and persistence in brain and placental tissue. Emerg Infect Dis 2017;23(3). http://dx.doi.org/10.3201/eid2303.161499.

56. Cugola FR, Fernandes IR, Russo FB, et al. The Brazilian zika virus strain causes birth defects in experimental models. Nature 2016;534(7606):267–71.

57. Miner JJ, Cao B, Govero J, et al. Zika virus infection during pregnancy in mice causes placental damage and fetal demise. Cell 2016;165(5):1081–91.

58. Li C, Xu D, Ye Q, et al. Zika virus disrupts neural progenitor development and leads to microcephaly in mice. Cell Stem Cell 2016;19(5):672.

59. Wu KY, Zuo GL, Li XF, et al. Vertical transmission of zika virus targeting the radial glial cells affects cortex development of offspring mice. Cell Res 2016;26(6): 645–54.

60. Tabata T, Petitt M, Puerta-Guardo H, et al. Zika virus targets different primary human placental cells, suggesting two routes for vertical transmission. Cell Host Microbe 2016;20(2):155–66.

61. Jurado KA, Simoni MK, Tang Z, et al. Zika virus productively infects primary human placenta-specific macrophages. JCI Insight 2016;1(13):e88461.

62. Dang J, Tiwari SK, Lichinchi G, et al. Zika virus depletes neural progenitors in human cerebral organoids through activation of the innate immune receptor TLR3. Cell Stem Cell 2016;19(2):258–65.

63. Tang H, Hammack C, Ogden SC, et al. Zika virus infects human cortical neural progenitors and attenuates their growth. Cell Stem Cell 2016;18(5):587–90.

64. Anaya JM, Ramirez-Santana C, Salgado-Castaneda I, et al. Zika virus and neurologic autoimmunity: the putative role of gangliosides. BMC Med 2016; 14:49.
65. Shao Q, Herrlinger S, Yang SL, et al. Zika virus infection disrupts neurovascular development and results in postnatal microcephaly with brain damage. Development 2016;143(22):4127–36.
66. Rasmussen SA, Jamieson DJ, Honein MA, et al. Zika virus and birth defects–reviewing the evidence for causality. N Engl J Med 2016;374(20):1981–7.
67. Pacheco O, Beltran M, Nelson CA, et al. Zika virus disease in Colombia—preliminary report. N Engl J Med 2016. [Epub ahead of print].
68. Kleber de Oliveira W, Cortez-Escalante J, De Oliveira WT, et al. Increase in reported prevalence of microcephaly in infants born to women living in areas with confirmed zika virus transmission during the first trimester of pregnancy—Brazil, 2015. MMWR Morb Mortal Wkly Rep 2016;65(9):242–7.
69. Brasil P, Pereira JP Jr, Raja Gabaglia C, et al. Zika virus infection in pregnant women in Rio de Janeiro preliminary report. N Engl J Med 2016;375(24): 2321–34.
70. Soares de Souza A, Moraes Dias C, Braga FD, et al. Fetal infection by zika virus in the third trimester: report of 2 cases. Clin Infect Dis 2016;63(12):1622–5.
71. Cuevas EL, Tong VT, Rozo N, et al. Preliminary report of microcephaly potentially associated with zika virus infection during pregnancy—Colombia, January–November 2016. MMWR Morb Mortal Wkly Rep 2016;65:1409–13.
72. Brasil P, Pereira JP Jr, Moreira ME, et al. Zika virus infection in pregnant women in Rio de Janeiro. N Engl J Med 2016;375(24):2321–34.
73. Russell K, Oliver SE, Lewis L, et al. Update: Interim guidance for the evaluation and management of infants with possible congenital zika virus infection—United States, August 2016. MMWR Morb Mortal Wkly Rep 2016;65(33):870–8.
74. Moore CA, Staples JE, Dobyns WB, et al. Characterizing the pattern of anomalies in congenital zika syndrome for pediatric clinicians. JAMA Pediatr 2016; 171(3):288–95.
75. Russell LJ, Weaver DD, Bull MJ, et al. In utero brain destruction resulting in collapse of the fetal skull, microcephaly, scalp rugae, and neurologic impairment: the fetal brain disruption sequence. Am J Med Genet 1984;17(2):509–21.
76. Franca GV, Schuler-Faccini L, Oliveira WK, et al. Congenital zika virus syndrome in Brazil: a case series of the first 1501 livebirths with complete investigation. Lancet 2016;388(10047):891–7.
77. Sarno M, Aquino M, Pimentel K, et al. Progressive lesions of central nervous system in microcephalic fetuses with suspected congenital zika virus syndrome. Ultrasound Obstet Gynecol 2016. [Epub ahead of print].
78. Ventura CV, Maia M, Travassos SB, et al. Risk factors associated with the ophthalmoscopic findings identified in infants with presumed zika virus congenital infection. JAMA Ophthalmol 2016;134(8):912–8.
79. de Paula Freitas B, de Oliveira Dias JR, Prazeres J, et al. Ocular findings in infants with microcephaly associated with presumed zika virus congenital infection in Salvador, Brazil. JAMA Ophthalmol 2016. [Epub ahead of print].
80. Leal MC, Muniz LF, Ferreira TS, et al. Hearing loss in infants with microcephaly and evidence of congenital zika virus infection—Brazil, November 2015-May 2016. MMWR Morb Mortal Wkly Rep 2016;65(34):917–9.
81. Brasil P, Calvet GA, Siqueira AM, et al. Zika virus outbreak in Rio de Janeiro, Brazil: clinical characterization, epidemiological and virological aspects. PLoS Negl Trop Dis 2016;10(4):e0004636.

82. Dirlikov E, Ryff KR, Torres-Aponte J, et al. Update: Ongoing zika virus transmission—Puerto Rico, November 1, 2015-April 14, 2016. MMWR Morb Mortal Wkly Rep 2016;65(17):451–5.

83. Duffy MR, Chen TH, Hancock WT, et al. Zika virus outbreak on Yap Island, Federated States of Micronesia. N Engl J Med 2009;360(24):2536–43.

84. Arzuza-Ortega L, Polo A, Perez-Tatis G, et al. Fatal sickle cell disease and zika virus infection in girl from Colombia. Emerg Infect Dis 2016;22(5):925–7.

85. Azevedo RS, Araujo MT, Martins Filho AJ, et al. Zika virus epidemic in Brazil. I. Fatal disease in adults: clinical and laboratory aspects. J Clin Virol 2016;85: 56–64.

86. Parra B, Lizarazo J, Jimenez-Arango JA, et al. Guillain-Barre syndrome associated with zika virus infection in Colombia. N Engl J Med 2016;375(16):1513–23.

87. Cao-Lormeau VM, Blake A, Mons S, et al. Guillain-Barre syndrome outbreak associated with zika virus infection in French Polynesia: a case-control study. Lancet 2016;387(10027):1531–9.

88. Dos Santos T, Rodriguez A, Almiron M, et al. Zika virus and the Guillain-Barre syndrome—case series from seven countries. N Engl J Med 2016;375(16): 1598–601.

89. Mecharles S, Herrmann C, Poullain P, et al. Acute myelitis due to zika virus infection. Lancet 2016;387(10026):1481.

90. Carteaux G, Maquart M, Bedet A, et al. Zika virus associated with meningoencephalitis. N Engl J Med 2016;374(16):1595–6.

91. Vinhaes ES, Santos LA, Dias L, et al. Transient hearing loss in adults associated with zika virus infection. Clin Infect Dis 2016;64(5):675–7.

92. Goodman AB, Dziuban EJ, Powell K, et al. Characteristics of children aged <18 years with zika virus disease acquired postnatally—U.S. States, January 2015-July 2016. MMWR Morb Mortal Wkly Rep 2016;65(39):1082–5.

93. Nogueira ML, Estofolete CF, Terzain AC, et al. Zika Virus Infection and Solid Organ Transplantation: A New Challenge. Am J Transplant 2017;17(3):791–5.

94. Rabe IB, Staples JE, Villanueva J, et al. Interim guidance for interpretation of zika virus antibody test results. MMWR Morb Mortal Wkly Rep 2016;65(21): 543–6.

95. Oduyebo T, Igbinosa I, Petersen EE, et al. Update: Interim guidance for health care providers caring for pregnant women with possible zika virus exposure—United States, July 2016. MMWR Morb Mortal Wkly Rep 2016; 65(29):739–44.

96. Hurwitz ES, Nelson DB, Davis C, et al. National surveillance for Reye syndrome: a five-year review. Pediatrics 1982;70(6):895–900.

97. Guideline: infant feeding in areas of zika virus transmission. Geneva (Switzerland): World Health Organization; 2016.

98. Pfaender S, Vielle NJ, Ebert N, et al. Inactivation of zika virus in human breast milk by prolonged storage or pasteurization. Virus Res 2016;228:58–60.

99. Abbink P, Larocca RA, De La Barrera RA, et al. Protective efficacy of multiple vaccine platforms against zika virus challenge in rhesus monkeys. Science 2016;353(6304):1129–32.

100. NIH news releases. Phase 2 Zika Vaccine Trial Begins in US, Central and South America. Available at: https://www.niaid.nih.gov/news-events/phase-2-zika-vaccine-trial-begins-us-central-and-south-america. Accessed May 2, 2017.

101. Grant GB, Reef SE, Dabbagh A, et al. Global progress toward rubella and congenital rubella syndrome control and elimination—2000-2014. MMWR Morb Mortal Wkly Rep 2015;64(37):1052–5.

102. Cetron M. Revision to CDC's zika travel notices: minimal likelihood for mosquito-borne zika virus transmission at elevations above 2,000 meters. MMWR Morb Mortal Wkly Rep 2016;65(10):267–8.

103. Ndeffo-Mbah ML, Parpia AS, Galvani AP. Mitigating prenatal zika virus infection in the Americas. Ann Intern Med 2016;165(8):551–9.

104. U.S. Department of Commerce, ITA, National Travel and Tourism Office (NTTO). 2016. Available at: http://Tinet.ita.doc.gov/outreachpages/download_data_table/2015_US_Travel_Abroad.pdf. Accessed December 15, 2016.

105. CDC. Congenital microcephaly case definitions. Available at: http://Www.cdc.gov/zika/public-health-partners/microcephaly-case-definitions.html. Accessed December 1, 2016.

106. Miranda-Filho Dde B, Martelli CM, Ximenes RA, et al. Initial description of the presumed congenital zika syndrome. Am J Public Health 2016;106(4):598–600.

107. de Fatima Vasco Aragao M, van der Linden V, Brainer-Lima AM, et al. Clinical features and neuroimaging (CT and MRI) findings in presumed zika virus related congenital infection and microcephaly: retrospective case series study. BMJ 2016;353:i1901.

108. Miranda HA 2nd, Costa MC, Frazao MA, et al. Expanded spectrum of congenital ocular findings in microcephaly with presumed zika infection. Ophthalmology 2016;123(8):1788–94.

109. PAHO/WHO. Case definitions. Updates. 2016. Available at: http://Www.paho.org/hq/index.php?option=com_content&view=article&id=11117:2015-zika-case-definitions-&Itemid=41532&lang=en. Accessed December 1, 2016.

Management of Refugees and International Adoptees

Linda A. Waggoner-Fountain, MD

KEYWORDS

- International adoption • Refugee • Immigrant health

KEY POINTS

- Refugee children and international adoptees have special medical considerations that must be addressed.
- Providers must be aware of the immigration history — where and under what circumstances the child lived and migrated to the United States.
- Federal guidelines exist regarding which infections should be screened for and how and when and which vaccines should be administered.

When caring for children who arrive from other countries, it is important to establish whether these children are immigrants or refugees. Children who arrive as refugees are required to undergo a physical examination prior to entering the United States and are required to have a physical evaluation after arrival in the United States. If a child enters the United States as an immigrant, it is important to understand whether he or she is an undocumented immigrant, given that this can impact on what types of infectious diseases should be screened for.

In all cases, it is important to know the countries and situations children were in when they left their native country and began their journey to their new home. Issues of communicable diseases, vaccine delivery, sanitation, nutrition, and the potential for sexual abuse are all important in consideration of infectious diseases. This article addresses screening tests for immigrants and refugees first, next addresses international adoptees who fall under the first category but can potentially have some other

Disclosure Statement: The author denies conflict of interest or any relationship with a commercial company that has a direct financial interest in subject matter or materials discussed in article or with a company making a competing product.

Department of Pediatrics, Division of Infectious Diseases, University of Virginia School of Medicine, 3601 Hospital Drive, Charlottesville, VA 22908, USA

E-mail address: law4q@virginia.edu

infectious issues given their unique background, and then addresses screening tests for migrants without premigration medical examination.

IMMIGRANTS AND REFUGEES

For immigrants and refugees entering the United States, the Centers for Disease Control and Prevention (CDC) is responsible for providing the instructions for medical examination performed by identified civil surgeon and panel physicians. These instructions were developed to enforce the Immigration and Nationality Act regulations regarding the health-related grounds for inadmissibility of persons applying for admission into the United States. The purpose of the medical examination is to identify applicants with inadmissible health-related conditions for the Department of State and US Citizenship and Immigration Services (USCIS). The infectious diseases–related grounds for inadmissibility include persons who have a communicable disease of public health significance and those who fail to present documentation of having received vaccination against vaccine-preventable diseases (**Table 1**).

Communicable diseases of public health significance in all immigrants include tuberculosis (TB), syphilis, gonorrhea, and Hansen disease. In addition to these 4 specific diseases, screening by history and physical examination includes evaluation for quarantinable diseases designated by any presidential executive order. Current diseases include cholera, diphtheria, plague, smallpox, yellow fever, viral hemorrhagic fevers, severe acute respiratory syndrome (SARS), and influenza caused by novel or re-emergent influenza (pandemic flu). In addition to these infectious diseases, other infectious diseases are reportable as a public health emergency of international concern to the World Health Organization (currently polio, smallpox, SARS, and influenza) and other public health emergencies of international concern (recently includes Ebola virus).

As part of the medical examination for immigration, all immigrants are required to have an assessment for the following vaccine-preventable diseases: polio, tetanus, diphtheria toxoids, pertussis, *Haemophilus influenzae* type B, rotavirus, mumps, measles, rubella, hepatitis A, hepatitis B, meningococcal disease, varicella, influenza, and pneumococcus.

Persons already in the United States applying for adjustment of status for permanent residency, including refugees, are also required to be assessed for these vaccine-preventable diseases. For vaccines requiring a series, only a single dose is required for immigration purposes with a plan to complete the necessary series of

Table 1
Who is required to have a medical examination for migration to the United States?

Category	Medical Examination	Examination Site	Examination Location
Immigrants	Yes	Panel physicians	Overseas
Refugees	Yes	Panel physicians	Overseas
Status adjusters	Yes	Civil surgeons	United States
Nonimmigrants	No	—	—
Short-term transit	No	—	—
Others[a]	No	—	—

[a] Others include migrants who entered the United States without inspection, including those who entered with and without proper documentation.
Courtesy of US Department of Homeland Security.

vaccinations. Individuals who want to obtained a personal belief waiver (based on religious or moral conviction) from the vaccine requirements can apply for this with a separate application process.

A list of civil surgeons and medication documentation needs for individuals applying for permanent status is available on the USCIS Web site: http://www.uscis.gov/portal/site/uscis.

The information regarding medical documentation required for individuals applying for immigrant visas is available at the Department of State Web site: http://www.travel.state.gov/visa/visa_1750.html. General information concerning civil surgeons and the medical examination required for immigration purposes is also available at www.uscis.gov.

The blanket designation of health departments as civil surgeons applies only to the vaccination assessment and only to refugees. Also, only health departments that have a physician or physicians meeting the legal definition of civil surgeon can participate in this designation, and accepting the designation is entirely voluntary on the part of health departments. A civil surgeon is legally defined as a licensed physician with greater than 4 years of professional experience. The completed I-693 medical examination form must contain the official stamp or seal of office and be given to a refugee in a sealed envelope for presentation to the USCIS. The vaccine series that must be completed is available from the CDC.

Overseas medical examinations of aliens are valid for variable amounts of time, as discussed later, for specific infectious illnesses.

Medical examinations are valid for 6 months for individuals with the following conditions:

- No class (ie, no apparent defect, disease, or disability)
- Class A other than TB
- Class B2 latent TB infection
- Class B3 TB (contact evaluation)

Medical examinations are valid for 3 months for individuals with the following conditions:

- Class A TB with waiver
- Class B1 TB, pulmonary
- Class B1 TB, extrapulmonary
- HIV infection

The American Academy of Pediatrics recommends that medical screening should be conducted as soon as possible after entry, and refugees should be assured ongoing primary care.

A general medical examination should include a history outlining nutrition and growth with a dietary history, reviewing previous vaccines, history of diseases, and a general physical examination. On physical examination, anthropometric indices of weight, length or height, and head circumference should be obtained.

Previous vaccinations should be recorded into a computerized state vaccination database as well as history of disease (eg, varicella and mumps) or laboratory evidence of immunity (eg, hepatitis B and rubella). The author recommends that any series of vaccinations that has been started should be completed and not repeated if given as recommended by the Advisory Committee on Immunization Practices. If a patient has no documentation, it must be assumed the patient has not been vaccinated unless laboratory evidence of immunity indicates otherwise.

Regarding all refugees, little screening laboratory work is suggested; however, the following is a potential algorithm to consider when evaluating these patients.

Laboratory Recommendations for all Refugees

- Perform pregnancy test as indicated.
- Perform complete blood cell count with differential to be able to look for evidence of anemia and an absolute eosinophil count.
- Some specialists recommend a urinalysis but this is optional in patients unable to provide a clean-catch specimen.
- Consideration of tuberculosis screening.

The 4 most commonly queried categories of infectious illnesses are addressed, specifically given the frequency at which they are encountered when caring for immigrants, migrants, and refugees. These 4 groups of illnesses include TB, malaria, and parasitic infections and sexually transmitted infections (STIs).

Tuberculosis

The current TB screening requirements, called the Technical Instructions for Tuberculosis Screening and Treatment Using Cultures and Directly Observed Therapy, were most recently updated in 2009. These requirements were first created, however, in 1991 and have been updated throughout the years. These technical instructions have been implemented on a country-by-country basis since 2007 and have been used by all countries that screen immigrants and refugees coming to the United States. These instructions include tests and procedures for diagnosing TB more quickly and more accurately. Factors that affect the choice of TB tests for children include their age, whether they have a known HIV infection, and if they have signs or symptoms of tuberculous disease.

TB screening varies by both age and HIV status. In children less than 2 years of age without HIV infection, no TB screening tests need to be performed unless a child has signs or symptoms suggestive of TB or has been in contact with a person with TB. In children between 2 years and 14 years of age without HIV infection, a screening tuberculin skin test (TST) or interferon-gamma release assay (IGRA) is indicated followed by a chest radiograph if either is positive. If the screening radiograph is indicative of TB diseases, then sputum smear and subsequent cultures are obtained and drug susceptibility tests are performed in individuals with positive smears. In teens over 15 years of age, a chest radiograph is required in all patients with subsequent sputum smear and culture and drug susceptibility testing as indicated. If a patient has symptoms of TB, even with negative TST/IGRA and chest radiograph results, sputum tests are indicated.

All children and adolescents with known HIV infection undergo evaluation for TB regardless of symptoms. It is well documented that HIV infection is one of the most common risk factor to cause latent (inactive) TB infection to become (active) TB disease. For children less than 15 years of age, a TST or IGRA is obtained as well as chest radiograph, sputum smear, and culture regardless of the results of the TST or IGRA. For adolescents over 15 years of age, a chest radiograph and sputum smear and cultures and susceptibility testing is proceeded to directly, without need for TST or IGRA.

The different TB tests include the TST, IGRA, sputum sample, sputum smear, sputum culture, and drug susceptibility testing (**Table 2**). The TST is considered positive in children less than 4 years of age if it measures greater than 5 mm of induration regardless of bacillus Calmette-Guérin vaccination status. Some practitioners consider a measurement of 10 mm or greater as a positive in children. In these situations, a chest radiograph must be obtained and if a child is symptomatic, sputum samples via sputum induction or early morning gastric aspirate is required. These samples are examined for acid-fast smears and cultures that are held for 8 weeks. If a positive sputum culture is obtained, drug susceptibility testing is essential. It is also critical to

Table 2
Tuberculosis screening tests and turnaround time for tests

Tuberculosis Screening Tests	Turnaround Time for Testing Results
TST	48–72 h
IGRA	<7 d depending on laboratory
Chest radiograph	Same day
Sputum smears	3 d after last sputum collection
Sputum culture	8 wk
Drug susceptibility test	2–4 wk

find the adult who transmitted the disease to the child, although in refugees this may not be possible if a child is separated from parents or adults who cared for the patient prior to entrance to the United States. If children have active TB disease, they usually are treated with directly observed therapy for at least 6 months. For children who have TB infection, this is typically not directly observed therapy but with physician follow-up at intervals and the end of therapy is appropriate.

Malaria

Refugees who arrived from sub-Saharan Africa (SSA) countries that are endemic for *Plasmodium falciparum* and who do not have a contraindication should be assumed to have received predeparture presumptive antimalarial therapy with artesunate combination therapy. Tests for refugees who require postarrival testing or presumptive treatment include polymerase chain reaction (PCR) testing, traditional blood films, and/or a rapid antigen test. The most sensitive test for persons with subclinical malaria is PCR; when PCR is not available, traditional blood films and/or a rapid antigen test may be used but have limited sensitivity in asymptomatic persons.

In refugees from SSA, who did not receive presumptive treatment prior to departure or refugees from a malaria-endemic country with signs or symptoms of infection should receive a thorough evaluation. Individuals who do not receive presumptive therapy include children weighing less than 5 kg at the time of departure, pregnant or lactating women, or those for whom presumptive treatment was contraindicated. Any refugee from a malaria-endemic country with signs or symptoms of infection should receive a thorough evaluation. Refugees from SSA who receive presumptive treatment prior to departure and asymptomatic refugees from malaria-endemic countries outside the SSA do not require postarrival testing or presumptive treatment on arrival.

Parasites

Postarrival screening for endoparasites depends on the region of departure and predeparture presumptive therapy received.

Currently, all refugees without contraindications from the Middle East, South and Southeast Asia, and Africa receive a single dose of albendazole prior to departure. In addition, all SSA refugees without contraindications receive treatment with praziquantel for schistosomiasis. The only population currently receiving presumptive therapy for *Strongyloides* is refugees from Myanmar, who receive ivermectin if they do not have contraindications.

For those who have contraindications or who did not receive complete predeparture therapy, the following screening is recommended.

All refugees who received no predeparture treatment or partial predeparture treatment or for whom their treatment status is unknown should be provided presumptive treatment or screened for roundworms and *Strongyloides*. All SSA refugees should be screened for schistosomiasis if not treated with praziquantel. An absolute eosinophil count should be reviewed in the complete blood cell count.

Sexually transmitted infections

STIs should be screened for in refugees if there is a history of sexual abuse, if an adolescent is sexually active, if a patient's mother tested positive for an STI, or if a patient has symptoms consistent with an STI.

If screening tests are positive for syphilis, then a confirmation test should be performed as well, because there are some countries that are endemic for other treponemal subspecies besides syphilis (eg, yaws, bejel, and pinta)

As of 2010, refugees are no longer tested for HIV infection prior to arrival in the United States; however, refugees less than 12 years of age can be screened unless their parents opt out or a mother's HIV status can be confirmed as negative and there is no history of potential high-risk exposures (blood transfusions and sexual abuse). Screening should be repeated 3 and 6 months after resettlement for those who had recent exposure or are at high risk.

Children less than 18 months of age who test positive for HIV antibodies should be tested with DNA or RNA assays. Results of positive antibody tests in this age group can be unreliable because they may detect persistent maternal antibodies. All individuals who are confirmed as HIV-infected should be referred to infectious diseases specialists who care for these children. As for children born in the United States, the provider should initiate prophylactic trimethoprim/sulfamethoxazole for all children born to or breastfed by an HIV-infected mother, beginning at 6 weeks of age and continuing until they are confirmed uninfected.

INTERNATIONAL ADOPTEES

The medical examination process for an adopted child typically begins overseas with an evaluation by a physician affiliated with the adoption agency. These medical records, including immunization records, can range from very useful and accurate, to scant or difficult to read, to belonging to another patient. They must be looked at with scrutiny, and parents frequently ask for an opinion of the health of the child based on an assessment of these medical records, a photo, or brief video. When parents make a decision to adopt a child, they visit a Department of State–designated medical doctor (panel physician) who performs medical examinations overseas for international adoptees as well as other immigrants and refugees coming into the United States. Panel physicians are located in many countries in the world and must refer to CDC guidelines on medical examinations. As with documented refugees, the purpose of the overseas medical examination is to identify applicants with class A conditions. Children with these conditions must be treated or get a waiver before they can get a visa to come to the United States. Again, this visa medical examination includes physical examination, vaccines, TB screening, and a blood test for syphilis in children greater than 15 or with concerns for infection. Some adopted children can receive a waiver to have their vaccinations delayed until after they arrive in the United States. The Immigration and Nationality Act requires that all immigrant visa applicants, including adopted children, show proof of having received certain vaccinations named in the law as well as others recommended by the Advisory Committee on Immunization Practices before they may be granted an immigrant visa. Vaccination requirements depend on the age of the child. The age-appropriate vaccinations the child may require can be found in the vaccination schedules for children and Web sites about vaccinations for international adoptions. The US Consulate informs the parents whether the waiver was granted. If the waiver is granted, the child receives a visa. If a waiver is granted, the adoptee must begin receiving the required vaccines once arriving in the United States. At the author's international adoption clinic, families are asked to request a second copy of the sealed packet so that these medical examination forms can be given to the child's personal physician. After arrival to the United States, if the child is doing well, a physical examination with the child's personal physician within several weeks of arrival in the United States is recommended. If a child is symptomatic, immediate evaluation should be performed by the child's personal physician.

If a child is found to have a class A condition, parents should talk to the panel physician and the US Consulate to find out if it is possible to get a waiver. Thus, all tests must be completed and read by the panel physician before a class can be assigned. The USCIS within the Department of Homeland Security makes the final decision to approve or deny the waiver. This is with an opinion from the CDC to USCIS or the American Embassy about a patient's infectious situation.

The point of the physical examination and laboratory testing performed in the country of origin is to identify class A conditions, which include the following infections: TB, syphilis, gonorrhea, Hansen disease, cholera, diphtheria, plague, smallpox, yellow fever, viral hemorrhagic fevers, SARS and novel influenza (eg, pandemic flu), polio, and other potential public health emergencies of international concern. The class A condition that is most relevant for international adoptees is TB. Individuals with class A conditions are to be treated with their country of origin; however, in patients with TB whose medical situations suggest that they would benefit from receiving their TB treatment in the United States, the Department of Homeland Security may grant a waiver (also called a class A waiver), allowing them to travel to the United States before the end of the TB treatment. This is often the case in poor, overcrowded orphanage settings.

MIGRANTS WITHOUT PREMIGRATION EVALUATION

This group of children and adolescents, migrants without premigration evaluation, brings up all the same concerns plus other potential risk factors for infections but they often present in challenging settings, such as a free medical clinic or emergency department, or are new to a practice. There are often language barriers and sometimes there is a reluctance to share a child's entire story for concerns of immigration status or judgment of the care providers who may not be the child's parents. There are often challenges associated with payment for services and treatment as well. Providers need to ensure culturally sensitive care for refugees and ensure the competence of interpreters and bilingual staff to provide language assistance to patients/families with limited English proficiency. Finally, these children often present with progression of disease rather than infection being discovered with screening laboratories.

All the diseases discussed previously can present in these patients and it remains important to consider financial concerns in these patients who may only be able to come to the physician at certain times. At times, it may be more prudent to treat presumptively rather than screen for extensive infections when considering parasitic infections. The local health department is designed to aid in these situations where individuals cannot afford medications that are a concern for the well-being of the community (eg, TB).

SUMMARY

With an ever-evolving geopolitical climate, it is important to understand where refugees, immigrants, migrants, and adoptees may come from as they enter the United

States. Depending on their country of origin and their path to the United States or Canada, different infectious diseases may be of concern when evaluating each child. The more common infectious issues of concern for children and adolescents include TB, malaria, parasitic infection, and STI. There are both governmental requirements that must be followed for legal entry into a country as well as medical issues that should be addressed depending on a child's underlying health, country of origin, circumstances of travel, and current signs and symptoms. All these factors allow practitioners the unique opportunity of caring for these patients and to be a part of their individual journey.